AMERICAN COLLEGE OF PHYSICIANS

MKSAP®14
MEDICAL KNOWLEDGE *Self-Assessment Program*®

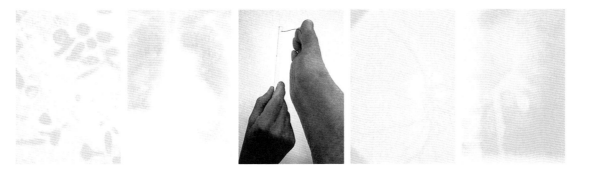

General Internal Medicine

General Internal Medicine

Contributors

Kurt Kroenke, MD, MACP, Book Editor [2]
Professor of Medicine
Research Scientist, Regenstrief Institute
Indianapolis, Indiana

Jack Ende, MD, FACP, Associate Editor [1]
Professor of Medicine
University of Pennsylvania School of Medicine
Chief, Department of Medicine
Penn Presbyterian Medical Center
Philadelphia, Pennsylvania

Richard M. Hoffman, MD, MPH, FACP [1]
Professor of Medicine
New Mexico VA Health Care System
University of New Mexico School of Medicine
Albuquerque, New Mexico

Jeffrey L. Jackson, MD, MPH, FACP [1]
Associate Professor of Medicine
Program Director, General Medicine Fellowship
Division Director, General Internal Medicine
Walter Reed Army Medical Center and
  Uniformed Services University of the Health Sciences
Bethesda, Maryland

Valerie A. Lawrence, MD, MSc, FACP [1]
Professor of Medicine
Audie L. Murphy Division/South
  Texas Veterans Health Care System
Division of General Medicine
University of Texas Health Science Center at San Antonio
San Antonio, Texas

Lia Logio, MD [1]
Assistant Professor of Medicine
Program Director, Internal Medicine Residency
Indiana University School of Medicine
Indianapolis, Indiana

Patrick G. O'Malley, MD, MPH, FACP [1]
Professor of Medicine
Division of General Internal Medicine
Walter Reed Army Medical Center and
  Uniformed Services University of the Health Sciences
Bethesda, Maryland

Marilyn M. Schapira, MD, MPH [1]
Associate Professor of Internal Medicine
Center for Patient Care and Outcomes Research
Medical College of Wisconsin
Milwaukee, Wisconsin

Laura Zakowski, MD [1]
Associate Professor of Medicine
University of Wisconsin School of Medicine and Public Health
Madison, Wisconsin

Co-Editors-in-Chief

Patrick C. Alguire, MD, FACP [1]
Director, Education and Career Development
American College of Physicians
Philadelphia, Pennsylvania

Paul E. Epstein, MD, FACP [1]
Clinical Professor of Medicine
University of Pennsylvania School of Medicine
Philadelphia, Pennsylvania

ACP Staff

Sean McKinney, Director, Self-Assessment Programs [1]
Charles Rossi, Managing Editor [1]
Margaret Wells, Senior Staff Editor [1]

---

1 Has no relationships with any proprietary entity that provides health care goods or services, with the exception of non-profit or government organizations and non–health care–related companies.

2 Has disclosed relationship(s) with any proprietary entity that provides health care goods or services, with the exception of non-profit or government organizations, and non–health care–related companies.

Disclosure of Relationships with any Proprietary Entity that Provides Health Care Goods or Services, with the Exception of Non-Profit or Government Organizations, and Non–Health Care–Related Companies

Kurt Kroenke, MD, MACP
Research Grants/Contracts
Eli Lilly, Pfizer, Wyeth
Honoraria
Eli Lilly, Wyeth

Principal Staff

Senior Vice President, Medical Education and Publishing
Steven Weinberger, MD, FACP

Vice President, Medical Education and Publishing
D. Theresa Kanya, MBA

Director, Self-Assessment Programs
Sean McKinney

Managing Editor
Charles Rossi

Senior Staff Editors
Charlotte Fierman
Becky Krumm
Ellen McDonald, PhD, ELS
Margaret Wells

Staff Editor
Amanda Neiley

Production Administrator
Sheila O'Steen

Program Administrator
Valerie Dangovetsky

Editorial Coordinators
Katie Idell
Karen Williams

Developed by the American College of Physicians

Acknowledgements

The American College of Physicians (ACP) gratefully acknowledges the special contributions to the development and production of the 14th edition of the Medical Knowledge Self-Assessment Program® of Scott Thomas Hurd (systems analyst/developer), Ricki Jo Kauffman (senior systems analyst/developer), and Michael Ripca (graphics technical design administrator). The CD-ROM and Online versions are developed within the Electronic Product Development department by Steven Spadt (Director) and Christopher Forrest, John McKnight, Sean O'Donnell, and Elijah Odumosu (software developers). Computer scoring and reporting are being done by ACT, Iowa City, Iowa. The College also wishes to acknowledge that many other persons, too numerous to mention, have contributed to the production of this program. Without their dedicated efforts, this program would not have been possible.

Continuing Medical Education

The American College of Physicians is accredited by the Accreditation Council for Continuing Medical Education (ACCME) to provide continuing medical education for physicians.

The American College of Physicians designates this educational activity for a maximum of 150 *AMA PRA Category 1 Credits*™. Physicians should only claim credit commensurate with the extent of their participation in the activity.

The American Medical Association has determined that physicians not licensed in the United States who participate in this CME activity are eligible for *AMA PRA Category 1 Credit*™.

Credit is available from December 29, 2006 to July 31, 2009.

Learning Objectives

The learning objectives of the Medical Knowledge Self-Assessment Program are to assess the current state of your knowledge in clinical medicine, update your knowledge in key areas of internal medicine, apply new clinical problem-solving skills to improve the health of your patients, compare your performance on the self-assessment tests with that of your peers, and pursue in-depth study using critically reviewed evidence-based references.

Target Audience

- General internists and primary care physicians
- Subspecialists who need to remain up-to-date in internal medicine
- Residents preparing for the certifying examination in internal medicine
- Physicians participating in maintenance of certification in internal medicine (recertification)

Educational Disclaimer

The editors and publisher of Medical Knowledge Self-Assessment Program 14 recognize that the development of new material offers many opportunities for error. Despite our best efforts, some errors may persist in print. Drug dosage schedules are, we believe, accurate and in accordance with current standards. Readers are advised, however, to ensure that the recommended dosages in MKSAP 14 concur with the information provided in the product information material. This is especially important in cases of new, infrequently used, or highly toxic drugs.

The primary purpose of MKSAP 14 is educational. Information presented, as well as publications, technologies, products, and/or services discussed, are intended to inform subscribers about the knowledge, techniques, and experiences of the contributors. A diversity of professional opinion exists, and the views of the contributors are their own and not those of the ACP. The ACP disclaims any and all liability for damages and claims, which may result from the use of information, publications, technologies, products, and/or services discussed in MKSAP 14.

Publisher's Information

ISBN: 1-930513-78-X

Printed in the United States of America.

For order information in US or Canada call 800-523-1546, extension 2600, all other countries call 215-351-2600. Fax inquiries to 215-351-2799, or email to custserv@ acponline.org.

DISCLOSURE

It is the policy of the American College of Physicians (ACP) to ensure balance, independence, objectivity, and scientific rigor in all its educational activities. To this end, and consistent with the policies of the ACP and the Accreditation Council for Continuing Medical Education (ACCME), contributors to all ACP continuing medical education activities are required to disclose all financial relationships they have with proprietary entities producing health care goods or services, with the exception of non-for-profit or government organizations and non–health care–related companies. Contributors are required to use only generic names in the discussion of therapeutic options and are required to identify any unapproved or investigative use of commercial products or devices. If trade-name products manufactured by companies with whom they have relationships are discussed, contributors are asked to provide evidence-based citations in support of the discussion. The information is reviewed by the committee responsible for producing this text and by a separate group of outside physician reviewers. If necessary, adjustments to topics or contributors' roles in content development are made to balance the discussion. Further, all readers of this text are asked to evaluate the content for evidence of commercial bias so that future decisions about content and contributors can be made in light of this information.

Contributors' disclosure information can be found at the beginning of this book.

Table of Contents

General Internal Medicine

ROUTINE CARE OF THE HEALTHY PATIENT

RECENT ADVANCES

- **Abdominal aortic aneurysm screening in men**
- **Abnormal TSH levels as a marker for subclinical thyroid disease**

Age-specific Screening Recommendations

Routine care of the healthy patient includes screening for asymptomatic disease and assessing potential risk factors that contribute to disease or other health problems (**Table 1**). Cancer screening is a large component of preventive health, but other behaviors and important diseases also warrant discussion. Cancer screening recommendations include routine testing for breast, cervical, and colorectal cancer (see Hematology and Oncology Syllabus). Lifestyle screening includes evaluation and counseling on tobacco use, alcohol use, seat belts, domestic violence, sun exposure, diet, and exercise. Significant nonmalignant diseases subject to screening include heart disease, diabetes mellitus, *Chlamydia trachomatis* infection, hepatitis C infection, and osteoporosis. Generally, recommendations are age-specific, with consideration for susceptible subgroups. The United States Preventive Services Task Force (USPSTF) is an independent panel of experts who regularly review the available evidence on the efficacy of clinical preventive services with summaries available at http://www.ahrq.gov/clinic/uspstfix.htm.

The routine physical examination should include periodic height and weight measurement and blood pressure monitoring every 2 years. Patients with a calculated body mass index (BMI) >30 should receive obesity counseling. Education on a healthy diet should be provided to all patients, with emphasis on intake of limited saturated fat and adequate intake of fruits, vegetables, and whole grain foods, in addition to a recommendation for regular physical activity. Measurement of serum lipid cholesterol is suggested for patients 20 years of age or older (1), although the USPSTF recommends beginning this type of screening in middle-aged adults.

Preventive health care of adolescents and young adults includes a detailed sexual history and risk assessment for sexually transmitted diseases (STDs). Risk factors for STDs include promiscuity, unprotected sexual intercourse, and history of venereal infection. Individuals should receive screening about safe sex practices and the benefits of barrier-method contraception. Sexually active women younger than the age of 25 years should undergo screening for chlamydial infection given its implication in pelvic inflammatory disease and subsequent infertility. Periodic HIV testing and syphilis serology should be offered to those at risk for these diseases. There is insufficient evidence to recommend routine screening of the general population or even high-risk subgroups for hepatitis C infection (2).

In addition to motor vehicle accidents, homicide and suicide contribute significantly to the mortality of adolescents and young adults; therefore, depression screening may be appropriate in this population and should include open-ended questions about whether patients feel threatened in any of their relationships. Knowledge of any firearms in the house and safety practices with vehicles (motorcycle, bicycle, all-terrain vehicles, boats, and cars), including helmet use, should be discussed. Questions about substance abuse are helpful in identifying drug-related health problems.

In women, a Papanicolaou (Pap) test should be performed at least every 3 years, beginning when the patient becomes sexually active until age 65 years (or until hysterectomy is performed in women with benign conditions). It is unclear whether the use of liquid-based cytology is superior to the conventional methodology for Pap testing, but there is evidence that the former is as accurate (3). There is insufficient evidence to screen routinely for human papillomavirus (HPV) as an adjunct to or substitute for the Pap smear, although some recent data suggest that HPV-DNA testing as a follow-up to finding low-grade atypia is a sensitive method for detecting high-grade lesions (4). By the age of 30 years, women should receive encouragement to ingest adequate dietary calcium and partake in regular physical activity. All women anticipating a pregnancy should take folic acid supplementation beginning at preconception and continuing until delivery. HIV screening is recommended in all pregnant women. There is no consensus on the routine use of mammography in women ages 40 to 50 years. The USPSTF recommends that women receive a mammogram once every 1 to 2 years after age 40 years and cites good evidence for annual testing after age 50 years. Breast examination, performed by the patient or provider, has not been found to have any effect on outcome. Nonetheless, women's physical examinations should include a breast examination, which provides a unique opportunity to sensitize patients to breast cancer issues.

Bone health becomes a concern for women nearing menopause but should be considered earlier in both women and men with risk factors for osteoporosis, including prolonged hyperthyroidism, celiac sprue, anorexia nervosa and

TABLE 1 USPSTF-Recommended Interventions for the General Population

Screening

Height and weight (periodically)

Blood pressure (every 2 y)

Problem drinking

Depression

Diabetes mellitus

Total and HDL cholesterol (men age ≥35 y; women age ≥45 y; others with cardiovascular risk factors, every 5 y)

Colorectal cancer screening (men and women age ≥50 y)

Mammogram ± clinical breast exam (every 1 to 2 y for women age ≥40 y)

Papanicolaou test (at least every 3 y until age 65 y)

Chlamydia (sexually active women age ≤25 y, and older at-risk women)

Bone mineral density test (women age ≥65 y and at-risk women ages 60-64 y)

AAA screening (men age 65 to 75 y who ever smoked)

Vision screening (age ≥65 y)

Assess for hearing impairment (age ≥65 y)

Sexual Behavior

Contraception for unintended pregnancy

STD prevention (educate about avoiding high-risk behavior, condoms/female barrier protection with spermicide)

Injury Prevention

Lap/shoulder belts

Motorcycle/bicycle/ATV helmets

Smoke detectors

Safe storage/removal of firearms

Dental Health

Regular visits to dental care provider

Floss, brush with fluoride toothpaste daily

Counseling–Substance Abuse

Tobacco cessation

Reduce at-risk or harmful alcohol use

Avoid alcohol/drug use while driving, swimming, and boating

Counseling–Diet and Exercise

Limit saturated fat, maintain caloric balance, emphasize grains, fruits, and vegetables

Adequate calcium intake (women)

Regular physical activity

Chemoprevention

Multivitamin with folic acid (women planning pregnancy)

Discuss benefits and harms of aspirin for prevention of MI in middle-aged adults and others at increased risk for heart disease

CRF = cardiac risk factors; AAA= abdominal aortic aneurysm; HDL = high-density lipoprotein; STD = sexually transmitted diseases; ATV = all-terrain vehicle; MI = myocardial infarction.

other digestive disorders, hypogonadism, early menopause, history of androgen-deprivation (for example, prostate cancer treatment), and history of long-term corticosteroid therapy. A family history of osteoporosis, low body weight, and personal history of fracture are also indicators for early bone-density studies.

Older adults become more susceptible to certain types of cancer and require more vigilant screening. Colon cancer screening is appropriate beginning at age ≥50 years and earlier in those at higher risk for this disease considering evidence that screening reduces mortality from colorectal cancer. Options for colorectal cancer screening include colonoscopy, fecal occult blood testing, flexible sigmoidoscopy, or barium enema used alone or in combination for screening. The USPSTF reports each of these screening methods as equally effective. New virtual colonoscopy options (two- and three-dimensional CT or colonography) are being developed but have marked interoperator variability (5). Virtual colonoscopy currently requires a similar laxative bowel preparation and a colonoscopy for the definitive biopsy of any abnormality. Use of fecal DNA testing to identify colorectal cancer–related DNA mutations in stool has promise, with a sensitivity of 52% and specificity of 94% (6), but this testing modality needs further refinement before being widely used (7).

The USPSTF has not found evidence supporting the use of prostate cancer screening. Serum prostate-specific antigen (PSA) levels are neither sensitive nor specific for cancer. Nine systematic reviews have failed to provide evidence that prostate cancer screening lowers morbidity or mortality from prostate cancer (8). When offering PSA testing to patients, practitioners should discuss with them in detail the potential benefits and harms of such screening. Randomized controlled trials in Europe and the United States are ongoing in this area.

Routine screening for skin cancer using a total body skin examination is not recommended. The USPSTF found insufficient evidence that routine skin examination was effective at reducing the morbidity and mortality from cutaneous melanoma, basal cell carcinoma, or squamous cell carcinoma. Patients with high cumulative levels of sun exposure and those with prior skin cancers should be encouraged to wear sunscreen and protective clothing, although the benefit of such counseling is unknown.

Evidence has shown that screening for cancer of the bladder, ovary, lung, mouth, and pancreas is ineffective. CA-125 measurement and vaginal ultrasonography can detect ovarian cancer at an earlier stage than physical exam alone; however, screening-related early detection has been shown to have only a small effect on mortality. The harms of ovarian cancer screening in the general population have been found to outweigh the benefits because of the disease's low prevalence and the invasiveness of diagnostic testing in patients with positive screening results; therefore, ovarian cancer screening in the general population is not recommended (9).

In the United States, the biggest contributors to overall mortality in the 1990s were cardiovascular disease, malignant neoplasms, cerebrovascular disease, and accidents, followed by chronic lower respiratory tract disease and diabetes mellitus. Statistical projections for developed countries indicate that ischemic heart disease, cerebrovascular disease, and major depression will be the top three causes of disability in 2020. Given this burden of disease, screening measures and counseling efforts may be warranted for these conditions.

Adults older than 50 years require more attention to abnormal serum lipid levels and unhealthy lifestyle habits, including excessive daily fat intake, smoking tobacco, and a sedentary routine (see Hyperlipidemia section). The Framingham Risk Index and other simple calculators can help estimate individual 5- and 10-year cardiac risk to guide recommendations for the use of aspirin for cardioprotection (see also http://hin.nhlbi.nih.gov/atpiii/calculator.asp). Patients identified at risk for coronary artery disease (CAD) require more aggressive counseling about diet and tobacco use than those without such risk. There is strong evidence that counseling interventions less than 3 minutes in duration are effective in changing smoking behavior. Pharmacologic adjuncts and behavioral classes can further strengthen the effect on smoking cessation. Counseling to stop tobacco use is particularly important in pregnant women. Routine use of nutritional counseling to improve outcomes is less established in healthy patients but has significant benefit for those at risk for CAD, stroke, and diabetes.

Routine screening for CAD is not recommended. Resting electrocardiography, exercise treadmill testing, and electron-beam CT may identify some patients with asymptomatic disease, but these strategies lack supportive evidence. A complete risk factor assessment should be the basis for making decisions about further cardiac testing. Patient preferences must also be considered but should be balanced with available evidence suggesting that results of expensive tests likely do not change at-risk lifestyle factors.

Routine monitoring of blood pressure in adult patients is recommended. A single elevation in blood pressure does not define hypertension but warrants continued follow-up to identify a trend. Hypertension is a commonly undertreated condition. Management of patients with hypertension consists of defining specific blood pressure goals, identifying contributing risk factors, and prescribing tailored, benefit-maximizing antihypertensive medications. Informing patients of their goal blood pressure and educating them about the benefits of maintaining it are also appropriate.

Routine screening for diabetes beginning in patients 45 years of age has been recommended by some but not the USPSTF. Benefits of screening are greater in patients with additional cardiac risk factors, including hyperlipidemia and hypertension. A family history of diabetes might also be an indicator for more liberal diabetes screening.

Routine screening for carotid arterial stenosis by physical examination or ultrasonography is unfounded. Risk factors for cerebrovascular disease should be addressed in high-risk patients who have a significant medical or family history and risk factors for atherosclerosis. New guidelines from the USPSTF support one-time screening for abdominal aortic aneurysm by ultrasonography in men aged 65 to 75 years who have ever smoked, with fair evidence to support this practice (10). There is no evidence to support screening in women or in male nonsmokers for this condition.

Depression occurs commonly in internal medicine patients and frequently goes undetected. Although several depression screening tools have been developed, asking the following two questions has been found to increase the detection rate of patients with major depression: "Over the past 2 weeks have you felt down, depressed, or hopeless?" and "Over the past 2 weeks, have you felt little interest or pleasure in doing things?" Patients who answer yes to either question screen positively for depression and should receive appropriate treatment and ongoing follow-up.

Screening asymptomatic patients for thyroid disease is an area of debate. Some guidelines suggest periodic measurement of serum thyroid-stimulating hormone (TSH) levels in postmenopausal and postpartum women, patients with diabetes or Down's syndrome, and the elderly. Abnormal TSH levels can help to identify patients with subclinical thyroid disease, but evidence about the efficacy of treating such patients is inconclusive (11).

Screening for alcohol misuse is recommended for adults, including pregnant women. Brief screening tools can identify patients with alcohol-related problems and risky patterns of alcohol consumption. Pregnant women should routinely be advised to stop drinking. Patients who screen positively for alcohol-related problems may respond to even simple counseling by physicians. Other behavioral counseling and group support networks can provide additional help to patients attempting to decrease their alcohol use (See Foundations of Internal Medicine Syllabus).

Screening for tuberculosis might be considered in high-risk groups, including immigrants, health care workers, anyone who has recently been in contact with someone who has had tuberculosis, homeless patients, and alcoholics.

Screening for hearing and vision impairment in the elderly can detect correctible problems before these patients become isolated and lose their independence. Screening for hearing impairment can be easily accomplished with the use of a portable audioscope, screening questionnaire, or both (see Geriatrics section).

KEY POINTS

- Patients with a calculated BMI >30 should receive obesity counseling.
- Risk factors for STDs include promiscuity, unprotected sexual intercourse, and history of venereal infection.
- Sexually active women younger than the age of 25 years should undergo screening for chlamydial infection.
- Women should receive a Papanicolaou test at least every 3 years, beginning with the onset of sexual activity until age 65 years.
- Women should receive a mammogram once every 1 to 2 years after age 40 years, with annual testing after age 50 years.
- Colon cancer screening is appropriate beginning at age ≥50 years and earlier in those at higher risk for this disease.
- The harms of ovarian cancer screening in the general population have been found to outweigh the benefits of screening.
- Counseling interventions less than 3 minutes in duration are effective in changing smoking behavior.
- The USPSTF supports one-time screening for abdominal aortic aneurysm by ultrasonography in men aged 65 to 75 years who ever smoked.
- Abnormal thyroid-stimulating hormone levels can help to identify patients with subclinical thyroid disease, but evidence about the efficacy of treating such patients is inconclusive.
- Screening for alcohol misuse is recommended for adults, including pregnant women.

Immunization

Immunization is one of the most cost-effective preventive care services available, helping minimize the morbidity and mortality caused by many infectious diseases. Routine vaccines available to adult patients provide protection against infection from influenza, pneumococcal disease, hepatitis A and B, tetanus, measles, mumps, rubella, varicella, polio, and meningococcal disease (12).

Health factors and age are the predominant determinants in choosing appropriate vaccinations, but lifestyle and occupational factors, immunization history, and any known reactions to previous vaccines are also considerations (**Table 2** and **Table 3**).

TABLE 2 Recommended Immunization Schedule for Adults by Age

Age	Recommended Schedule
Teenagers/young adults	• Completion of all childhood primary immunizations • Hepatitis B for those not immunized in childhood • Td booster
50 y	• Completion of all primary immunizations • Td booster • Assessment of risk factors indicating need for pneumococcal or influenza vaccine
≥65 y	• Completion of primary immunizations • Yearly influenza vaccine • Pneumococcal vaccine

Td = diphtheria tetanus vaccine. Data from Adult Immunization Schedule (Reference 12).

TABLE 3 Routine Immunizations Available to Adults

Vaccine	Recommendation
Influenza	• Yearly for all adults age ≥65 y • Younger adults with risk factors (chronic heart disease, chronic pulmonary disease [COPD and asthma], diabetes mellitus, renal dysfunction, hemoglobinopathies, immunosuppression) • Offer to other younger adults with pregnancy or occupational risk (health care workers, employees of long-term care facilities)
Pneumococcal	• All adults age ≥65 y • Younger adults with risk factors (cardiovascular disease, COPD, diabetes mellitus, chronic liver disease, chronic renal failure, nephritic syndrome, functional/anatomic asplenia, immunosuppressive conditions, chemotherapy) • Re-immunization every 5 y
Hepatitis A	• Occupational (travelers or food handlers) • Chronic liver disease • Men who have sex with men • Users of illicit drugs
Hepatitis B	• Sexually active young adults • High-risk groups (healthcare workers, public safety workers, injection drug users, those demonstrating promiscuity, men who have sex with men, those with any recently acquired STD) • Assess serologic response in adults age ≥30 y
Td	• Completion of primary (three-dose) series • Booster every 10 y
MMR	• Adults born after 1956 without proof of immunity • Two doses for special risk groups
Varicella	• High-risk groups (health care workers, family contacts of immunosuppressed persons, teachers and child care providers, residents and staff in institutional settings)
Polio	• Only if primary series not completed
Meningococcal	• Exposed during recent outbreak • Complement deficiencies • Functional asplenia • Travelers, college dormitory residents

Td = diphtheria and tetanus vaccine; MMR = measles mumps rubella vaccine; STD = sexually transmitted disease; COPD = chronic obstructive pulmonary disease.

The influenza vaccine is offered annually to individuals at risk for complications from the flu, including patients older than 65 years, those with chronic disease, those who are immunocompromised, and pregnant women whose last two trimesters coincide with the influenza season (late December through mid-March). Other groups in whom influenza vaccine administration might be considered are health care providers, day care workers, college students, nursing home residents, and prisoners. The efficacy of the vaccine depends on host factors; it is less effective in elderly patients but still provides them with considerable protection. Patients with documented fever, a known prior severe reaction, or an allergy to eggs should not be immunized. The main vaccine used in the United States is a trivalent inactivated virus, but an intranasally administered vaccine from a trivalent live-attenuated virus is also available for patients aged 5 to 49 years. The live vaccine is contraindicated in immunocompromised persons and pregnant women, and its use should be delayed in patients who have received any antibody-containing products.

The pneumococcal polysaccharide vaccine (PPV-23) consists of polysaccharides from 23 antigen types of streptococcal pneumonia. It is recommended for use in patients 65 years of age and older; in those with chronic disease, particularly diabetes and alcoholic cirrhosis; in immunocompromised hosts; in patients with sickle cell disease; and in those who have undergone surgical splenectomy. It has been found to be 60% efficacious in protecting against bacteremic disease, the single largest cause of morbidity in patients with pneumococcal disease. Immunity likely wanes 5 or more years after initial vaccination, with a single booster dose recommended for those continually at risk. Local site reactions are common with PPV-23, but serious reactions are rare.

Two forms of hepatitis A vaccinations are available in the United States. The hepatitis A vaccine is primarily indicated in persons traveling to developing countries that have a high prevalence of this disease and can be administered in combination with immunoglobulin when more immediate immunity is needed. Administration of the hepatitis A vaccine should also be considered in food handlers, men who have sex with men, injection drug users, and patients with chronic liver disease. This vaccine is not recommended in health care workers or nursing home residents. Two doses of the hepatitis A vaccine administered 6 months apart are recommended. Local site reactions with soreness and tenderness are the most common side effects of this vaccine.

In addition to the populations for whom the hepatitis A vaccine is recommended, the hepatitis B vaccine is recommended for adolescents and young adults who have not previously been immunized, anyone with a history of STDs, immunocompromised hosts, prisoners of long-term correctional facilities, patients born outside of the United States, health care providers, and patients with end-stage renal disease receiving chronic hemodialysis (13). Administration of this vaccine consists of three doses, with the second and third doses given at 1 and 6 months after the initial dose. In previously vaccinated individuals, evidence of serologic immunity is warranted at 10-year intervals, with a single booster dose appropriate for those with undetectable levels of hepatitis B surface antibody.

Tetanus is a rare disease in the United States because of the effectiveness of the tetanus vaccine. All adolescents and adults should receive a documented tetanus/diphtheria (Td) vaccine, with administration of booster doses recommended every 10 years. At the time of lacerations and puncture wounds, it is reasonable to provide a booster dose for further prevention even if the timing of this vaccine is earlier than otherwise recommended. Some patients born outside of the United States who have not received the primary series of three doses of tetanus should receive their complete series given as a first dose followed by a second and third dose administered 1 and 6 months after the initial dose.

The measles vaccine is usually administered as the MMR and includes the mumps and rubella vaccine. It is recommended for adults born after 1956 without evidence of immunity or prior infection. A booster should be given to adolescents and young adults because of recent outbreaks in colleges and other institutional settings. Immigrants who have not received their primary series of vaccination should receive at least one dose of the MMR. Groups at high risk for contracting these diseases include health care workers, international travelers, and day care providers. Women of childbearing age should be tested for evidence of immunity and given the vaccine if results of rubella serology are negative. The MMR is contraindicated in pregnant women; therefore, rubella testing should be done during the preconception phase. During an outbreak of measles in institutions, all persons at risk who have no evidence of two prior doses or serologic immunity should be vaccinated. Fever is common after the first vaccine. Encephalopathy, encephalitis, and thrombocytopenic purpura are rare, but reported consequences, of MMR.

The varicella vaccine is indicated in all susceptible adults and adolescents. Since 1995, it has been routinely administered to children. Administration of this vaccine should be considered in high-risk groups, including health care workers, family contacts of immunocompromised persons, immigrants, international travelers, teachers and day care employees, nonpregnant women of childbearing age, and residents and staff of institutional settings, such as colleges and prisons. The varicella vaccine is contraindicated in pregnant women and immunocompromised patients, including those who are taking chronic corticosteroid therapy at a dose higher than 20 mg/day. Avoiding close contact with immunosuppressed patients within 4 weeks after vaccination is advised, although viral shedding is most likely to occur in those with a rash developing as a complication to the injection.

Polio vaccination is not routinely recommended for adults but might be indicated in those who have never received or completed a primary series of vaccinations. Meningococcal vaccine is also not administered to adults routinely considering the low risk for this infection but is recommended for those at risk. The main groups at risk for polio include travelers, especially to sub-Saharan Africa, and college freshman living in dormitories. Immunization during local outbreaks might also be useful.

KEY POINTS

- The influenza vaccine is offered annually to patients >65 years, those with chronic disease, those who are immunocompromised, and pregnant women whose last two trimesters coincide with the influenza season.

- The PPV-23 is recommended for patients ≥65 years, in those with chronic disease, in immunocompromised hosts, in those with sickle cell disease, and in those who have undergone surgical splenectomy.

- The hepatitis A vaccine is indicated in persons traveling to developing countries with a high prevalence of this disease and can be administered in combination with immunoglobulin when more immediate immunity is needed.

- The hepatitis B vaccine is recommended for adolescents and young adults who have not previously been immunized, persons with a history of STDs, immunocompromised hosts, prisoners of long-term correctional facilities, patients born outside of the United States, health care providers, and patients with end-stage renal disease receiving chronic hemodialysis.

- All adolescents and adults should receive a documented tetanus/diphtheria vaccine, with administration of booster doses every 10 years.

- The MMR is recommended for adults without evidence of immunity or prior infection, with a booster administered to adolescents and young adults.

- The varicella vaccine is routinely administered to children and should be considered for high-risk groups, including health care workers, family contacts of immunocompromised persons, immigrants, international travelers, teachers, and day care employees.

References

1. **National Cholesterol Education Program.** Third Report of the Expert Panel on Detection, Evaluation, and Treatment of High Blood Cholesterol in Adults (Adult Treatment Panel III). [The National Heart, Lung, and Blood Institute Web site]. Available at: http://www.nhlbi.nih.gov/guidelines/cholesterol/atp3full.pdf. Accessed on July 5, 2007.

2. **United States Preventive Services Task Force.** Systematic Evidence Review. Screening for Hepatitis C [Agency for Healthcare Research and Quality Web site]. March 2004. Available at: http://www.ahrq.gov/downloads/pub/prevent/pdfser/hep-cser.pdf. Accessed June 1, 2006.

3. **Mattosinho de Castro Ferraz Mda G, Nicolau SM, Stavale JN, Focchi J, Castelo A, Dores GB, et al.** Cervical biopsy-based comparison of a new liquid-based thin-layer preparation with conventional Pap smears. Diagn Cytopathol. 2004;30:220-6. [PMID: 15048954]

4. **Andersson, Sonia, Dillner, Lena, Elfgren, Kristina, Mints, Miriam, Persson, Maria & Rylander, Eva.** A comparison of the human papillomavirus test and Papanicolaou smear as a second screening method for women with minor cytological abnormalities. Acta Obstetricia et Gynecologica Scandinavica. 2005;84(10): 996-1000.

5. **Mulhall BP, Veerappan GR, Jackson JL.** Meta-analysis: computed tomographic colonography. Ann Intern Med. 2005;142:635-50. [PMID: 15838071]

6. **Imperiale TF, Ransohoff DF, Itzkowitz SH, Turnbull BA, Ross ME.** Fecal DNA versus fecal occult blood for colorectal-cancer screening in an average-risk population. N Engl J Med. 2004;351:2704-14. [PMID: 15616205]

7. **Woolf SH.** A smarter strategy? Reflections on fecal DNA screening for colorectal cancer [Editorial]. N Engl J Med. 2004;351:2755-8. [PMID: 15616212]

8. **Harris R, Lohr KN.** Screening for prostate cancer: an update of the evidence for the U.S. Preventive Services Task Force. Ann Intern Med. 2002;137:917-29. [PMID: 12458993]

9. **Menon U.** Ovarian cancer screening. CMAJ. 2004;171:323-4. [PMID: 15313987]

10. **Fleming C, Whitlock EP, Beil TL, Lederle FA.** Screening for abdominal aortic aneurysm: a best-evidence systematic review for the U.S. Preventive Services Task Force. Ann Intern Med. 2005;142:203-11. [PMID: 15684209]

11. **Helfand M.** Screening for subclinical thyroid dysfunction in nonpregnant adults: a summary of the evidence for the U.S. Preventive Services Task Force. Ann Intern Med. 2004;140:128-41. [PMID: 14734337]

12. **Adult Immunization Schedule.** Centers for Disease Control and Prevention Web site. Available at: http://www.cdc.gov/nip/recs/adult-schedule.htm. Accessed June 20, 2006.

13. **Summary of Recommendations for Adult Immunization.** Immunization Action Coalition and Hepatitis B Coalition Web site. Available at: http://www.immunize.org/catg.d/p2011b.pdf. Accessed on June 20, 2006.

COMMON SYMPTOMS

RECENT ADVANCES

- Behavioral therapy in migraine and tension headache
- β-Blockers and tricyclic antidepressants in headache prophylaxis
- The placebo effect in IBS
- Efficacy of tegaserod in IBS
- Bisphosphonates in complex regional pain syndrome
- Efficacy of nonpharmacologic treatment of chronic pain
- Efficacy of guaifenesin in acute cough
- Eszopiclone in chronic insomnia
- Effectiveness of cognitive behavioral therapy in primary insomnia
- Diagnostic value of B-type natriuretic peptide in dyspnea
- Short-term prednisolone therapy in adhesive capsulitis
- Efficacy of duloxetine in fibromyalgia syndrome

Epidemiology of Common Symptoms

Physical symptoms account for at least half of all outpatient visits. Overall, 40% to 50% of these symptoms are pain complaints, 30% are upper respiratory symptoms, and 20% to 25% are nonpain, nonrespiratory symptoms. Two thirds of patients have musculoskeletal pain (back, neck, hip, knee, and other joints) and one third have nonmusculoskeletal pain (most commonly headache, abdominal pain, and chest pain). Physical symptoms are even more prevalent in the community, with less than 25% of symptomatic patients visiting a health care provider.

Most physical symptoms occur 25% to 50% more commonly in women than in men, the reasons for which are not well elucidated but are probably multifactorial in nature. Older age is not associated with increased symptom reporting in clinical practice. Possible explanations include age differences in the reasons for seeking care (for example, older patients often are evaluated for routine follow-up of stable medical conditions, whereas younger patients more commonly seek acute care for symptomatic problems); "normalization" of symptoms that may occur with aging; and a lower prevalence of depressive and anxiety disorders in older patients. The influence of race/ethnicity and other sociodemographic variables on symptom reporting is less clear.

At least one third of somatic symptoms in primary and specialty care and population-based studies are medically unexplained. Also common are syndromes manifested by constellations of symptoms, such as irritable bowel syndrome, fibromyalgia, chronic fatigue syndrome, temporomandibular joint disorder, tension headache, and interstitial cystitis. These syndromes overlap in terms of symptoms, functional impairment, psychiatric comorbidity, and response to cognitive behavioral therapy and antidepressants. Patients with one syndrome have at least a 30% to 50% chance of having one or more of the other syndromes (1).

Two thirds of depressed patients are evaluated exclusively for physical complaints, and half report multiple, unexplained somatic symptoms (2). Factors that increase the likelihood of an underlying depressive or anxiety disorder include medically unexplained symptoms, the total number of symptoms, physical symptom severity, and physician-rated "difficulty" of the encounter. Anxiety and somatoform disorders, a history of sexual or physical abuse, recent stress, and other psychosocial factors also substantially increase the likelihood of somatic symptom reporting.

Less than 5% of symptoms are caused by acutely serious conditions. In another 70% to 75% of patients, symptoms are self-limited, improving over 2 to 6 weeks, whereas approximately 20% to 25% of patients have chronic or recurrent symptoms (3). Upper respiratory tract symptoms have the lowest rate of chronicity, whereas pain complaints, especially headache, back pain, and other musculoskeletal symptoms, have the highest rate of persistence.

Certain symptoms (chest pain, dyspnea, or acute abdominal pain) may require initial testing more often than others (back pain, headache, fatigue, or dizziness). The presence of "red flags" or signs of a potentially serious underlying cause of symptoms on history or physical examination typically dictates whether immediate diagnostic evaluation is warranted. History and physical examination help to establish the ultimate diagnosis in more than 75% of cases. Follow-up is preferable to an initial and expensive workup in many patients; a 2- to 6-week period of watchful waiting can clarify whether symptoms will be self-limited or persistent. Studies of both specific and general types of symptoms have shown that physicians' initial judgment is quite accurate, and when disease is thought unlikely to be serious at the index visit, serious disease is unlikely to emerge with long-term follow-up.

Studies have shown the benefit of addressing patients' symptom-specific concerns and expectations, which commonly include an explanation of the symptom's cause and prognosis and a desire for specific physician actions, such as medication prescribing, test ordering, subspecialty referral, or administrative action (4). Screening for potentially treatable depression and anxiety is warranted in patients whose unexplained physical symptoms persist at 2- to 6-week follow-up visits, or in those in whom psychosocial factors are suspected at the initial visit.

KEY POINTS

- **Most physical symptoms occur 25% to 50% more commonly in women than in men.**
- **At least 30% of somatic symptoms are medically unexplained.**

Headache

Population-based studies have found that up to 30% of individuals experience a migraine or tension headache at some time in their life, with more than half seeking medical attention for this symptom. In the United States, 87% of those with headaches report disability, with 25% having at least four disabling episodes per month. Migraine headaches alone cost the United States $1 billion per year in direct medical costs, with $13 billion per year in lost productivity. The total cost to society is close to that of diabetes and exceeds that of asthma.

The International Headache Society has developed criteria for various headache types (5). Although the list is complete and the criteria simple to apply, they are too cumbersome for everyday use and were designed primarily to standardize definitions for research purposes. Most patients with headaches who are evaluated in primary care settings have three types of headaches: migraine, tension, and cluster headaches (6).

Headaches are classified as either primary or secondary. Primary headaches are those in which an underlying cause cannot be determined. Secondary headaches are due to other processes and include several diagnoses that are of immediate danger to the patient, including infection, metastatic disease, and subdural or intracranial hemorrhage. Red flag features include recent onset (<6 months); headaches beginning after age 50 years; headaches that are acute (thunderclap) in onset; signs of infection; the presence of a rash; a history of malignancy, HIV or pregnancy; markedly elevated blood pressure; recent head trauma; or nonresolving neurologic deficits. One popular instrument for headache screening is the Brief Headache Screen, which consists of the following questions:

- How often do you get severe headaches (that is, without treatment, how often do you find it difficult to function)? *Any patient with severe episodic headaches should be assumed to have migraine headaches.*
- How often do you get other (milder) headaches? *Patients with daily headaches should be evaluated for worrisome symptoms. Daily headache is often due to medication overuse.*
- How often do you take headache relievers or pain pills? *Use of medication for more than 3 days/week represents medication overuse.*
- Has there been any recent change in your headaches? *Headaches occurring for >6 months have very low likelihood of secondary cause.*
- How often do you miss work (or leisure activities) because of headache? *The answer to this question can help to determine the impact of headaches on patients' lives.*

Most patients with headaches whom primary care physicians evaluate have primary headaches, and most of these are migraines, although episodic tension headaches are more common in the community, occurring in up to 50% or more of the population (7). This is because tension headaches are usually less severe than migraine headaches and are self-managed by patients. The exception is when a tension headache becomes a chronic daily headache.

Migraine headaches are more prevalent in women. In many patients, they are misdiagnosed as sinus or tension headaches. Tension and migraine headaches tend to gradually increase in intensity, reaching a peak over several minutes to hours. Headache caused by intracranial bleeding is often described as a "thunderclap," constituting the most severe headache of a patient's life, with acute onset, whereas severe headaches that occur episodically should be assumed to be migraine. Other features suggestive of migraine headaches include worsening with activity, unilateral or throbbing pain, and an association with nausea and/or sensitivity to light or sound.

Cluster headaches are repetitive headaches that occur for weeks to months at a time, followed by periods of remission.

They occur more commonly in men. The pain in cluster headaches is always unilateral, but it can switch sides during subsequent bouts and is associated with ipsilateral lacrimation and redness of the eye, stuffy nose, rhinorrhea, sweating, pallor, and Horner's syndrome. Other focal neurologic symptoms occur rarely in patients with cluster headaches. A typical cluster headache lasts from 30 minutes to 3 hours (mean duration 45 to 60 minutes).

Although the presence of a daily headache may be a sign of a potentially serious underlying condition, many headaches are induced by medication overuse. Up to a third of chronic daily headaches in primary care patients are caused by the overuse of analgesics, ergotamine, or triptans (8); in headache clinics, up to 80% of chronic daily headaches are caused by the overuse of these agents (9). Because almost all anti-headache drugs, including analgesics, ergots, triptans, and combination medications containing barbiturates, tranquilizers, codeine, or caffeine, can result in medication-overuse headaches (10), the use of such drugs should be limited to no more than 3 days per week. Some data suggest that triptans can cause daily headaches at shorter durations and lower monthly doses (1.7 years with 18 average monthly doses) than ergots (2.7 years with 37 average monthly doses) or analgesics (4.8 years with 114 average monthly doses). Medication-overuse headaches originate as tension or migraine types. Patients whose original headache type was migraine have a "transformed" migraine headache.

Treatment of headaches is abortive, and treatment for acute headaches is prophylactic, intended to reduce the frequency, duration, or intensity of headaches. Patients usually self-manage acute-onset tension headaches with over-the-counter medications and often seek medical care when headaches become chronic, although patients with more severe tension headaches may also seek medical attention. For acute treatment, analgesics, such as acetaminophen and other NSAIDs, are first-line therapy (11). Combination drugs that contain butalbital, caffeine, ergotamine, or narcotics, may also be effective, but their use should be limited to no more than 3 days per week.

Effective abortive treatment of cluster headaches includes 100% oxygen, triptans (sumatriptan and zolmitriptan), or ergots (cafergot and DHE 45 [dehydroergotamine]); indomethacin and other NSAIDs may also be effective. Effective drugs for acute migraine headaches include NSAIDs, acetaminophen, triptans, ergotamines, combination drugs that contain butalbital or caffeine, and antiemetics (intravenous or intramuscular administration only; oral antiemetics are ineffective). The triptans are considered specific treatment for migraine headaches, and all have been demonstrated to be effective.

Some patients respond to simple analgesics or combination drugs, but these agents are associated with transformation of episodic migraine headaches to chronic daily headaches; therefore, their use should be limited to no more than 3 days per week, although there is no evidence to guide safe dosing frequencies.

All patients with cluster headaches should receive prophylactic treatment for at least a few months to decrease or prevent recurrent attacks; verapamil, lithium, ergotamine, methysergide, cyproheptadine, and indomethacin are all effective preventive therapies in patients with cluster headaches. Both migraine and tension headaches appear to respond equally well to prophylactic therapy. Behavioral treatments, including relaxation therapy, biofeedback, and cognitive behavioral therapy (CBT), have resulted in a 35% to 55% improvement in migraine and tension headache, with effects persisting up to 7 years, the longest reported follow-up duration (12, 13). Spinal manipulation has not been found to be effective (14) in preventing headache. Medications well supported by evidence for headache prophylaxis include β-blockers (15) (but not pindolol), tricyclic antidepressants, valproate, calcium channel blockers (but not dihydropyridines), and gabapentin (16). The selective serotonin reuptake inhibitors appear to be no more effective than placebo in preventing migraine headaches and not as effective as tricyclic antidepressants in preventing tension headaches (17). Recent randomized controlled trials have suggested that ACE inhibitors or angiotensin receptor blockers may also be effective in headache prophylaxis, although larger trials are needed before the use of these agents can be recommended (18, 19).

Chronic daily headaches only respond to cessation of daily analgesics, but discontinuing such medication can be difficult for those with severe daily headaches. Patients who have been misusing codeine, barbiturates, or tranquilizers may experience withdrawal from these medications and may require hospitalization. For patients deemed sufficiently motivated and in whom outpatient withdrawal is safe, a reasonable approach is initiation of a prophylactic regimen before beginning drug withdrawal. Some physicians also administer a 1-month course of prednisone to patients before drug withdrawal. Valproate has been shown useful in treating analgesic-induced daily headaches (see also Reference 10). Paradoxically, ergotamines or long-acting analgesics can be used for triptan withdrawal, as can triptan and the long-acting analgesics for ergotamine withdrawal and ergotamine or triptans for analgesic-withdrawal headaches. The daily use of these drugs for 2 to 3 weeks during the period of withdrawal headaches does not produce subsequent withdrawal headaches when they are stopped.

Chronic Abdominal Pain

Abdominal pain is among the most common physical complaints, accounting for more than 12 million clinic visits in the United States each year. A major decision for physicians is whether the pretest probability of an urgent and/or treatable cause (for example, obstructive, infectious, inflammatory, or ischemic) for acute abdominal pain warrants expedited evaluation, such as blood and urine testing, radiologic imaging, endoscopy, or surgical consultation. Chronic abdominal pain, which can be persistent or recurrent, requires a different diagnostic approach from that used for acute abdominal pain. Although there is no a consensus on the definition, "chronic" abdominal pain is commonly characterized as pain persisting for 6 or more months.

The epidemiology of abdominal pain in primary care is not well characterized, but three descriptive studies totaling more than 1200 patients suggest some preliminary conclusions. The cause of pain in 50% to 75% of patients with abdominal pain who are evaluated in a primary care setting (versus in the emergency department) is solely functional (for example, irritable bowel syndrome or nonulcer dyspepsia) or idiopathic. Most (>80%) of the specific diagnoses are established early in care, and few patients (<10%) with an initial "nonorganic" diagnosis (that is, functional or idiopathic causes) have an occult, more serious disorder. Because the age

TABLE 4 Common Categories of Chronic Abdominal Pain (Excluding Malignant and Gynecologic Causes)

Category	Comments on Evaluation and/or Treatment
Peptic ulcer	• Epigastric pain 1 to 3 hours after eating or nocturnal pain relieved by acid suppressive medications or food • *Helicobacter pylori* testing and, if positive, antibiotic treatment • Endoscopy, particularly if negative for *H. pylori* or on treatment failure
Gastroesophageal reflux	• Substernal reflux, regurgitation, and heartburn exacerbated when supine or consuming certain foods (for example, citrus fruits), typically relieved by acid-suppressive medications • Acid suppression – H_2-blockers or PPI • Endoscopy if weight loss, anemia, dysphagia
Gallstones (biliary)	• Ultrasonography (if postcholecystectomy, consider ERCP or MRCP)
Chronic pancreatitis	• Lipase and amylase often normal (versus acute pancreatitis) • Opiates often necessary; role of ERCP is uncertain
Inflammatory bowel disease	• If pain is the predominant symptom, Crohn's disease is more common than ulcerative colitis • Consider complete blood count, ESR, CT, colonoscopy
Irritable bowel syndrome	• Usually bowel symptoms (diarrhea and/or constipation) • Young age of onset, and more common in women
Nonulcer dyspepsia	• H_2-blockers or PPI, but evidence for efficacy is uncertain • Refractory symptoms may require endoscopy
Nonvisceral	• Muscles, lower ribs, ventral hernia, psychologic, idiopathic

PPI = proton pump inhibitor; ERCP = endoscopic retrograde cholangiopancreatography; MRCP = magnetic resonance cholangiopancreatography; ESR = erythrocyte sedimentation rate.

of the average patient in these studies ranges from 40 to 47 years, these results must be extrapolated cautiously in older patients, in whom cancer, intestinal ischemia, and other serious diseases increase in frequency.

Table 4 highlights some common diagnoses in patients with chronic abdominal pain. Dyspepsia has been interpreted in many ways but should not include heartburn or indigestion and is best defined as persistent or recurrent abdominal pain or discomfort centered in the upper abdomen.

The four cardinal findings characterizing chronic pancreatitis include pain (90% to 95%), diabetes mellitus, steatorrhea, and pancreatic calculi. Periods of pain may be irregular, with weeks to months of remission. A third to half of patients with pancreatitis may become pain-free, but this may take years. Pancreatic enzymes are often ineffective for pain, and many patients require chronic opiates. Refractory pain in these patients sometimes necessitates sphincterotomy, stenting, or

TABLE 5 Important Causes of Chronic Lower Abdominal Pain in Women of Childbearing Age

Cause	Age of Onset	Comments
Primary dysmenorrhea	Early 20s	• Menstrual pain (first 1 to 3 days); decreases with age • Treatment includes NSAIDs or oral contraceptives
Endometriosis	Late 20s	• Premenstrual pain (few days to 1 to 2 weeks before menses) • Diagnostic tests include ultrasound and/or laparoscopy • Treatment includes oral contraceptives or surgery
Chronic pelvic pain	25 to 35 y	• Often multiple other chronic physical symptoms • Previous sexual or physical abuse increases risk
Fibroids (leiomyoma)	Late 30s to 40s	• Diagnosis made by physical examination, ultrasonography • Often regress postmenopause • Surgery required with severe anemia, persistent pain, compression of other pelvic structures (e.g., bowels or bladder)
Ovarian cancer	>40 y (peaks in 60s)	• Diagnosis typically includes CT

surgical resection, although evidence confirming the efficacy of these procedures is limited.

Although right upper-quadrant colic is a classic symptom of gallbladder disease, the relationship between dyspepsia and gallstones is less certain (20). The prevalence of gallstones is 8% in patients older than 40 years, increasing to 20% in patients older than 60 years. Most (90%) patients with gallstones remain asymptomatic. At the same time, 25% of the population seeks care for dyspepsia. Thus, a causative versus coincidental relationship between gallstones and dyspepsia can be difficult to ascertain. Acalculous biliary pain can be caused by microscopic crystals ("sludge") or sphincter of Oddi dysfunction, but this type of pain also would be manifested as right upper-quadrant colic rather than dyspepsia. Finally, 20% or more of patients continue to experience pain after cholecystectomy.

Abdominal wall pain may account for approximately 10% of chronic idiopathic abdominal pain in patients evaluated by gastroenterologists as recently summarized in the literature (21). Abdominal wall pain is characterized by very localized pain in which the most intense component can be covered by a fingertip, superficial tenderness to the depth of the rectus abdominus, and/or increased point tenderness with abdominal wall muscle tensing. Small trials, largely uncontrolled, suggest local anesthetic/corticosteroid injections may be beneficial in these patients, but further study is required.

Cancer is present in only a few patients with abdominal pain, but signs such as weight loss, decreased appetite or early satiety, abdominal swelling or masses, blood loss (overt or occult), unexplained anemia, nocturnal or refractory pain, and older age (>40 to 50 years) are worrisome and heighten the suspicion for malignancy (see Hematology and Oncology Syllabus). Chronic abdominal pain in premenopausal women, especially when located in the lower abdomen, may be caused by gynecologic disorders (see Women's Health Section) (**Table 5**). A history of sexual or physical abuse has been found to be a strong risk factor for chronic, unexplained abdominal or pelvic pain in women. Finally, intestinal

ischemia and adhesions are important considerations in the evaluation of patients with acute abdominal pain, but they may also be occasional causes of chronic or recurrent abdominal pain (for example, abdominal "angina" manifested by postprandial pain and weight loss in older patients with vascular disease or recurrent pain in patients who have adhesions from prior surgery).

Radiologic imaging is often performed in patients with unexplained or persistent abdominal pain. CT is the preferred method for imaging the bowel, including for conditions such as appendicitis, diverticulitis, and pneumoperitoneum, but it has some limitations in visualizing common bile duct stones and the female pelvic organs. MRI is a less rapid testing approach than CT and requires greater patient cooperation. This test is helpful in viewing parenchymal lesions, especially in the liver. Magnetic resonance cholangiopancreatography is a noninvasive option to endoscopic retrograde cholangiopancreatography for evaluating biliary or pancreatic abnormalities (22). CT is preferable for the assessment of possible urolithiasis, because MRI does not detect calcium well. Ultrasonography is a rapid, inexpensive option, which is particularly useful in diagnosing gallbladder disease, including common bile duct stones. It is more operator dependent than other imaging techniques and may have poor resolution in obese patients.

Treatment of chronic abdominal pain varies with specific disorders; because this type of pain is frequently functional or idiopathic, attention to pain management and psychologic factors is important (23).

The conventional precaution against using opioid analgesics in patients with undiagnosed abdominal pain has recently been questioned in a literature synthesis (24). Although these results are mainly applicable to the management of patients with acute abdominal pain, the question arises frequently enough to warrant mentioning here. Of the eight trials reviewed, none reported an association between opioid analgesia use and diagnostic impairment or dangerous masking of the findings on physical examination. Although the reviewed studies had several methodologic limitations, the authors concluded that "a practice of judicious provision of analgesia appears safe, reasonable, and in the best interests of patients with pain."

KEY POINTS

- Findings indicative of chronic pancreatitis include relapsing-remitting pain, diabetes mellitus, steatorrhea, and pancreatic calculi.
- Right upper-quadrant colic is a classic symptom of gallbladder disease.
- Weight loss, decreased appetite or early satiety, abdominal swelling or masses, blood loss, unexplained anemia, nocturnal or refractory pain, and older age are signs suspicious for malignancy.
- A history of sexual or physical abuse is a strong risk factor for chronic, unexplained abdominal or pelvic pain in women.
- CT is the preferred method for imaging the bowel, including for appendicitis, diverticulitis, and pneumoperitoneum, but it has limitations in visualizing common bile duct stones and the female pelvic organs.
- No association has been found between opioid analgesia use and diagnostic impairment or dangerous masking of the findings on physical examination in patients with undiagnosed abdominal pain.

Irritable Bowel Syndrome

Irritable bowel syndrome (IBS) is common, present in approximately 12% of individuals worldwide (25). Most individuals with IBS do not seek medical treatment (26). Patients seeking medical care for IBS often have comorbidities; many have depression, anxiety, or somatoform disorders, and more than half also have fibromyalgia, chronic fatigue syndrome, temporomandibular joint disorder, or chronic pelvic pain (27). Although patients with IBS who are evaluated by primary care physicians tend to be younger and are more likely to be women (2:1 predominance), population-based studies have found IBS to be common in young and elderly patients and in both men and women. There are no studies of the natural history of IBS.

The pathophysiology of IBS is unclear. Putative factors include abnormal gastrointestinal motility, visceral hypersensitivity, and small bowel overgrowth (28). IBS symptoms worsen with stress. Heredity and environmental factors have also been implicated in the pathophysiology of this syndrome.

IBS lacks a biologic marker; it is a symptoms-based diagnosis. Although formal criteria for the diagnosis of IBS exist, most clinicians are unaware of them (29), and the American College of Gastroenterology recommends diagnosis based on the presence of "abdominal discomfort associated with altered bowel habits" (see also Reference 25). The most recent formal criteria are the Rome II criteria, which require the presence of at least two of three symptoms occurring for 3 months (not necessarily consecutive) during a 12-month period. These symptoms include pain relieved with defecation, onset associated with change in stool frequency, or onset associated with change in the consistency of the stool. In clinical practice, these criteria have a positive predictive value of 98% (30). In the absence of alarm symptoms, such as hematochezia, weight loss greater than 4.5 kg (10 lb), family history of colon cancer, recurring fever, anemia, or chronic severe diarrhea, most experts recommend no further diagnostic evaluation in patients presenting with IBS symptoms beyond a careful history and physical examination, because additional tests have a diagnostic yield of 2% or less (see also Reference 30). Some experts suggest testing for the presence of IgA endomysial antibodies to rule out celiac sprue among patients with chronic diarrhea, especially in those who are at increased risk for this disease (Northern European descent, family history for celiac sprue, type 1 diabetes mellitus).

In clinical practice, IBS tends to have three different forms: diarrhea-predominant, constipation-predominant, and pain-predominant (31). Alternating between diarrhea and constipation or changing from constipation predominance to diarrhea predominance (or vice versa) over time is not uncommon. The management of IBS focuses on managing symptoms rather than on cure (32).

Because mental disorders are common in patients with IBS, screening and treating patients for depression and anxiety is indicated. Nonpharmacologic treatments for IBS include dietary modification, exercise, relaxation therapy, biofeedback, hypnotherapy, cognitive behavioral therapy (CBT), and psychotherapy. Pharmacologic approaches to treatment of this syndrome include antispasmodic agents, bulking agents, antidiarrheal agents, tricyclic antidepressants, the $5HT_4$ receptor agonist tegaserod, and the $5HT_3$ receptor antagonist alosetron.

Several studies have found that up to 50% of patients with IBS experience significant improvement from placebo (33). Because of the implication of the placebo effect in these studies, full evaluation of the effectiveness of any intervention must be done using blinded methods, which makes it difficult to assess the effects of many common treatment modalities, including dietary modification and nonpharmacologic treatments because these interventions cannot be blinded. In the absence of lactose intolerance or celiac sprue, studies of dietary modification have been largely disappointing. Some clinicians recommend lower-fat diets in the management of patients with IBS because lipids amplify gut sensations and motor reflexes. Stress reduction may be helpful in patients with this syndrome and has been shown to reduce clinical visits, if not IBS symptoms. No trials have proven unequivocally that behavioral therapies are efficacious in IBS, although several have shown some improvement in individual IBS symptoms with relaxation therapy, biofeedback, hypnotherapy, CBT, or psychotherapy in these patients (34).

The antispasmodic agents, antidiarrheal agents, and tricyclic antidepressants have not been found helpful in treating overall IBS symptoms or improving the quality of life, but all of these agents have been shown useful in treating specific IBS symptoms. Antispasmodic agents and tricyclic antidepressants can help reduce pain among patients with pain-predominant IBS (35). In patients with diarrhea-predominant IBS, the antidiarrheal agent loperamide is useful; bulking agents have also been suggested for use in these patients, although the data do not suggest they are effective (36). Antidiarrheal agents exacerbate constipation-predominant diarrhea, bulking agents can lead to bloating and abdominal discomfort—even while improving constipation—and the tricyclic antidepressants have a myriad of side effects; therefore, none of these is a panacea.

The $5HT_4$ receptor agonist tegaserod is Food and Drug Administration–approved for use in patients with constipation-predominant IBS and has been found helpful in several randomized controlled trials in reducing both specific and overall IBS symptoms and in improving quality of life (37). Because it is expensive, its use should be reserved for patients who do not respond to bulking and antispasmodic agents. Similarly, the $5HT_3$ receptor antagonist alosetron has FDA approval for use in patients with diarrhea-predominant IBS and has been shown to improve global IBS symptoms in several well-constructed randomized controlled trials (38). There is concern, however, about the risk for ischemic colitis with use of alosetron, which has occurred in approximately 1 in 700 patients who took this drug. Alosetron was temporarily withdrawn from the market, but, after advocacy groups lobbied for its reinstitution, was reintroduced to the marketplace, and is currently available. This drug should be used cautiously if at all.

KEY POINTS

- IBS is characterized by pain relieved with defecation, a change in stool frequency, or a change in stool consistency.
- The presence of two of three IBS symptoms occurring for 3 not-necessarily-consecutive months during a 12-month period has a positive predictive value for IBS of 98%.
- In the absence of alarm symptoms, most patients with IBS symptoms require only a physical examination and history.
- Testing for celiac sprue may be appropriate in individuals with chronic diarrhea, particularly in those at increased risk for this disease.
- Half of patients with IBS experience significant improvement from placebo.
- Screening for depression and anxiety is appropriate in patients with IBS symptoms.
- Tegaserod is a Food and Drug Administration (FDA)–approved drug for treatment of constipation-predominant IBS, but its use should be reserved for patients who do not respond to therapy with bulking and antispasmodic agents.
- Alosetron is an FDA-approved drug for use in diarrhea-predominant IBS but is associated with ischemic colitis.

Nonulcer Dyspepsia

Nonulcer dyspepsia (NUD), also known as functional dyspepsia, is defined as nonspecific upper abdominal discomfort or nausea not attributable to peptic ulcer disease and is one of the most common forms of dyspepsia in the primary care setting. The etiology and pathophysiology of NUD are unclear, but this disorder may have multifactorial causes, including dysmotility, visceral hypersensitivity, *Helicobacter pylori* infection, acid-peptic disease, psychosocial factors, or an interaction among multiple processes.

Current ROME criteria for the diagnosis of NUD are 12 weeks' duration of dyspepsia (not necessarily consecutive) occurring within the past year, no evidence of irritable bowel syndrome, and no apparent organic explanation for the symptoms. It is difficult to establish a diagnosis and manage patients with NUD because not everyone can undergo endoscopy to exclude organic pathology, and this disorder is often recalcitrant to therapeutic interventions. The symptoms of NUD are similar to those of peptic ulcer disease, gastroesophageal reflux, and gastric malignancy, and it is difficult to differentiate NUD from such other diseases with high specificity based on clinical information derived by noninvasive means. In comparing various diagnostic approaches, results from one decision analysis concluded that a "test and treat" approach using urea breath testing and *H. pylori* eradication was the most cost-effective strategy compared with performing initial endoscopy, double-contrast barium, empirical eradication therapy, empirical antisecretory therapy, or sequential testing (laboratory serology followed by urea breath testing if positive) in achieving symptomatic cure in these patients (39). In the same decision analysis, more cases of early gastric malignancy are diagnosed in patients older than 45 years who are evaluated for dyspepsia (regardless of other symptoms or comorbidities) when endoscopy is used as the initial approach compared with other approaches.

Drug treatment for NUD is limited and only marginally effective. There is a small benefit to eradicating *H. pylori* infection in patients with NUD (summary relative risk for persistent or worse symptoms after eradication: 0.91% CI, 0.86 to 0.95) (40). Ineffective treatments of NUD studied in clinical trials include antacids, sucralfate, and bismuth. Effective treatments of NUD include tricyclic antidepressants, H_2-receptor antagonists, and proton pump inhibitors, although the acid suppression effects are modest, and whether these treatments are actually treating subgroups of patients with GERD is uncertain. NUD treatments undergoing investigation include gastric fundus relaxation therapies (buspirone and sumatriptan), prokinetic agents (tegaserod), and visceral analgesic medications (octreotide, fedotozine, and serotonin receptor antagonists).

Psychologic interventions, such as cognitive behavioral therapy, hypnosis, and relaxation therapy, are generally not helpful in patients with NUD (41); however, these patients have a higher prevalence of depression, anxiety, and somatoform disorders than patients without NUD. Screening patients with NUD for these disorders and providing necessary treatment is appropriate (42).

Up to 86% of primary care patients with dyspepsia continue to be symptomatic up to 1 year after initial presentation and persist in using high levels of medical resources (43); therefore, a strategy of care similar to that used in managing patients with other unexplained physical symptoms is appropriate in patients with NUD. This management approach consists of monitoring symptoms with regular follow-up visits, addressing psychosocial stressors, and enabling patients to cope with their illness while still being attentive to the development of other potential causes for this disorder.

KEY POINTS

- Current ROME criteria for the diagnosis of nonulcer dyspepsia (NUD) are 12 weeks' duration of dyspepsia (not necessarily consecutive) within the past year, no evidence of irritable bowel syndrome, and no apparent organic explanation.

- Urea breath testing and *Helicobacter pylori* eradication was the most cost-effective strategy compared with performing initial endoscopy, double-contrast barium, empirical eradication therapy, empirical antisecretory therapy, or sequential testing in achieving symptomatic cure in patients with suspected NUD.

- There is a small benefit to eradicating *H. pylori* infection in patients with NUD.

- Effective treatments of patients with NUD include tricyclic antidepressants, H_2-receptor antagonists, and proton pump inhibitors.

Chronic Pain Management

Chronic pain is an extremely common problem in primary care, accounting for substantial health care utilization. It is generally undertreated, possibly because of concerns about overtreatment, toxicity, and addiction. Although no specific taxonomy or definition for chronic pain has been defined, one accepted definition is pain that persists for longer than 3 months.

Chronic pain can be categorized as malignant or oncologic (see Foundations of Internal Medicine syllabus), neuropathic (central nervous system [phantom limb or poststroke]; peripheral diabetic neuropathy; trigeminal neuralgia; postherpetic neuralgia; compressive neuropathy; and reflex sympathetic dystrophy), or nonmalignant non-neuropathic (idiopathic pain syndromes; degenerative joint or disk disease; or musculoskeletal disease pain). The focus of diagnosis and evaluation of chronic pain should be on reversible causes of the pain. Exhaustive workups are often not necessary and are unlikely to identify a reversible cause of the pain when the symptoms have been chronic.

Drug treatment is largely dependent on type of chronic pain syndrome (nonmalignant pain versus malignant pain with expanding tumor burden). Even among patients with nonmalignant (degenerative arthritis, neuropathic pain) or idiopathic pain syndromes (low back pain, irritable bowel, or chronic headache), syndrome-specific treatments are available for which there is supporting randomized trial evidence.

For nonmalignant non-neuropathic pain syndromes, a step-wise approach is the most efficacious and least toxic strategy, similar to that illustrated in the World Health Organization Analgesic Ladder (see Foundations of Internal Medicine Syllabus). This approach suggests an initial dose of acetaminophen (up to 1 g four times daily), followed by NSAIDs, with progression first to mild-potency narcotics such as codeine and then to moderate high-potency narcotics such as morphine. Weaker analgesic agents, such as tramadol and topical capsaicin, are generally used as adjunctive therapies for chronic pain. Surgical options such as joint replacement should be discussed with patients who have advanced degenerative joint or disk disease and in whom pain is refractory to medical therapy, side effects of medical therapy are not acceptable, or surgery versus pharmacologic therapy is favored.

For neuropathic pain, the same strategy of step-wise medications is appropriate, although tricyclic antidepressants or anticonvulsant therapies may be appropriate for use earlier than they would be to treat other pain syndromes given their efficacy in this setting. For postherpetic neuralgia and diabetic neuropathy, tricyclic antidepressants are particularly efficacious and should be considered as first-line therapy, although they are not Food and Drug Administration–approved for pain treatment. For trigeminal neuralgia, carbamazepine is a first-line agent for pain control.

Combination therapy with multiple modalities and drugs from different classes may offer synergistic efficacy while minimizing dosing and side effects. Other chronic pain therapies that are being developed include neuronal transmission modulators (epibatidine and conotoxins) and cannabinoids.

Chronic pain management becomes complicated in the elderly or during end-of-life situations in which multiple comorbidities and polypharmacy may result in drug–drug interactions and side effects. Patients with chronic renal insufficiency or end-stage renal or liver disease require special attention and monitoring because of the variable toxicity and clearance of pain medications in these settings. Central pain syndromes, such as phantom limb pain, are notoriously difficult to treat and are not responsive to the typically efficacious agents used in treating neuropathic pain. Patients with comorbid addictions can be difficult to treat with narcotics or other controlled substances but can be successfully managed with close follow-up, formal contracting with a single prescriber, use of limited prescription quantities, drug screens, and pill monitoring. Complex regional pain syndrome, also known as reflex sympathetic dystrophy, is a unique chronic pain syndrome defined as chronic pain of the extremities often characterized by swelling, vasomotor instability, skin changes, and patchy bone demineralization. This syndrome frequently begins after an injury, surgery, or a vascular event. Although the general principles of pain management apply, patients with complex regional pain syndrome also respond to bisphosphonates, presumably because of bone-associated effects on nociception (44).

Several long-acting agents are available for patients with chronic pain requiring narcotic analgesia (**Table 6**) (45). Because

TABLE 6 Long-acting Analgesics		
Generic Name	**Analgesic Dose**	**Typical First Dose**
Codeine		
Oral	30 mg every 3–4 h	30 mg every 3–4 h
Parenteral	10 mg every 3–4 h	10 mg every 3–4 h
Fentanyl†	25 µg/h	25 µg/h
Patch	Patch every 72 h*	Patch every 72 h†
Hydrocodone‡		
Oral	NA	10 mg every 3–4 h
Parenteral	NA	NA
Hydromorphone		
Oral	7.5 mg every 3–4 h	2-4 mg every 3–4 h
Parenteral	1.5 mg every 3–4 h	1.5 mg every 3–4 h
Levorphanol		
Oral	4 mg every 6–8 h	4 mg every 6–8 h
Parenteral	2 mg every 6–8 h	2 mg every 6–8 h
Meperidine		
Oral	300 mg every 2–3 h	100 mg every 3 h
Parenteral	100 mg every 3 h	100 mg every 3 h
Methadone		
Oral	20 mg every 6–8 h	5 mg every 8–12 h
Parenteral	10 mg every 6–8 h	5 mg every 8–12 h
Morphine		
Oral	30 mg every 3–4 h	15 mg every 3–4 h
Parenteral	10 mg every 3–4 h	10 mg every 3–4 h
Morphine SR		
Oral	NA	15 mg every 8–12 h
Parenteral	NA	NA
Oxycodone‡		
Oral	NA	5 mg every 3–4 h
Parenteral	NA	NA
Oxycodone CR		
Oral	NA	10 mg every 8–12 h
Parenteral	NA	NA

*The information is adapted from The Massachusetts General Hospital Handbook of Pain Management. Equivalent doses of opioids vary markedly according to source. A low dose of an opioid should be used to start and gradually increased until a dose is established that combines maximal analgesia with minimal adverse effects. A short-acting opioid should be used when the patient's pain is occasional, and a long-acting opioid when the pain is constant or frequent. A short-acting opioid can be added to a long-acting opioid to treat breakthrough or incidental pain, but in the treatment of chronic pain the use of nonmedical strategies to treat breakthrough pain is preferable. Rapid or frequent increases in dose should be avoided. Opioid rotation may be useful when dose escalation fails. The new opioid can be started at one half to one quarter of the calculated equivalent dose of the previously prescribed opioid.

NA denotes not applicable.

†This is the lowest available dose. There is a risk for overdose in patients unaccustomed to opioid therapy.

‡There are combinations of formulations (with acetaminophen or aspirin) that have limited usefulness in the treatment of chronic pain.

Reprinted with permission by: Ballantyne JC, Mao J. Opioid therapy for chronic pain. N Engl J Med. 2003;349:1943-53.

all are equally efficacious, the choice of agent should be based on cost, although a trial of these drugs may be necessary to determine which achieves the most acceptable balance of benefits and side effects. The less-expensive, long-acting narcotics are morphine sulfate and methadone, whereas the more expensive agents include oxycodone and fentanyl patches, the latter of which offer the benefit of dosing once every 72 hours. Committing to a chronic opioid analgesia regimen requires a systematic approach involving only one prescriber and pharmacy, with a well-defined plan and goals as well as appropriate documentation.

There are numerous nonpharmacologic and invasive treatments available for chronic pain management, each of which have variable efficacy depending on the cause of the chronic pain; these include transcutaneous electrical nerve stimulation, spinal injections (corticosteroids, methylmethacrylate for vertebral compression fractures), acupuncture, hypnosis, and cognitive behavioral therapy (46–49). The screening and treatment of comorbid depression and anxiety disorders, in addition to identification and addressing of psychosocial stressors, can help to modulate chronic pain.

KEY POINTS

- A step-wise approach, such as that illustrated in the World Health Organization Analgesic Ladder, is appropriate for management of nonmalignant, non-neuropathic pain syndromes.
- Tricyclic antidepressants are effective in treating postherpetic neuralgia and diabetic neuropathy, although they are not FDA approved for these uses.
- In additional to general pain management therapy, patients with complex regional pain syndrome also respond to bisphosphonates.
- Screening for and treatment of comorbid depression and anxiety disorders is helpful in the management of patients with chronic pain.

Acute Cough

Acute cough is one of the most common presenting complaints in primary care and is usually self-limiting. Common causes include upper respiratory tract infections, which are most often viral; bacterial sinusitis; rhinitis due to allergens or environmental irritants; acute tracheobronchitis; pneumonia (viral or bacterial); influenza; exacerbations of chronic pulmonary disease or left ventricular failure; malignancy; aspiration or foreign body; medication reactions; and, less commonly, pulmonary embolism.

Acute cough is typically defined as cough lasting fewer than 3 weeks, with subacute and chronic cough conventionally defined as cough lasting 3 to 8 weeks and longer than 8 weeks, respectively (50). However, acute viral airway infection can result in protracted bronchial hyperreactivity, with secondary coughing lasting for weeks to months. Also, women have a lower cough threshold than do men in controlled trials of locally applied irritants and a higher rate of cough due to ACE inhibitors (see also Reference 50).

Viral upper respiratory tract infection is the most common cause of acute cough. Airway cough receptors are located in the larynx, trachea, and bronchi, and cough in the setting of rhinitis, rhinosinusitis, and pharyngitis is attributed to reflex stimulation from postnasal drainage or throat clearing. Viral rhinitis or rhinosinusitis (the common cold) usually is characterized by rhinorrhea, sneezing, nasal congestion, and postnasal drainage with or without fever, headache, tearing, and throat discomfort, and the chest examination in these patients is normal. Bacterial pneumonia develops in approximately 5% to 10% of adults with acute tracheobronchitis.

Patients with viral pneumonia often have initial influenza-like symptoms followed by more severe cough, fever, and respiratory distress. Patients with community-acquired pneumonia usually have symptoms of acute bronchitis, including cough; however, because cough receptors are located only in the larynx, trachea, and bronchi, pneumonia may be associated with significant alveolar fluid accumulation without significant cough.

Viral influenza usually is characterized by the sudden onset of fever and malaise, followed by cough, headache, myalgia, and nasal and pulmonary symptoms. Patients with this infection may initially have symptoms similar to those associated with the common cold, but they quickly begin experiencing constitutional symptoms. Clinical criteria for influenza from the Centers for Disease Control and Prevention include fever ≥ 37.7 °C (≥ 100.0 °F) (although fever may not be high in the elderly or debilitated) and a minimum of at least one of cough, sore throat, or rhinorrhea. A diagnosis of influenza can be established by analysis of viral cultures or secretions or results of several rapid diagnostic tests (immunofluorescence, polymerase chain reaction, and enzyme immunoassays).

Management of acute cough is directed toward the presumptive cause of cough and includes nasal decongestants for viral rhinitis and rhinosinusitis, antihistamines and nasal corticosteroids for allergies, β-agonists for asthma, treatment of exacerbations of chronic obstructive pulmonary disease or heart failure, and antibiotics when indicated. The over-the-counter market for cough and cold symptoms is responsible for several billion dollars in sales annually in the United States, yet efficacy of the various over-the-counter cough treatment modalities is uncertain. Classes of cough medications include antitussives, expectorants, mucolytics, antihistamines, and nasal anticholinergics. **Table 7** lists examples of antitussive agents; guaifenesin acts as both an expectorant and mucolytic. The main indications for therapy are sleep disruption, painful cough, debilitating cough in frail, elderly patients, and reassurance for patients that action is being taken. Elderly patients are the most vulnerable to the adverse

TABLE 7 Centrally and Peripherally Acting Antitussives

Centrally Acting Antitussives

Opioids	Codeine (hydrocodone, hydromorphone, methadone, and morphine have been used as antitussives but usually only in patients who are terminally ill or have very severe cough)
Non-narcotic opioid derivative	Dextromethorphan: may cause confusion but does not cause constipation, nausea, sedation, or addiction associated with opioids
γ-Aminobutyric receptor activator in brain stem cough center	Baclofen: appears effective for idiopathic and ACE inhibitor–associated cough

Peripherally Acting Antitussives

Local anesthetics	Benzonatate: the only oral local anesthetic in common use for cough, given as aerosol or lozenge

KEY POINTS

- Clinical criteria for influenza are fever ≥37.7 °C (≥100.0 °F) and a minimum of at least one of cough, sore throat, or rhinorrhea.
- A diagnosis of influenza can be established by analysis of viral cultures or secretions or results of rapid diagnostic tests.
- Evidence from two trials suggested benefit in patients with acute cough who took guaifenesin.
- β-Agonists should be used in patients with wheezing but are of unclear benefit in those with acute bronchitis without wheezing.
- In patients with protracted cough for weeks to months, evaluation for other causes, such as asthma, postnasal drip, gastroesophageal reflux disease, and malignancy, is warranted.

effects of antitussive agents, including confusion, nausea, and constipation. In addition, the effect of placebo appears to be almost equal to that of antitussive agents in randomized, blinded trials (51). Recent systematic reviews indicate that no one antitussive agent is clearly superior to or effective than the other in treating acute cough in adults (52, 53). Among antitussives, codeine was no more effective than placebo, and evidence was mixed for dextromethorphan. Evidence from two trials suggested benefit in patients who took guaifenesin. For antihistamine–decongestant combinations, one trial of loratadine (5 mg/pseudoephedrine 120 mg twice daily for 4 days) was no more effective than placebo for treating cough and was associated with more dry mouth, headache, and insomnia. In an additional trial, a combination of dexbrompheniramine (6 mg/pseudoephedrine 120 mg twice daily for 7 days) was associated with significantly less severe cough than placebo but was associated with more dizziness and dry mouth. This evidence base is limited by small studies of overall poor quality and few trials in each drug category; positive studies were more frequently industry supported.

β-Agonists should be used in patients with wheezing but are of unclear benefit in those with acute bronchitis without wheezing. A recent systematic review of β-agonists found conflicting results, but careful examination of patient subgroups suggested that these drugs improve acute cough in studies that enrolled more patients with wheezing or airflow limitation versus studies that enrolled patients without these symptoms (54). In patients with protracted cough for weeks to months, evaluation for other causes, such as asthma, postnasal drip, gastroesophageal reflux disease, and malignancy, is warranted (See Chronic Cough section).

Chronic Fatigue and Chronic Fatigue Syndrome

Chronic fatigue, defined as disabling fatigue lasting for longer than 6 months, is a common symptom in primary care settings, occurring in up to 10% of patients. Of these, only a few patients (1 in 7) meet criteria for chronic fatigue syndrome (CFS). Most cases of CFS are unrecognized. The core clinical features of this syndrome are physical and mental fatigue exacerbated by physical and mental effort. These are subjective phenomena and are often less evident on objective testing.

The precise etiology of CFS remains unknown. A wide range of causative factors have been proposed, but none have been unequivocally established. One etiologic model suggests that a variable combination of environmental factors and individual vulnerability initiates a series of social, psychologic, and biologic processes that eventually lead to the development and perpetuating nature of CFS. Factors that have been positively associated with CFS include genetics, abuse, socioeconomic status, education, infection (Epstein–Barr virus, Q fever, viral meningitis and hepatitis), stress, illness beliefs (specifically, attribution of symptoms to physical causes and low self-efficacy), behavioral factors (fear, avoidance, and decreased activity, which lead to deconditioning), and lack of social support.

Although the Centers for Disease Control and Prevention published criteria for CFS in 1994 based on an international consensus, there is evidence that a more parsimonious definition—impairing chronic fatigue not due to a known cause—is more clinically useful (55, 56). CFS is associated with more severe symptoms, more disability, more unemployment (as high as 50%), worse functioning, more associated symptoms, more psychologic distress, higher levels

TABLE 8 Common Medical Causes of Fatigue

1. Mental disorders: depression, anxiety
2. Chronic disease: COPD, heart failure, cancer, chronic liver disease, chronic kidney disease, autoimmune disease
3. Anemia
4. Drugs
5. Thyroid disease: hypothyroidism, apathetic hyperthyroidism
6. Sleep disturbance: sleep apnea, narcolepsy, idiopathic insomnia, poor sleep hygiene
7. Chronic infection: endocarditis, osteomyelitis, occult abscess

COPD = chronic obstructive pulmonary disease.

of health care utilization, and twice the rate of depression than chronic fatigue that does not meet the criteria for CFS (57). Demographic factors associated with CFS include female sex (2:1), age 30 to 50 years, lower socioeconomic status, less education, and Western nationality (58).

The prognosis for patients with CFS is variable and typically has a fluctuating-chronic course (59). Fifty percent of patients who do not undergo rehabilitative therapy achieve gradual improvement, but with few returning to premorbid levels of functioning. Prospective studies in the general population report that approximately 50% of patients with CFS have partial or complete remission at 2 to 3 years after initial diagnosis. Factors associated with persistence of symptoms include older age, longer illness duration, use of sedating medications, less education, unemployment, worse mental health, lack of social support, and somatic attributions.

Chronic fatigue and CFS require the same management approach. Effective management of patients with possible CFS requires consideration of alternative medical and psychiatric diagnoses and that patients receive a comprehensive assessment on which to collaboratively plan management. The common medical diagnoses characterized by chronic fatigue can be established though a standard history, physical examination, and basic laboratory studies (**Table 8**). If there are no specific indications for performing special investigations, the following screening tests are appropriate: serum thyroid-stimulating hormone measurement (low levels in hyperthyroidism high levels in hypothyroidism); erythrocyte sedimentation rate measurement (sensitive for polymyalgia rheumatica and any condition characterized by systemic inflammation, such as rheumatologic conditions and chronic infections); complete blood count; basic serum chemistries; toxicology screen; and screening for medication withdrawal (particularly for sedating medications).

Immunologic and virologic tests are generally unhelpful as routine investigations and remain research tools in patients with chronic fatigue. Sleep studies can be useful in excluding obstructive sleep apnea and narcolepsy.

A systematic review of interventions for CFS reported that only two interventions, cognitive behavioral therapy (CBT) and graded exercise, were found to be beneficial in improving, but not curing, symptoms (60); therefore, a rehabilitative outpatient program based on appropriately managed increasing activity levels as graded exercise therapy or as CBT is the therapy of choice. The aim of CFS therapy is to maximize functioning and quality of life while minimizing the risk for iatrogenic harm.

Antidepressant drug treatment is a reasonable consideration in the setting of CFS because as many as 75% of all patients with this syndrome also meet the criteria for depression and/or anxiety syndromes. These agents also have a specific role in reducing pain and improving sleep; however, evidence suggesting an overall improvement in symptoms with the use of these agents is mixed. Because sedation is a common side effect of these medications, nonsedating antidepressants should be tried before sedating antidepressants. Amphetamines and other stimulants (for example, methylphenidate) have been used in CFS, but evidence on their efficacy is insufficient, and these drugs confer a risk for dependency.

KEY POINTS

- A systematic review identified only two interventions, cognitive behavioral therapy and graded exercise, as beneficial in improving, but not curing, symptoms of chronic fatigue syndrome (CFS).

- Antidepressant drug treatment is a reasonable consideration in the setting of CFS because most patients with this syndrome also meet the criteria for depression and/or anxiety syndromes.

- Prescribing nonsedating antidepressants before sedating drugs is appropriate in patients with CFS.

Dizziness

Dizziness accounts for an estimated 7 million clinic visits in the United States each year and is a common reason for referrals to neurologic and otolaryngologic practices.

Several factors make dizziness a challenging symptom. First, precise classification of the cause is often difficult. Second, patients and clinicians alike may worry about a serious cardiac or neurologic cause for dizziness. Third, specific therapy is not available for many patients with dizziness. Fourth, in at least 50% of patients, dizziness may be related to multiple potentially causative factors (61).

Approximately half the time, dizziness is described as vertigo, a sensation of rotation or movement, and in most cases representing vestibular dysfunction (62). The three most common specific peripheral vestibular disorders are benign positional vertigo (BPV), labyrinthitis, and Meniere's disease. BPV consists of brief episodes (5 to 15 seconds) that are aggravated or elicited by changes in position, such as turning, rolling over or getting in and out of bed, or bending over (63). Labyrinthitis, sometimes called vestibular neuronitis, occurs acutely, lasts for several days, and resolves spontaneously. Although typically a single episode, labyrinthitis may be recurrent in a few patients. Meniere's disease is characterized by repeated episodes of tinnitus, fluctuating hearing loss, and severe vertigo accompanied eventually by a progressive sensorineural hearing loss. Nausea and vomiting frequently accompany labyrinthitis, Meniere's disease, and other severe vertiginous attacks.

Central vestibular disorders account for a few cases of vertigo; these include cerebrovascular disease, brain tumors, multiple sclerosis, and rarer central causes. Vertigo of vascular origin is usually preceded or accompanied by other neurologic deficits in the distribution of the posterior circulation. Tumors are found in less than 1% of dizzy patients and are slightly more prevalent (2% to 3%) in older patients who are referred to neurologists. The most common tumor associated with dizziness is acoustic neuroma, for which cochlear symptoms (tinnitus and hearing loss) often predominate. Unilateral cochlear symptoms are one marker for acoustic neuroma, whereas bilateral symptoms typically represent presbycusis rather than a tumor. Although vertigo may accompany migraine headache, acephalgic migraine, which is isolated vertigo in the absence of pain, is a controversial diagnosis.

Presyncope is the sensation of near fainting, which, in contrast to true syncope, is often due to postural change (such as orthostatic hypotension) rather than due to more serious cardiac causes (such as electrical [tachy- or bradyarrhythmias] or structural [especially aortic outflow obstruction] causes). Disequilibrium is a sensation of unsteadiness when standing, or, in particular, when walking. Typically occurring in older patients, disequilibrium can be caused by multiple factors, including chronic vestibulopathies, visual problems, arthritis, and neurologic deficits, such as neuropathies, history of stroke, Parkinson's disease, or dementia.

Lightheadedness is a vaguer sensation than the three more discrete types of dizziness sensations—vertigo, presyncope, or disequilibrium. In the vernacular of patients, these latter three sensations may be experienced as "spinning," "fainting," or "falling." Although any cause of dizziness may occasionally produce a nondescript "lightheaded" type of sensation, the two most prominent considerations are psychiatric (primarily depressive, anxiety, or somatoform disorders) or idiopathic causes, which together account for up to a third of all cases of dizziness.

Table 9 outlines key steps in the evaluation of the dizzy patient. The history and physical examination alone help to establish a diagnosis in more than 75% of the cases in which a diagnosis can be established, with the history yielding most of these diagnoses. Four cardinal questions in the evaluation of the dizzy patient are the following:

1. Is the dizziness characterized by spinning, fainting, or falling?

2. What is the effect of position?

3. What are the associated symptoms?

4. Did the onset of dizziness coincide with initiation of a new medication?

Syncope is a particularly important associated symptom with dizziness because the actual loss of consciousness involves a very small subset of dizzy patients in whom early cardiac evaluation may be warranted. Tinnitus or hearing changes are associated with certain vestibular disorders such as Meniere's disease or, rarely, acoustic neuroma. Nausea and,

TABLE 9 Evaluation of the Dizzy Patient

Evaluation	Key Steps
History	• Clarify sensation (spinning, fainting, falling). A sensation of "spinning" suggests vertigo, of "fainting" makes presyncope more likely, and of "falling" makes disequilibrium a stronger consideration • Positional effects: Does dizziness worsen with head movements (e.g., benign positional vertigo), standing up (e.g., orthostatic hypotension), or ambulating (e.g., disequilibrium) • Associated symptoms (syncope, nausea/vomiting, hearing or ear symptoms, ataxia or focal neurologic deficits, multiple somatic complaints) • Medications (especially if initiated around the time of onset of dizziness)
Physical examination	• Orthostatic blood pressure and pulse • Nystagmus exam: gaze-evoked, head shaking, Hallpike maneuver • Brief cardiovascular (murmurs, abnormal rhythm) and neurologic (cerebellar or focal deficits) examination
Early testing or referral	• Certain "red flags" might prompt an earlier work-up • If true syncope, follow guidelines for syncope evaluation • If other cardiovascular abnormalities, consider selected testing (e.g., a suspicious murmur may warrant echocardiography, an abnormal cardiac rhythm on examination may prompt electrocardiography and, if indicated, further dysrhythmia evaluation) • If vertical-beating nystagmus or neurologic abnormalities are present, consider neuroimaging and/or neurologic or otolaryngologic referral
Later testing or referral	• In the few patients with persistent (>4 to 6 weeks) unexplained dizziness, further testing may be needed for diagnostic reasons and/or patient reassurance • Reconsider psychogenic causes, especially depressive, anxiety, and somatoform disorders • Referral for formal vestibular testing (e.g., electronystagmography) or vestibular rehabilitation

in particular, vomiting, suggest vertigo. Patients with a central cause for dizziness seldom have isolated dizziness and instead also have neighboring neurologic symptoms. Patients with psychogenic dizziness typically have associated symptoms, such as mood disturbances, fatigue, insomnia, and pain.

Aspects of the physical examination most diagnostically useful are outlined in Table 9. The four screening maneuvers described below are used to identify a vestibular cause for dizziness and share the objective of detecting nystagmus:

- Primary position. The patient looks straight ahead while the physician tries to detect the presence of nystagmus.

- Gaze-evoked. The patient looks to the right, left, upwards, and downwards, holding each position for 5 to 10 seconds. The finding of more than three to five beats of nystagmus is abnormal.

- Dix-Hallpike test. While seated on the examination table, the patient is asked to lie down quickly, first with one ear turned toward the table, and then with the other ear turned toward the table. The finding of 10 to 20 seconds of nystagmus (and possibly vertigo) is abnormal. The test is positive in about half of patients with BPV, usually those with symptoms of recent onset.

- Head-shaking. The patient closes the eyes while rapidly shaking the head back and forth for 10 seconds, and then opens the eyes. The physician tries to detect the presence of nystagmus.

Nystagmus resulting from peripheral causes usually is represented by horizontal beating. Vertical nystagmus (that is, upward or downward beating) is uncommon and warrants early evaluation for central causes of dizziness with neuroimaging, formal vestibular testing, or neurologic or otolaryngologic referral.

Diagnostic testing is useful in only a few dizzy patients (64). Simple laboratory tests, including complete blood cell counts, serum electrolyte measurement, plasma glucose measurement, serum creatinine measurement, thyroid function, and serologic tests for syphilis, have a very low yield. Audiometry may be helpful in patients with cochlear symptoms, such as tinnitus or asymmetric hearing loss. Although vestibular testing most commonly involves electronystagmography, this test has variable sensitivity and cannot readily distinguish between central and peripheral causes of dizziness. Other vestibular tests include brain stem auditory–evoked responses, rotatory chair, and dynamic posturography, although the value of these diagnostic tests is not well established. An electrocardiogram is commonly obtained in older patients with cardiovascular risk factors but has a low diagnostic value in patients with a normal cardiac examination and nonsyncopal dizziness. Other tests helpful in evaluating syncope, ischemia, or valvular disease (for example, Holter and event monitors, echocardiography, stress testing, tilt-tables, and electrophysiologic stud-

TABLE 10 Management of Potentially Treatable Causes of Dizziness	
Type of Dizziness	**Management**
Acute vertigo	• Meclizine (and, if needed benzodiazepine), especially for peripheral vestibular causes, such as labyrinthitis or Meniere's disease
Benign positional vertigo	• Reassurance and follow-up (gradually resolves in most patients) • Habituation exercises • Canalith repositioning (Epley's) maneuver
Meniere's disease	• Symptomatic treatment (see Acute Vertigo) for acute episodes • Prophylaxis (salt restriction, diuretics) if frequent recurrences • Refer to otolaryngologist to consider surgery for refractory cases
Orthostatic hypotension	• Correct reversible causes (e.g., volume depletion, medication-related) • Treat irreversible causes (such as autonomic neuropathies, aging): fludrocortisone, compression stockings, β-blockers, depending on particular cause
Disequilibrium	• Take measures to prevent falls (e.g., canes, walker) in elderly • Vestibular rehabilitation
Depressive or anxiety disorder	• Antidepressants • Cognitive behavioral therapy
Chronic dizziness	• Vestibular rehabilitation (consisting primarily of home exercises)

ies) have not been shown to be useful in evaluating isolated dizziness.

Neuroimaging should usually be reserved for patients with signs suggesting potentially serious underlying conditions, such as cerebellar or focal neurologic symptoms or vertical-beating nystagmus. Although CT is the procedure of choice for detecting strokes, MRI is better able to provide an image of the posterior fossa structures. However, a community-based study of older individuals found a similar prevalence of MRI abnormalities in dizzy and nondizzy patients (65).

In up to half of patients, dizziness spontaneously resolves or substantially improves within 2 weeks. Evidence-based treatments pertain to only a modest proportion of dizzy patients. Types of dizziness for which specific management strategies may be helpful are summarized in **Table 10**. Vestibular rehabilitation is a promising treatment for chronic dizziness that includes a 30- to 45-minute instructional session that can be administered by a nurse and a manual detailing standard head and eye exercises that can be performed at home (66).

About 20% to 25% of dizzy patients experience chronic or recurrent symptoms, especially those with disequilibrium, psychiatric disorders, or a vestibulopathy other than BPV or labyrinthitis. Chronic dizziness is more common in the elderly and, although not a risk factor for mortality, is associated with an increased risk for falling, worse self-rated health, and depression.

KEY POINTS

- **The history and physical examination alone help to establish a diagnosis in more than 75% of patients with dizziness in whom a diagnosis can be established, with the history yielding most of these diagnoses.**
- **Patients who experience dizziness with associated syncope may require cardiac evaluation.**
- **Tinnitus or hearing changes are associated with certain vestibular disorders, such as Meniere's disease or, rarely, acoustic neuroma.**
- **The presence of vertical nystagmus is uncommon and warrants early evaluation for central causes of dizziness.**
- **Vestibular rehabilitation is a promising treatment for chronic dizziness.**

Insomnia

The American Psychiatric Association's Diagnostic and Statistical Manual of Mental Disorders (DSM-IV) defines insomnia as a complaint about the quantity or quality of sleep, occurring at least three times per week for at least 1 month (67). In the Western industrialized countries, it is estimated that 30% to 40% of the population have at least occasional sleep disturbances and that 10% to 15% have chronic insomnia lasting at least 1 year (68, 69). Risk factors for insomnia include female sex, family history of insomnia, increased age, existing medical or psychiatric illness, and substance abuse.

Restless legs syndrome is characterized by an impulse to move the lower extremities and dysesthesias that occur at rest; this syndrome occurs most commonly in the evening or at bedtime. Many of these patients also have periodic limb movement during sleep. Both restless legs syndrome and periodic limb movement are common disorders (2% to 4%) that may contribute to insomnia. Pregnancy is also associated with restless legs syndrome. Approximately half of patients with sleep disorders have idiopathic insomnia, and the remainder have insomnia associated with various chronic medical conditions, such as peripheral neuropathies, uremia, diabetes mellitus, Parkinson's disease, or iron-deficiency anemia.

Insomnia often goes unrecognized because most patients do not mention this problem to their physicians. A focused sleep history includes previous attempts at treatment for insomnia; current medications used for insomnia; and associated symptoms, including fatigue, low motivation, diminished concentration, impaired mood and memory, irritability, and problems with interpersonal relationships. The focused physical examination of patients with insomnia includes an

TABLE 11 Causes of Secondary Chronic Insomnia

Psychiatric Disorders
Major depression
Anxiety disorders
Posttraumatic stress disorder
Psychoses
Personality disorder
Medical or Neurologic Disorders
Chronic pain
Chronic obstructive pulmonary disease
Cardiac disease
Gastroesophageal reflux disease
Irritable bowel syndrome
Benign prostatic hyperplasia
Allergies
Medications
Decongestants
β-Agonists
Corticosteroids
β-Blockers
Diuretics
Antidepressants (fluoxetine or bupropion)
H_2-blockers
Sleep–Wake Schedule Disorders
Shift-work sleep disorder
Primary Sleep Disorders
Sleep apnea
Periodic limb movement disorder

evaluation of cardiac, pulmonary, gastrointestinal, and neurologic disease. Polysomnography is reserved for patients with symptoms of a sleep-related breathing disorder, narcolepsy, sleepwalking, or those employed as pilots or truck drivers.

Short-term insomnia refers to symptoms of less than 1-month's duration. Short-term insomnia may be stress related and caused by interpersonal, academic, or employment circumstances. Reassurance and counseling on healthy sleep-related behaviors may be adequate treatment for those with short-term insomnia.

Chronic insomnia can be secondary to five types of conditions (**Table 11**). Idiopathic insomnia with no identifiable precipitating factors is present in 15% to 20% of patients with chronic insomnia. Persons with this disorder have higher rates of somatic complaints, medical office visits, and hospitalization. Chronic medical conditions, such as hypertension, chronic pulmonary disease, arthritis, chronic pain or

TABLE 12 FDA-Approved Insomnia Medications

Medication	Dose (mg)*	Half-life (h)	Approved Duration	Side Effects
Benzodiazepines*				
Temazepam	7.5–30.0	8–15	7–10 d	Drowsiness/dizziness/incoordination
Estazolam	0.5–2.0	10–24	7–10 d	Drowsiness/dizziness/incoordination
Triazolam	0.125–0.25	2–5	7–10 d	Above plus amnesia
Benzodiazepine-receptor agonist				
Eszopiclone	1–3	5–7	Chronic	Unpleasant taste, dry mouth, drowsiness, dizziness
Zolpidem	5–10	3	7–10 d	Drowsiness, dizziness, occasional amnesia
Zaleplon	5–20	1	7–10 d	Drowsiness
Melatonin-receptor agonist				
Ramelteon	8	2–5		Drowsiness, dizziness, increased prolactin levels

Adapted from Silber MH. Chronic Insomnia. N Engl J Med 2005:353:803-10.

*All of these agents are contraindicated in pregnancy. They should not be combined with alcohol and should be used only with caution in patients taking other central nervous system depressants. Lower doses should be used in the elderly, in debilitated patients, and in those with hepatic insufficiency. FDA = Food and Drug Administration.

headache, and diabetes, occur at higher than expected rates in these patients. Untreated insomnia may be a risk factor for the new onset of psychiatric disorders, including major depression, anxiety, and substance abuse.

Three meta-analyses support the efficacy of nonpharmacologic therapy for chronic insomnia (see also Reference 69). Good sleep hygiene involves the avoidance of alcohol, tobacco, caffeine, large meals, daytime napping, or vigorous exercise close to bedtime. Sleep-disturbing factors, such as pets, television, or other noise, should be removed from the bedroom, and adherence to a regular sleep schedule is recommended. Cognitive behavioral therapy (CBT) is a group of techniques that addresses the underlying factors causing insomnia. CBT techniques include stimulus-control, sleep-restriction, and relaxation therapies. Meta-analyses have found CBT to be efficacious in reducing time until sleep onset and the number and duration of awakenings (70–72). In most clinical trials, CBT has been administered by psychologists for an average of six sessions. Performing fewer sessions and self-administered treatments with the use of videotapes or written materials have also proved to be effective.

Medications that are Food and Drug Administration (FDA) approved for the treatment of insomnia are summarized in **Table 12**. The primary classes of therapy are the benzodiazepines, benzodiazepines-receptor agonists, and melatonin-receptor agonists (Table 12). Recently, the FDA has given the first approval for chronic treatment of insomnia with the benzodiazepine-receptor agonist eszopiclone (Lunesta™). The approval of eszopiclone for the long-term treatment of insomnia was based on a clinical trial in which the efficacy of the medication did not abate during the course of the 6-month trial. Eszopiclone is an intermediate-acting agent and is indicated primarily for sleep-maintenance insomnia. The major side effects of this drug are an unpleasant taste, dry mouth, drowsiness, and dizziness.

Many trials support the efficacy of benzodiazepines and benzodiazepine-receptor agonists in improving short-term insomnia. Shorter-acting agents have the most effect on sleep latency (time until sleep), but longer-acting agents have the most effect on total sleep time. The major side effects of long-acting benzodiazepines are daytime sleepiness, dizziness, and incoordination. Shorter-acting benzodiazepines may lead to rebound insomnia on discontinuation of the drug or anterograde amnesia (Table 12). No rebound insomnia has been noted with use of the benzodiazepine-receptor agonists. Sleep history is an important consideration in choosing a sleep medication. If a patient has middle-of-the night awakening, then a longer half-life medication may be indicated. Older persons who use benzodiazepines are at risk for falls and confusion, especially with use of the longer-acting agents; therefore, a small dose may be appropriate in these patients.

Antidepressants (most commonly trazodone), antipsychotics, and antihistamines are used as off-label treatments for insomnia but with a lack of evidence-based data available on their efficacy. Antihistamines cause drowsiness at bedtime, but their half-life of up to 8 hours may cause residual daytime sedation. Tolerance may develop rapidly with the use of antihistamines, and side effects include dry mouth, constipation, and urinary retention. There are no evidence-based data to support the use of herbal preparations and other over-the-counter sleeping aids for the treatment of insomnia.

Untreated insomnia is associated with adverse effects, including impaired quality of life, impaired cognitive function, and impaired occupational functioning. Insomnia may also predispose to depression, posttraumatic stress disorder, and other illnesses. Close follow-up monitoring of patients with insomnia is necessary to identify the effectiveness of therapeutic interventions and detect the emergence of new diagnoses related to chronic insomnia.

KEY POINTS

- Polysomnography is reserved for patients with symptoms of sleep-related breathing disorders, narcolepsy, sleepwalking, or those employed as pilots or truck drivers.
- Reassurance and counseling on healthy sleep-related behaviors may be adequate treatment for those with short-term insomnia.
- Untreated insomnia may be a risk factor for the new onset of major depression, anxiety, and substance abuse.
- Good sleep hygiene involves the avoidance of alcohol, tobacco, caffeine, large meals, daytime napping, or vigorous exercise close to bedtime.
- Eszopiclone is the first Food and Drug Administration–approved drug for the chronic treatment of insomnia.
- Shorter-acting agents have the most effect on time until sleep, but longer-acting agents have the most effect on total sleep time.
- Long-acting benzodiazepines are associated with daytime sleepiness, dizziness, and incoordination, whereas shorter-acting benzodiazepines are associated with rebound insomnia on discontinuation of the drug or anterograde amnesia.
- A small dose of benzodiazepines may be appropriate in older patients.

Dyspnea

Dyspnea or breathlessness is a common symptom in adults. The subjective sensation of difficulty breathing has a broad differential diagnosis, including various pulmonary or pleural diseases, heart failure or valvular incompetency, anemia, hyperthyroidism, or psychogenic causes. Determining whether dyspnea is acute or chronic is an important distinction in establishing its cause. History and physical examination findings provide further diagnostic clues in the evaluation of patients with dyspnea.

A very rapid onset of dyspnea can indicate a pneumothorax, an asthma attack, acute pulmonary edema secondary to a myocardial infarction, or a pulmonary embolism. A more progressive onset of symptoms generally indicates disease of the lung parenchyma (that is, pneumonia, alveolitis, or pleural effusions). Chronic pulmonary diseases, including interstitial fibrosis and chronic obstructive pulmonary disease (COPD), usually have an even slower course of progression than that associated with disease of the lung parenchyma.

The history in patients with dyspnea should focus on identifying specific characteristics of the symptom, including whether it occurs at rest or with exertion, any associated positional or circadian variation, and the presence of associated chest pain. Chest pain occurs most commonly with acute coronary syndromes, pulmonary embolism, traumatic effusions, and some types of pneumonia. Concomitant paroxysmal nocturnal dyspnea generally suggests a cardiac source but should not be confused with the nighttime symptoms of asthma. Risk factors for venous thromboembolic disease are important considerations in the evaluation of patients with dyspnea. Palpitations, generalized fatigue, and heat intolerance support a diagnosis of thyrotoxicosis, whereas fatigue, pallor, and any evidence of blood loss may indicate anemia. Aspiration, foreign-body airway obstruction, and neuromuscular disease are less likely sources of dyspnea but should not be overlooked as potential underlying causes. A productive cough, sore throat, fever, and chills support infectious etiologies (**Table 13**).

The physical examination is equally important in patients with dyspnea, with emphasis on vital signs, including temperature; position of trachea; the presence of abnormal lung sounds; cardiac murmurs; lower-extremity swelling; and inspection of chest wall mechanics. The general severity of the patient's illness is often a significant clue to the cause of dyspnea. Wheezing generally indicates airway obstruction most commonly caused by asthma or COPD but can also be caused by pulmonary edema (known as "cardiac asthma"). Volume overload in the lung normally produces coarse crackles and jugular venous distention. Dry crackles are found in patients with interstitial fibrosis. Percussion of the lung helps to establish the differential diagnosis in these patients. Dullness to percussion with rhonchi may be suggestive of pneumonia, while dullness to percussion without rhonchi raises the suspicion for a malignant or traumatic effusion.

The initial diagnostic workup for dyspnea should include pulse oximetry and electrocardiography followed by a complete blood count and posterioanterior and lateral chest radiography. Additional studies for acute dyspnea might include blood gas studies, D-dimer assay, helical CT, or ventilation-perfusion scan. In patients with chronic dyspnea, pulmonary function tests, with or without methacholine challenge, may be helpful. The newest test in the armamentarium to evaluate dyspnea is the serum b-type natriuretic peptide (BNP) (73). Many patients

TABLE 13 Evaluation of Dyspnea

Diagnosis	Characteristics
Pulmonary Disease	
Asthma COPD Pulmonary embolism Pneumonia Interstitial pulmonary fibrosis Pulmonary hypertension Pneumothorax Pleural effusion/ hemothorax Systemic sclerosis Pulmonary toxins	• Known asthma, smoking • Risk factors for thromboembolism • Risk factors for pneumonia/aspiration • Exposure to toxic/irritant inhalation • Known cardiothoracic disease • Trauma • Barrel-chested, cyanosis, clubbing • Position of trachea • Respiratory examination findings • Body habitus, oxygen saturation, +/- JVD • Joint/skin findings
Cardiac Disease	
Congestive heart failure Systolic dysfunction Diastolic dysfunction Aortic or mitral stenosis Mitral regurgitation Intracardiac shunt Pericardial disease	• History of CAD, hypertension, heart failure • Alcohol use • Known valvular disease or malignancy • Chest pain • Vital signs, pulsus parodoxus, JVD • Character of pulse (e.g., water hammer) • Cardiac examination, displaced PMI, S_3, murmurs • Hepatojugular reflux, peripheral edema • ECG
Other	
Anemia Thyroid disease Neuromuscular disease Deconditioning Psychogenic	• Pallor, known blood loss, signs of hemolysis • Palpitations, heat intolerance, weight loss, fatigue, insomnia, anxiety • Focal weakness, neurologic symptoms • Poor exercise tolerance • Evidence of anxiety/phobias

COPD = chronic obstructive pulmonary disease; JVD = jugular venous distension; CAD = coronary artery disease; ECG = electrocardiogram.

have both chronic pulmonary disease and congestive heart failure; however, elevated BNP levels are present in patients with heart failure and thereby help to differentiate heart failure from COPD (74). As a screening tool, BNP has a high sensitivity, negative predictive value, and accuracy (75). A recent study demonstrated BNP levels ≥100 pg/mL had an odds ratio (OR) of 21.4 (95% CI; 14.6 to 31.3) for predicting heart failure (76). In some settings, BNP is more readily available than echocardiography, although it cannot be used as a substitute for an estimate of left ventricular function or to evaluate for valvular disease (77) (**Table 14**).

Dyspnea is often a symptom of cardiopulmonary deconditioning. Encouraging patients to increase their aerobic exercise capacity is valuable when workups are otherwise normal. Physical deconditioning can be confirmed by cardiopulmonary stress testing, in which respiratory gas exchange is measured during a cardiac stress test. Calculations of the anaerobic threshold and the breathing reserve, if normal, rule out circulatory and ventilatory causes of dyspnea, confirming a deconditioned state (78). This is a valuable prognostic indicator in patients who also have systolic heart failure.

The management of patients with dyspnea depends on the underlying cause. For example, the dyspnea of anemia responds quickly to transfused packed erythrocytes, whereas the dyspnea of thyrotoxicosis or neuromuscular disease requires a specific approach for treating the underlying condition. If patients continue to experience the sensation of dyspnea after the underlying cause has been treated, this symptom may be indicative of another problem requiring a more thorough evaluation. For patients with intermittent dyspnea from chronic cardiac or pulmonary disease, anxiety is often present and should also be addressed.

For patients with hypoxia, supplemental oxygen should be used to decrease the work of breathing and prevent hypoventilation and respiratory failure. In using supplemental oxygen, careful monitoring of the respiratory rate in patients with chronic pulmonary disease helps to prevent hypercapneic respiratory acidosis and subsequent coma.

Left heart failure accounts for a considerable amount of dyspnea, especially in the aging population. Management of these patients includes education on a low-sodium diet, maximizing afterload reduction and rate control of any tachyarrhythmia, and aggressive diuresis with careful monitoring of renal function. In patients with evidence of diffuse volume overload, torsemide has better gastrointestinal absorption by the edematous bowel wall than furosemide.

Asthma and COPD constitute the other large component of underlying causes of dyspnea. Avoidance of any precipitating factors or allergens and smoking cessation are first-line measures to prevent exacerbations in these patients. Scheduled use of bronchodilators with or without inhaled corticosteroids is appropriate in patients with asthma and COPD, with education about the proper delivery of these medications.

Psychogenic dyspnea is a possible diagnosis when dyspnea occurs at rest but not with exertion. This type of

TABLE 14 Test Characteristics for Diagnosis of Heart Failure in Patients with Dyspnea

Test	Sensitivity, %	Specificity, %	LR +	LR -	Odds Ratio
Initial clinical judgment	61	86	4.4	0.45	
CXR with cardiomegaly	76	79	3.7	0.30	15.4
CXR with cephalization	41–54	96	10.7	0.65	15.4
CXR with interstitial edema	27–34	97	12.3	0.70	17.1
Orthopnea	58	67	1.8	0.63	2.6
JVD	38	91	4.5	0.67	5.5
S$_3$ gallop	13	99	9.5	0.88	9.1
Extremity edema	58	75	2.1-2.4	0.57	4.9
Abnormal ECG (atrial fibrillation)	58 (26)	78 (93)	2.66 (3.8)	0.54 (0.79)	4.9
BNP ≥100 pg/mL	90	75	3.66	0.14	26.2
BNP ≥250 pg/mL	89	81	4.6	0.14	

Adapted from Knudsen CW, et al. Diagnostic value of b-type natriuretic peptide and chest radiographic findings in patients with acute dyspnea. Am J Med. 2004; 116:363-368; and Wang, CS, Fitzgerald JM, Schulzer M, Mak E, Najib, TA. Does this dyspneic patient in the emergency department have congestive heart failure? JAMA. 2005;264:1944-1956.

CXR = chest radiograph; JVD = jugular venous distension; ECG = electrocardiogram; BNP = B-natriuretic peptide.

dyspnea often is accompanied by peripheral and periorbital paresthesias.

KEY POINTS

- Rapid onset of dyspnea can indicate a pneumothorax, an asthma attack, acute pulmonary edema secondary to a myocardial infarction, or a pulmonary embolism.
- The initial diagnostic workup for dyspnea should include pulse oximetry and electrocardiography followed by a complete blood count and posterioanterior and lateral chest radiography.
- A recent study demonstrated B-natriuretic peptide levels ≥100 pg/mL had an odds ratio of 21.4 (95% CI; 14.6 to 31.3) for predicting heart failure.
- Supplemental oxygen is appropriate for use in patients with hypoxia to decrease the work of breathing and prevent hypoventilation and respiratory failure.
- Psychogenic dyspnea is a possible diagnosis when dyspnea occurs at rest but not with exertion.

Syncope

Transient loss of consciousness not related to trauma may be caused by 1) syncope; 2) secondary impaired consciousness due to metabolic disorders (for example, hypoglycemia, hypoxia, or alcohol) or vertebrobasilar transient ischemic attack (TIA); or 3) disorders that resemble syncope but do not involve true loss of consciousness (for example, TIA of carotid artery distribution, psychogenic pseudosyncope, cataplexy, or drop attacks).

True syncope is abrupt, transient, caused by global cerebral hypoperfusion without focal neurologic deficit, and associated with spontaneous recovery. Carotid TIAs involve a focal neurologic deficit without loss of consciousness; vertebrobasilar TIAs may cause transient loss of consciousness but usually are associated with a focal neurologic deficit, such as hemianopsia or ataxia. Prodromal aura, secondary incontinence, slowness in regaining full consciousness (>5 minutes), and postictal disorientation are symptoms more characteristic of seizure, whereas prodromal nausea or sweating and rapid recovery are symptoms more characteristic of syncope. Patients with syncope may have jerking movements of very short duration that begin after loss of consciousness. Cataplexy, associated with narcolepsy, is characterized by a loss of muscle tone as a result of emotion, particularly laughter. Patients with cataplexy are conscious but unable to respond. Drop attacks are very brief spells of sudden falling without warning. These patients remember hitting the ground; therefore, loss of conscious in this setting is unlikely (79–80).

Syncope is responsible for 1% to 3% of emergency department visits. One-year cardiac mortality and sudden death are higher in patients with cardiac syncope than in those with noncardiac or idiopathic syncope. Patients with unexplained syncope have a higher all-cause mortality rate than patients without syncope, whereas vasovagal syncope

TABLE 15 Causes of Syncope

Cardiac

Arrhythmia
  Sinus node dysfunction
  Atrioventricular conduction disease
  Paroxysmal supraventricular and ventricular tachycardia
  Familial syndromes (e.g., long-QT syndrome, Brugada syndrome)
  Pacemaker of defibrillator malfunction
  Drug-induced
Structural cardiac or pulmonary disease
  Valvular disease
  Acute myocardial ischemia or infarction
  Hypertrophic obstructive cardiomyopathy
  Acute aortic dissection
  Atrial myxoma
  Pericardial disease or tamponade
  Pulmonary embolism or hypertension

Neurally mediated reflex syncopal syndromes

Vasovagal faint
Carotid sinus syndrome
Situational faint
  Cough, sneeze
  Gastrointestinal stimulation (swallowing, defecation, visceral pain)
  Micturition
  After exercise
  Acute hemorrhage
  Increased intrathoracic pressure (playing a brass instrument, weight lifting)
  Postprandial
Glossopharyngeal and trigeminal neuralgia
  Orthostatic Syncope
  Primary autonomic failure (pure autonomic failure, multiple system atrophy, Parkinson's disease)
  Secondary autonomic failure (diabetic, alcoholic, or amyloid neuropathy, drugs)
  After exercise
  Postprandial
  Hypovolemia (diarrhea, hemorrhage, adrenal insufficiency)
Cerebrovascular
  Vascular steal syndromes
No clear etiology

Adapted from Benditt DG, van Dijk G, Sutton R, Wieling W, Lin JC, Sakaguchi S, et al. Syncope. Current Problems in Cardiology. 2004;29: 145-229; and The Task Force on Syncope, European Society of Cardiology. Guidelines on management (diagnosis and treatment) of syncope – Update 2004. Executive Summary. Eur Heart J 2004;25:2054-72.

does not appear to be associated with increased mortality. Approximately 20% to 35% of patients with syncope have recurrent syncopal episodes (81–83).

Table 15 shows causes of syncope. In a recent study of 650 patients (mean age 60 years, range 18 to 93 years) who consecutively presented to an emergency department with syncope and were systematically evaluated, the cause was found to be neurally mediated in 38%, orthostatic hypotension in 24%, cardiac in 11%, neurologic in 5%, psychiatric in 2%, and unexplained in 14% (see also Reference 81). Usually, syncope has a single cause, but some patients may have interacting precipitants of syncope (for example, heart disease, orthostasis-causing medications, or bradycardia plus diabetes-induced autonomic dysfunction). Most patients with syncope can be evaluated as outpatients; hospitalization is indicated only when there is a high risk for life-threatening arrhythmias.

The history of patients with syncope should focus on precipitating or associated factors (for example, pain, standing quickly, exercise, straining at urination or defecation, or severe coughing); witnesses' observations of the syncopal episode (for example, seizure activity, incontinence, duration of unconsciousness, patient's color described as ashen or cyanotic, or mental status on regaining consciousness); neurologic symptoms; history of cardiac, neurologic, or psychiatric disease; family history of cardiac disease and sudden death; medications; and a detailed review of systems.

The initial evaluation of patients with syncope should include complete cardiovascular and neurologic examinations, orthostatic and bilateral arm blood pressures, and electrocardiography. To assess orthostasis, blood pressure should be taken while the patient is supine after 5 minutes of rest and then after standing for 3 minutes. Positive findings are a decrease of ≥ 20 mm Hg in systolic blood pressure or a decrease of ≥ 10 mm Hg in diastolic pressure or symptoms. Basic laboratory tests in patients with dyspnea are not indicated and are usually nondiagnostic, unless hypovolemia, severe anemia, or a metabolic disorder is suspected. Electrolyte abnormalities may be the result of volume depletion or the cause of seizure.

The initial evaluation results in a suspected diagnosis in $\geq 50\%$ of syncopal patients. Some patients with suspected diagnoses need no further evaluation for syncope, whereas others require specific confirmatory tests (**Table 16** and **Table 17**) (84).

If arrhythmia is the suspected cause of syncope but 24-hour ambulatory Holter electrocardiographic monitoring is not diagnostic, increasing monitoring to 72 hours does not appear to increase the diagnostic yield. Long-term (≥ 30 days) monitoring with continuous-loop recorders is recommended for those in whom suspicion of arrhythmia remains after a diagnosis has not been established by Holter monitoring. Continuous-loop recorders can monitor the heart rhythm for weeks to months but require that patients activate monitoring when symptoms occur. Readings are captured for the preceding several minutes and 60 seconds longer. Subcutaneously

TABLE 16 Findings Suggestive of Type of Syncope

Possible Diagnosis	Associated Findings
Vasovagal syncope	Sudden fear, pain, noxious sight, sound or smell, prolonged still standing, heavy exertion in an athlete without heart disease
Situational syncope	Micturition, defecation, cough, swallowing (especially very cold water)
Neurally mediated syncope with neuralgia	Throat or facial pain (glossopharyngeal or trigeminal neuralgia)
Carotid sinus syncope	Head turning, other pressure on carotid sinus (e.g., tumor, vascular dissection, tight collar, shaving)
Orthostatic hypotension	On standing from sitting or supine position, especially after a few moments or walking a short distance; drugs that can cause orthostatic hypotension or bradycardia
Arrhythmia	No prodrome but known coronary disease, palpitations, family history of sudden death, long-QT syndrome, Brugada syndrome, drugs that may cause long QT syndrome
Structural heart or lung disease	Syncope when supine or with exertion, angina, family history of sudden death
Atrial myxoma or thrombus	Syncope with position change (sitting to supine, bending, turning while supine)
Psychiatric syncope	Syncope (may be frequent) and somatic symptoms with no heart disease

TABLE 17 Diagnostic Approach Based on the Initial Evaluation of Syncope*

Classical vasovagal, situational, or orthostatic syncope	No further evaluation
Syncope associated with ECG evidence of acute ischemia or sinus bradycardia <40/min, repetitive sinoatrial blocks or pauses of 3 s in the absence of causative medicines, Mobitz II second- or third-degree atrioventricular block, alternating left and right bundle branch block, rapid paroxysmal supraventricular or ventricular tachycardia, and pacemaker malfunction	No further evaluation for syncope, treat cause
Unexplained syncope but risk factors for or known structural heart disease	Stress testing, echocardiography, prolonged electrocardiographic monitoring*, cardiac catheterization, then electrophysiologic studies if no diagnosis
Syncope with palpitations	Electrocardiographic monitoring and echocardiography
Angina before or after syncope	Stress testing, echocardiography, and electrocardiographic monitoring
Syncope during or after exertion	Echocardiography and stress testing
Recurrent syncope in young patients without evidence of heart or neurologic disease	Tilt testing
Older patients without evidence of heart or neurologic disease	Carotid sinus massage and tilt testing
Syncope associated with turning the neck	Carotid sinus massage
Syncope with autonomic failure or evidence of neurologic disease	Referral to neurologist
Frequent recurrent syncope with multiple somatic complaints, and stress, anxiety, or other possible psychiatric disorder	Referral to psychiatrist

ECG = electrocardiogram.

*Electrocardiographic monitoring includes Holter monitoring, external or implantable loop recorder.

implanted recorders can now monitor heart rhythms for up to 18 months.

If the evaluation is negative and arrhythmia is still suspected, electrophysiologic testing should be considered. The yield of electrophysiologic studies is higher in the presence of structural heart disease and tachyarrhythmias versus bradyarrhythmias. For patients with ischemic heart disease, signal-averaged electrocardiography can be useful in identifying patients at risk for ventricular tachycardia and who are therefore likely to have inducible ventricular tachycardia on electrophysiologic testing. It is not useful for identifying bradyarrhythmias as a cause of syncope.

Although reports of neurologic deficits after carotid massage are rare, this procedure should be avoided in patients with syncope and carotid bruits or known cerebrovascular disease unless carotid sinus sensitivity is highly suspected. In carotid massage, pressure with vigorous circular movement is applied where the carotid artery meets the angle of the jaw for 5 to 10 seconds, with the patient supine and standing, during continuous electrocardiographic and blood pressure monitoring. A positive result is a pause of ≥3 seconds, a decrease of

≥50 mm Hg in systolic blood pressure, or symptoms of presyncope or syncope. Tilt testing is usually performed without, then with, provocative drugs such as isoproterenol and nitroglycerin; the most common responses to these provocations are sudden hypotension, bradycardia, or both.

Patients in whom a suspected diagnosis is not established after the initial evaluation for syncope or after

TABLE 18 Driving Recommendations for Patients with Syncope

Cause of Syncope	Private Drivers	Professional Drivers
Cardiac Syncope		
Arrhythmia treated medically	After successful treatment	After successful treatment
Pacemaker placement	Within 1 week	Once appropriate function is established
Ablation	Successful treatment at 3 months	Successful treatment at 3 months
ICD	Controversial	Never
Neurally Mediated – Vasovagal, Carotid Sinus Syndrome, or Situational		
Mild	No restrictions	No restriction unless syncope occurred during high-risk activity
Severe	After symptoms controlled or effective therapy established	Never unless effective treatment established
Syncope of Uncertain Cause		
Mild	No restriction unless syncope occurred during high-risk activity	After diagnosis and effective therapy established
Severe	After diagnosis and effective therapy established	After diagnosis and effective therapy established

Adapted from The Task Force on Syncope, European Society of Cardiology. Guidelines on management (diagnosis and treatment) of syncope – Update 2004. Executive Summary. Eur Heart J. 2004;25:2054-2072.

ICD = implantable cardioverter defibrillator.

subsequent testing have unexplained syncope, which is most likely neurally mediated; evaluation in these patients should proceed to carotid massage and tilt testing. Patients with an unclear cause of syncope after cardiac evaluation but whose findings suggest arrhythmia or who have recurrent syncope resulting in injury should receive an implantable loop recorder. In patients in whom a full cardiac evaluation is nondiagnostic, a thorough examination for neurally mediated syncope is appropriate. Patients with initially suspected neurally mediated syncope but whose carotid massage and tilt tests are negative should undergo prolonged electrocardiographic monitoring. Patients with persistently unexplained syncope should undergo a full re-assessment, consisting of history, physical examination, and electrocardiography, to identify new findings.

Treating neurally mediated and orthostatic syncope comprises patient-based maneuvers, training, and medication when warranted. Patients should avoid factors precipitating syncope, such as suddenly rising, especially after long periods in bed; standing in one place for long periods; straining at the toilet; hot baths, showers or saunas; large meals; and severe exertion. Maneuvers to abort syncope include counter-pressure maneuvers of the legs (for example, crossing the legs at the thigh while standing or sitting) or arms (for example, isometric hand grip, or gripping one hand with the other and isometrically pushing the arms away from each other at the hands), squatting, bending over, and placing one foot on a chair while standing. Tilt training consisting of frequent tilting episodes with prolonged upright posture until the patient no longer has a positive result may also be effective. For patients with autonomic failure, sleeping with the upper part of the body and head raised is helpful. Treatment for orthostatic hypotension includes volume replacement, if needed, and reduction or cessation of implicated drugs. For autonomic dysfunction, options include waist-high support hose, abdominal binders, and increased salt and fluid intake in patients in whom there is no contraindication. For example, instructing a patient to quickly drink a half liter of fluid to induce an increase in blood pressure within several minutes may be effective, with an expected increase of 20-30 mm occurring within approximately 30 minutes (this increase should be sustained for approximately 1 hour). If these measures fail, fludrocortisone and then midodrine (5 g three times daily) may be beneficial. Randomized trials have shown that paroxetine, β-antagonists, and pacemakers for select patients with severe, recurrent syncopal symptoms and bradycardia on tilt testing appear effective (see also Reference 82). Driving recommendations for patients with syncope are listed in **Table 18** (see also Reference 84).

KEY POINTS

- Prodromal aura, secondary incontinence, slowness in regaining full consciousness, and postictal disorientation are more characteristic of seizure, whereas prodromal nausea or sweating and rapid recovery are more characteristic of syncope.
- Initial evaluation of patients with syncope should include complete cardiovascular and neurologic examinations, orthostatic and bilateral arm blood pressures, and electrocardiography.
- In patients with syncope, long-term (≥30 days) monitoring with continuous-loop recorders is recommended for those in whom suspicion of arrhythmia remains after a diagnosis has not been established by ambulatory electrocardiography (Holter monitoring).
- Carotid massage should be avoided in patients with syncope and carotid bruits or known cerebrovascular disease unless carotid sinus sensitivity is highly suspected.
- Patients with an unclear cause of syncope after cardiac evaluation but whose data suggest arrhythmia or who have recurrent syncope resulting in injury should receive an implantable loop recorder.
- Maneuvers to abort syncope include counter-pressure maneuvers of the legs or arms, squatting, bending over, and placing one foot on a chair while standing.
- Treatment for orthostatic hypotension includes volume replacement and reduction or cessation of implicated drugs.
- Paroxetine, β-antagonists, and pacemakers have been shown to be effective in select patients with severe, recurrent syncopal symptoms and bradycardia on tilt testing.

Chest Pain

In one study of the causes of chest pain in a primary care setting, musculoskeletal chest pain accounted for 20.4% of all diagnoses, followed by reflux esophagitis (13.4%), and costochondritis (13.1%) (85). Stable angina pectoris was the primary diagnosis in only 10.3% of episodes, and unstable angina or possible myocardial infarction in 1.5%. In this study, most resources evaluating chest pain were devoted to ruling out cardiac causes (86).

Other common causes of chest pain include esophageal spasm, herpetic neuralgia, anxiety (including panic disorder), and reactive airways. Panic disorder is present in more than 30% of patients evaluated in the hospital for chest pain and who are found to have no evidence of cardiovascular heart disease.

Patients with symptoms of ischemic heart disease present significantly differently depending on sex. In all types of acute coronary syndrome, women have significantly more back and jaw pain, nausea and/or vomiting, dyspnea, indigestion, and palpitations, but less chest pain than do men (87). Patients with chronic stable angina tend to be medically undertreated. In one analysis of a large cohort study of men with stable angina, 30% experienced angina more than twice weekly, of whom 22% received no antianginal medications such as nitrates, β-blockers, or calcium-channel blockers (see Cardiovascular Disease Syllabus), and of whom 33% received only one class of antianginal medication. Of those who received medications, 18% took no medications at the recommended therapeutic dose, and 50% received only one class of antianginal medication at the recommended therapeutic dose (88).

Among patients with chronic noncardiac chest pain, randomized placebo-controlled studies have shown that tricyclic antidepressants, β-blockers, ACE inhibitors, L-arginine, statins, and exercise may relieve symptoms (89). Empiric treatment with high-dose proton pump inhibitors may be helpful in patients with gastroesophageal reflux disease–related chest pain (90), and as-needed sublingual nitroglycerin or calcium-channel–blocker therapy may be appropriate for those with esophageal spasm.

KEY POINTS

- In all types of acute coronary syndrome, women have significantly more back and jaw pain, nausea and/or vomiting, dyspnea, indigestion, and palpitations, but less chest pain compared with men.
- Patients with chronic stable angina tend to be medically undertreated.
- Tricyclic antidepressants, β-blockers, ACE inhibitors, L-arginine, statins, and exercise may relieve symptoms in patients with chronic noncardiac chest pain.

Musculoskeletal Pain

Back Pain

Approximately two thirds of adults experience low back pain at some time during their lifetime. Back pain of less than 6 weeks' duration is defined as acute, whereas chronic back pain persists beyond 3 months. Low back pain is the fifth most common reason for visiting an internist and causes the most work-related disability in persons younger than age 45 years. Although 85% of patients with low back pain do not receive a specific diagnosis, most episodes are benign and self-limited (91), with a serious underlying systemic disease or neurologic disorder present in less than 5% of patients.

Low back pain can be categorized as mechanical (97%), nonmechanical (1%), or visceral (2%). Mechanical low back or leg pain is usually attributable to musculoligamentous injuries or age-related degenerative disease in the intervertebral disks

TABLE 19 Indications for Early Imaging in Patients with Back Pain

Clinical Finding	Rationale
Major trauma	Possible fracture
Corticosteroid use	Greater risk for osteoporotic fracture
Age >50 y	Greater risk for malignancy, osteoporotic fracture
History of cancer	Greater risk for underlying malignancy
Unexplained weight loss	Greater risk for malignancy or infection
Fever, immunosuppression, immunodeficiency, injection drug use, or active infection	Risk for spinal infection
Saddle anesthesia, bowel or bladder incontinence	Possible cauda equina syndrome
Severe or progressive neurologic deficit	Possible cauda equina syndrome or severe nerve root compression

and facet joints. Among the common mechanical causes associated with specific anatomic abnormalities in patients with low back pain are herniated intervertebral disks (4%), spinal stenosis (3%), osteoporotic compression fractures (4%), and spondylolisthesis (2%). Herniated intervertebral discs usually occur in adults aged 30 to 55 years. Sciatica, often associated with leg numbness or paresthesias, is a highly sensitive (95%) and specific (88%) finding for herniated disk; coughing, sneezing, and Valsalva maneuvers may exacerbate the pain in these patients. Spinal stenosis usually occurs in older adults and is characterized by neurogenic claudication—radiating back pain and lower extremity numbness—that is exacerbated by walking and spinal extension but improved by sitting.

Nonmechanical spinal conditions, which combined account for 1% of low back pain, include infections (0.01%), neoplasia (0.7%), and inflammatory arthritis (0.3%). Visceral causes for low back pain are also uncommon (2%), and the differential diagnosis for this type of pain includes pelvic organ dysfunction, renal disease, vascular disease, and gastrointestinal disease.

The initial evaluation of patients with low back pain should focus on whether a systemic disease is causing the pain, whether there are neurologic deficits that may require prompt surgical evaluation, and whether psychosocial factors are present that may impede treatment or prolong pain. The signs of a serious underlying cause, or red flags (92), for low back pain suggesting a need for early imaging and interventions are related to malignancy, spinal infection, fracture, and the cauda equina syndrome (**Table 19**). The cauda equina syndrome results when a massive midline herniation or tumor compresses the cauda equina, causing bowel or bladder problems, usually with urinary retention and overflow incontinence, and saddle anesthesia, bilateral sciatica, and leg weakness. Risk factors for primary or metastatic neoplasia include age older than 50 years, weight loss, history of cancer, and lack of response to conservative therapy. The presence of one or more of these factors has a positive likelihood ratio of 2.5, whereas the absence of these factors has a negative likelihood ratio of 0.0. Spinal infections are associated with fever, active urinary or skin infections, immunosuppression, immunodeficiency, injection drug use, or weight loss. A history of major trauma, osteoporosis, corticosteroid use, and age older than 70 years are associated with fractures; the likelihood ratio for fracture in patients with a history of corticosteroid use is 12.0.

Prolonged low back pain and poor response to therapy may be associated with a history of failed treatment, depression, and somatization. Substance abuse, job dissatisfaction, and ongoing litigation or compensation claims also predict poor outcomes in patients with low back pain.

In the absence of red flags, a brief neurologic and musculoskeletal examination is appropriate in the setting of low back pain. More than 95% of lumbar disk herniations occur at the L5 or S1 nerve roots; however, abnormal nerve-root findings are generally neither very sensitive nor specific. A straight-leg-raising test, performed with the patient supine or seated, is 80% sensitive but only 40% specific if sciatica is reproduced at an elevation of less than 60 degrees. Great-toe extensor weakness (L5 nerve root) has a positive likelihood ratio of 1.7. A positive crossed–straight-leg-raising (90%) and ankle plantar flexion weakness test (95%) are highly specific but insensitive findings. A wide-based gait (97%) and abnormal Romberg test (91%) are highly specific findings for spinal stenosis. Low back pain with axial loading or spinal rotation, sensory or motor deficits inconsistent with nerve-root distributions, general overreaction during examination, inconsistent seated and supine straight-leg-raising tests, and the presence of superficial or widespread tenderness are nonphysiologic findings that portend a poor response to treatment (93).

Radiographic imaging is reserved for patients with clinical findings suggesting cauda equina syndrome, systemic disease, or trauma, or in those in whom conservative treatment has failed (94). Suspected cauda equina syndrome is an indication for urgent CT or MRI. Guidelines for nonurgent imaging recommend first performing plain-film radiography; anteroposterior and lateral views are sufficient in patients without a history of previous back surgery. These imaging tests will identify fractures (although bone scans are necessary to determine acuity), but they are relatively insensitive for early cancer (60%) or infection (82%) and will not visualize herniated disks or spinal stenosis. Erythrocyte sedimentation rate measurement and a complete blood count may be helpful ancillary tests when systemic disease is suspected.

MRI is very sensitive in detecting spinal infections (96%) and cancer (83% to 93%), and CT and MRI are accurate in detecting herniated disks and spinal stenosis. These studies are appropriate when clinical findings suggest a high probability

TABLE 20 Evidence Levels for Back Pain Interventions

Evidence Level	Acute Low Back Pain	Chronic Low Back Pain
Evidence for benefit	• Behavioral therapy • Massage • Multidisciplinary (physical and psychosocial) rehabilitation program (subacute back pain) • Muscle relaxants • NSAIDs • Spinal manipulative therapy • Staying active	• Acupuncture • Analgesics • Antidepressants • Back school • Behavioral therapy • Massage • Multidisciplinary (physical and psychosocial) rehabilitation program • Muscle relaxants • NSAIDs • Exercise • Spinal manipulative therapy
Insufficient evidence to assess	• Acupuncture • Analgesics (opioids, acetaminophen) • Back school • Epidural corticosteroids • Lumbar supports • Temperature treatments • Traction	• Electromyographic feedback • Epidural corticosteroids • Local injections • Lumbar supports • Transcutaneous electrical nerve stimulation
Evidence for lack of efficacy	• Bed rest	• Facet joint injections • Traction

Adapted from Clinical Evidence, Cochrane Library.

for infection or cancer and when nonurgent surgery is being considered as treatment of herniated disks or spinal stenosis. However, CT or MRI imaging is not generally recommended for patients with acutely herniated disks in the absence of severe neurologic deficits because more than 90% of patients recover from this condition within 6 weeks, and these imaging studies have a low specificity. Additionally, incidental CT or MRI findings could be psychologically distressing and lead to unnecessary tests and treatments in these patients. A randomized trial comparing rapid MRI with plain-film radiography showed similar clinical outcomes, but rapid MRI was associated with higher costs and an increased likelihood for spinal surgery (95).

Treatment of low back pain depends on its severity and acuity. The cauda equina syndrome is a surgical emergency, and spinal infections and malignancies also require prompt treatment (**Table 20**). However, most patients with acute back pain, even those with sciatica, can be treated conservatively, and most are substantially improved within 1 to 3 months (see Table 20). Controlled trials demonstrate modest benefit with the use of NSAIDs, behavioral therapy, massage, spinal manipulative therapy, and muscle relaxants (96) in the treatment of low back pain. Maintaining normal activity improves pain control and functional status more than strict bed rest for acute low back pain, although not for sciatica. Exercise is not beneficial for patients with acute low back pain, and prolonged bed rest may delay recovery. Narcotic analgesics should be reserved for severe pain and used for only a limited time.

In the year after an episode of low back pain, 15% of patients still have severe pain. The estimated prevalence of chronic low back pain in the general population ranges from 5% to 8%. Tricyclic and tetracyclic antidepressants moderately reduce pain severity in patients with chronic low back pain but have an inconsistent effect on functional status (97, 98). These antidepressants control pain even in patients without depression. Trials of selective serotonin reuptake inhibitors have not shown benefits for reducing pain or improving function in patients with chronic low back pain. Other chronic low-back-pain treatments (see Table 20) with at least short-term benefit include acupuncture, analgesics (opioids, acetaminophen), behavioral therapy, back schools (systematic group instruction about back anatomy and function, ergonomics, and exercise), exercise, massage, muscle relaxants, NSAIDs, and spinal manipulative therapy (see also Reference 96). Conversely, there is no conclusive evidence for the efficacy of epidural steroid injections, electromyographic biofeedback, lumbar supports, or transcutaneous electrical nerve stimulation in the setting of low back pain. Randomized trial evidence suggests that traction and facet joint injections are ineffective in these patients.

Although conservative treatment is recommended for the initial management of patients with herniated disks, surgical referral is indicated in those with progressive or persistent sciatica or lower-extremity weakness (**Table 21**). Diskectomy more effectively relieves pain than conservative treatment through 4 years of follow-up, but longer-term benefits are uncertain (99). Progressive radiculopathy or disabling back or leg pain in patients with confirmed spinal stenosis is

TABLE 21 Indications for Surgery in Patients with Low Back Pain

Condition	Indications
Sciatica and probable herniated disk	• Cauda equina syndrome • Progressive or severe neurologic deficit • Persistent neuromotor deficit after 4 to 6 wk of conservative treatment • Persistent sciatica for 4 to 6 wk with consistent clinical and neurologic findings
Spinal stenosis	• Progressive or severe neurologic deficit • Persistent and disabling back and leg pain
Spondylolisthesis	• Progressive or severe neurologic deficit • Spinal stenosis with above referral indications • Severe back pain or sciatica with severe functional impairment that persists for ≥1 y

another indication for surgical referral. Cohort studies suggest that decompressive laminectomy relieves pain from spinal stenosis.

Neck Pain

Neck pain is a common reason patients seek medical advice, with a third of the adult population reporting neck pain within the previous year (100). This type of pain is often self-limited and responds to symptomatic treatment measures. Most patients with acute neck pain, with or without radicular symptoms, have musculoskeletal or degenerative disorders that do not require specific treatment. Chronic neck pain, defined as lasting more than 6 months, increases with age and affects approximately 14% of adults. The differential diagnosis for neck pain includes cervical strain; whiplash; cervical spondylosis; cervical radiculopathy secondary to intervertebral disc herniation; and more rare conditions, such as rheumatoid arthritis, spondyloarthropathy, and diffuse idiopathic skeletal hyperostosis (**Table 22**).

The history of patients with neck pain should focus on the duration and location of the pain. In patients with a history of blunt trauma, the presence of five clinical criteria can

TABLE 22 Differential Diagnosis and Treatment of Neck Pain

Diagnosis	Findings	Treatment
Mechanical neck disorders	• Associated headaches • Emotional and physical stress • Poor posture, poor sleep	• Analgesics and anti-inflammatory medication • Soft cervical collar • Massage, heat • Postural training • Muscle relaxants • Cervical traction • Antidepressants • Relaxation techniques • Strengthening and mobilization exercise
Whiplash (cervical strain)	• History of forced flexion/extension of the neck; pain often begins the day after the injury • Diffuse tenderness on exam • Normal radiograph	• Immobilization (until fracture ruled out) • Soft collar • Analgesic and anti-inflammatory medications • Ice in first 48 h, moist heat after initial period • Physical therapy for prolonged symptoms
Other cervical strain and/or acute torticollis	• Sudden onset of unilateral pain and spasm without trauma • History of prolonged odd position • Palpable spasm	• Intermittent heat • Analgesics • Soft collar
Radiculopathy	• Numbness and tingling down arm • Worse with cough/straining, standing or sitting; head tilting can make better or worse. • Unilateral, dermatomal • Hyporeflexia with C6 and C7	• Anti-inflammatory medications • Moist heat • Soft collars • Cervical traction (not in patients with RA, trauma, or signs of instability)
Cervical cord compression (from cervical disc protrusion, fracture, or neoplasm)	• Bilateral radiculopathy • Worse with neck flexion	• Immobilize ASAP with urgent neurosurgical consultation

RA = rheumatoid arthritis.

eliminate the need for cervical spine radiography, with a sensitivity of 99% and negative predictive value of 99.5%. These criteria consist of 1) an absence of midline cervical tenderness on direct palpation, 2) an absence of focal neurologic deficits, 3) normal alertness, 4) an absence of intoxication, and 5) no painful distracting injuries (101). Pain radiating down the arms, or any weakness, numbness, or paresthesias, usually suggests cervical radiculopathy. Identifying factors that relieve or precipitate the pain is important in combination with a thorough history of previous neck problems, including specific questions about injuries, stress, and positional effects.

Examination of patients with neck pain should include a thorough evaluation of any tender areas, including over the spine or any other trigger points. The motions and directions in which the movement is most restricted or painful should be noted, including flexion, extension, rotation, and leaning. Independent movement should be encouraged during the examination, and neurologic deficits elicited, including sensation, strength, and reflexes. Because neck pain can be caused by serious intracranial or intrathoracic disease, funduscopic and pulmonary examinations may be appropriate.

The report of bilateral radicular symptoms with or without involvement of the lower extremities should raise the suspicion for cervical cord compression syndrome. This syndrome can be caused by cervical disc protrusion, a fracture, or, occasionally, a neoplasm. Neck flexion usually exacerbates the symptoms of cervical cord compression syndrome; when this diagnosis is established, immediate cervical immobilization and neurosurgical consultation are required.

In patients with unilateral paresthesias or numbness, the pattern of symptoms can help to identify the cervical dermatome involved. The C6 nerve root involves the thumb and extends to the elbow on the lateral aspect of the forearm; C7 involves the mid-forearm on the dorsal and palmar surface; and C8 maps to the pinky digit along the medial forearm. Hyporeflexia may also be suggestive of a C6 or C7 nerve-root problem. Neck flexion reproduces or aggravates the distal symptoms if the root irritation is caused by a disc. Spurling's maneuver is a bedside exercise that causes foraminal compression. In this maneuver, a patient is asked to extend and rotate the head towards the affected side, which reproduces or intensifies the symptoms with or without external compression at the top of the head. This finding indicates degenerative arthritis with foraminal encroachment and nerve-root impingement. Treatment of this condition includes anti-inflammatory medications with moist heat; soft collars are also encouraged. Cervical traction might result in further improvement in patients with ongoing symptoms but is contraindicated in those with rheumatoid arthritis, acute trauma, instability, or decreased bone strength.

Sudden onset of unilateral pain and spasm without trauma is consistent with acute torticollis. On examination, diffuse tenderness is present on the involved side, with palpable spasm occurring in these patients. This condition usually resolves after a few days. Acute cervical strains usually begin after a sudden twist or prolonged abnormal posture, with tenderness localized to the specific area involved. For both torticollis and cervical strains, intermittent heat and analgesics can be helpful, with some additional benefit from the use of a soft cervical collar to unload the muscles and support the neck. In patients with chronic cervical dystonia, botulinum toxin type B therapy may be appropriate (102). A history of forced flexion/extension of the neck may be suggestive of cervical sprain or whiplash. The pain often begins the day after the injury, with diffuse tenderness on physical examination and normal radiography. In patients with acute cervical sprain or whiplash, immobilization is critical until radiography rules out a fracture, dislocation, or spinal cord injury. Treatment includes a soft collar; analgesics, including anti-inflammatory medications; and application of ice within in the first 48 hours of injury. Moist heat may be helpful after the initial period of ice application. Referral to a physical therapist may be warranted in patients with acute cervical sprain or whiplash when symptoms are severe or prolonged.

Chronic neck pain is usually caused by neck pain syndrome, a combination of pain and stiffness related to several factors, including muscle tension, incorrect posture, nerve-root irritation, and degenerative changes. Chronic neck pain results in a vicious cycle involving prolonged symptoms, and over time, a loss of flexibility. Limited range of motion and trigger points are noted on examination of patients with chronic neck pain. Comprehensive treatment is required depending on the precipitating factors but might include analgesics, anti-inflammatory medication, soft cervical collar, massage, heat, postural training, muscle relaxants, cervical traction, antidepressants, relaxation techniques, and strengthening and mobilization exercises. A recent Cochrane Systematic Review found strong evidence favoring a multimodal approach consisting of exercise, mobilization, or manipulation for subacute and chronic mechanical neck disorders (103, 104). Trigger point injections may also be effective in these patients.

Shoulder Pain

An estimated 7% to 34% of the general population has shoulder pain; it is the third most common musculoskeletal complaint of patients evaluated in primary care settings. Most shoulder pain arises from the periarticular structures of the shoulder, although 15% of shoulder pain is referred from the neck, thorax, or abdomen. Shoulder pain can impair activities of daily living and decrease general health-related quality of life. In younger adults, shoulder pain is usually related to athletic injuries, including muscle strain and subluxation of the glenohumoral joint. Rotator cuff tendonitis, partial or full-thickness tears, adhesive capsulitis (frozen shoulder), and osteoarthritis are more prevalent in middle-aged and older adults.

TABLE 23 Common Causes of Intrinsic Shoulder Pain

Cause	Clinical Features	Examination Signs
Rotator cuff tendonitis	Lateral shoulder pain, aggravated by reaching, raising arm overhead, lying on side	Subacromial pain to palpation and with passive/resisted abduction
Rotator cuff tear	Shoulder weakness, loss of shoulder function, tendonitis symptoms	Similar to tendonitis examination, plus weakness with abduction, external rotation; positive drop-arm test
Bicipital tendonitis/rupture	Anterior shoulder pain with lifting, overhead reaching, flexion; reduced pain after rupture	Bicipital groove tenderness; pain with resisted elbow flexion; "Popeye" lump in antecubital fossa following rupture
Adhesive capsulitis	Progressive decrease in range of motion, more from stiffness than pain	Loss of external rotation, abduction—unable to scratch lower back, fully lift arm straight overhead
Acromioclavicular syndromes	Anterior shoulder pain, deformity; usually from trauma or overuse.	Localized joint tenderness and deformity (osteophytes, separation), pain with adduction
Glenohumeral arthritis	Gradual onset of anterior pain, stiffness	Anterior joint-line tenderness, decreased range of motion, crepitation

Shoulder pain can be referred, traumatic, or intrinsic (**Table 23**); referred pain is likely when shoulder movement is normal and does not exacerbate pain. Potential underlying causes of referred shoulder pain include cervical radiculopathy, diaphragmatic irritation, pleural inflammation, hepatobiliary disease, or myocardial infarction. Traumatic injury to the shoulder can lead to dislocation, fracture, or a rotator cuff tear.

The most common cause of intrinsic shoulder pain is rotator cuff tendonitis, or impingement syndrome, which usually affects the supraspinatus tendon. Patients with this condition report diffuse lateral shoulder pain that often interferes with sleep and is exacerbated by overhead reaching. Subacromial tenderness is noted on examination and passive (painful arc) or resisted abduction of the glenohumoral joint may be painful. An inability to smoothly lower the arm after being raised (positive drop-arm test) is a very specific, though relatively insensitive, finding for rotator cuff tear. Adhesive capsulitis, characterized by global loss of shoulder range of motion due to stiffness more than pain, occurs in 10% of patients with rotator cuff tendonitis. Anterior humeral tenderness and pain with biceps flexion suggests bicipital tendonitis; rupture of the tendon causes a prominent bulge in the biceps.

Plain radiography has limited utility in the initial evaluation of shoulder pain in the absence of trauma or shoulder deformity. Imaging may be necessary in patients with severe or persistent pain and/or functional loss. Radiography can identify osteoarthritis or calcific tendonitis. MRI or ultrasonography can accurately detect partial and full-thickness rotator cuff tears; however, rotator cuff tears in asymptomatic patients are common, especially in patients older than age 60 years.

The goals of shoulder pain treatment are to relieve pain and improve or preserve range of motion. Systematic reviews of corticosteroid injections (105) and physiotherapy (106) for shoulder pain have concluded that insufficient evidence exists to guide treatment. Exercise and passive joint mobilization, although not ultrasound therapy, have been found to be effective for rotator cuff disease. Subacromial corticosteroid injections for rotator cuff disease provided slightly more short-term pain relief and functional improvement than placebo but no benefit when compared with NSAIDs. A randomized trial showed physiotherapy and corticosteroid injections to be similarly effective for new episodes of shoulder pain, although more patients in the injection group received additional interventions (107). Extracorporeal shock-wave therapy for calcific tendonitis improved shoulder pain and function at 12-month follow-up compared with sham treatment (108). Systematic reviews have not specifically assessed treatment for bicipital tendonitis, although it often coexists with rotator cuff tendonitis, and trials have not included patients with rotator cuff tears.

Intra-articular injections for adhesive capsulitis may provide small short-term benefits for pain and range of movement compared with placebo or physiotherapy. Prednisolone improved pain and disability in patients with adhesive capsulitis, but the benefits did not persist past 6 weeks (109).

Surgery may be necessary in patients with persistent severe rotator cuff pain despite conservative treatment or in younger patients with large, acute tears. Surgical repair of biceps tendon rupture may be indicated in younger patients who require full arm function. Surgical intervention is also a consideration when glenohumeral osteoarthritis is unresponsive to conservative treatment.

Elbow, Wrist, and Hand Pain

Elbow Pain

Epicondylitis is characterized by inflammation or pain at the extensor radii tendon that inserts on the lateral or medial epicondyle of the humerus. Lateral epicondylitis ("tennis elbow") is caused by repetitive overuse that involves pronation and supination with the wrist flexed. Medial epicondylitis ("golfer's elbow"), a much less common disorder, is caused by excessive, repetitive pronation. Treatment of epicondylitis consists of immobilization of the elbow with a sling and anti-inflammatory medications for 2 to 3 weeks. Recalcitrant symptoms can be treated with corticosteroid injections at the point of maximal tenderness. A forearm band, which consists of a simple strap that is wrapped around the forearm, can be used as a preventive measure to alter the dynamics of the extensor muscles of the forearm and lessen the strain on the point of insertion at the humeral head.

Olecranon bursitis is inflammation of the bursa, which lies in the posterior aspect of the elbow. This condition can result from repetitive trauma; systemic inflammatory conditions, such as rheumatoid arthritis, gout, or pseudogout; or infection from local extension of a soft-tissue infection. Treatment of olecranon bursitis consists of elbow rest with the use of a sling, anti-inflammatory medications, and antibiotics for suspected infection. For recalcitrant cases, corticosteroid injections may be used in the absence of infection.

Other less common causes of elbow pain include nerve entrapment, arthritis (rare), or forearm muscle pathology.

Wrist and Hand Pain

Tenosynovitis is inflammation of the extensor tendon of the wrist and generally is secondary to overuse syndromes involving repetitive motions of the wrist. In the absence of a history of overuse, inflammation may be caused by a systemic inflammatory condition. In patients with tenosynovitis, pain is exacerbated with extension of the tendon and with direct pressure on the affected area. DeQuervain's tenosynovitis involves the extensor tendon of the thumb, and a diagnosis is established by the finding of pain on extreme extension of the tendon (Finkelstein's test). Treatment includes splinting in the functional position, NSAIDs for 2 to 3 weeks (for example, ibuprofen 600 mg 3 to 4 times daily), and corticosteroid injection for persistent symptoms. When repeated trauma to the tendon sheaths of the extensor tendons occurs (typically involving the thumb), a tendon sheath nodule or granuloma can form, which disrupts tendon function and can cause the joint to remain in a fixed position. This is known as stenosing tenosynovitis, or "trigger finger," and is managed with splinting and corticosteroid injections.

Carpal tunnel syndrome (CTS) is a common cause of wrist and hand pain, typically caused by repetitive overuse of the wrist and resulting in soft-tissue entrapment of the median nerve within the carpal tunnel of the wrist. Other causes of CTS include medical conditions that cause soft-tissue expansion in the carpal tunnel, such as hypothyroidism, diabetes mellitus, fluid retention, trauma (for example, chronic sleeping on wrist under head), and arthritis of the wrist. The typical symptom of this syndrome is neuropathic pain radiating into the thumb and index finger, which can be induced by either hyperextension or flexion of the wrist. Nerve-conduction studies and electromyography are needed to confirm a diagnosis of CTS in patients who are considering surgical options or in those in whom symptoms fail to respond to empirical treatment. Empirical treatment includes the use of a cock-up wrist splint (especially at night), treatment of underlying disorders, and pain control. NSAIDs are frequently prescribed, but there is no evidence for their efficacy in CTS beyond pain control. For persistent symptoms, corticosteroid injection is more effective than surgical decompression, which is more effective than splinting (110–113).

Hip Pain

Hip pain may be indicative of musculoskeletal disease but may also be referred from the pelvis, intra-abdomen, or retroperitoneum. In most cases, physical examination and history, combined with the appropriate radiographic assessment, can lead to a diagnosis. True hip pain usually presents as groin pain but occasionally radiates to the knee. Thigh pain, buttock pain, and pain radiating below the knee are more often attributable to disorders of the lumbar spine or musculature than to the hip. History involving the hip, including surgery, developmental problems, and injections, as well as history of collagen vascular disease or malignancy, should be explored. Bone metastases to the hip should be considered in patients with a history of prostate, breast, lung, thyroid, and kidney cancer but may also be present in those with bladder cancer, osteosarcoma, melanoma, and adenocarcinoma of unknown primary site. Occupational and recreational activities are also important considerations in patients with hip pain, particularly any history of trauma.

Vital signs, including temperature, are important considerations in the physical examination of patients with hip pain, because hip pain with fever may be suggestive of septic arthritis; psoas abscess; prostatitis; pelvic inflammatory disease; or urinary tract calculi or infection. A lumbar spine examination and full neurologic assessment for motor, sensory, and lower-extremity reflexes is indicated in patients with hip pain. Pain at or below the knee with the straight-leg-raising test may suggest a lumbar spine origin of hip pain. Range-of-motion testing should include flexion, hyperextension, external rotation ("Figure 4 maneuver" with lateral ankle of one leg resting on top of knee of opposite leg), internal rotation, abduction, and adduction. Inspection of leg lengths may be useful in young patients. Hip radiography (anteroposterior and frog-leg lateral views) is indicated early in the evaluation of patients with hip pain because this joint is so inaccessible to palpation and frequently is involved in metastasis. Radiography of the hip is indicated in patients with significant trauma, bony tenderness or deep nonlocalizable pain, in older patients who are more likely to have degenerative conditions and/or neoplasm, or in patients with evidence of a distal radiculopathy. A bone scan is useful in confirming metastasis. A blood workup is usually reserved for investigating disease-specific diagnoses of hip pain, including rheumatoid arthritis, systemic lupus erythematosus, and septic arthritis.

TABLE 24 Differential Diagnosis of Hip Pain

Diagnosis	Description and Key Clinical Features
Spondyloarthropathies	• Reiter's syndrome, psoriatic arthritis, rheumatoid arthritis, ankylosing spondylitis, and inflammatory bowel disease • Inflammation of the SI joint • Pain over SI joint or referred to lower buttock and thigh • Pain with compression of pelvis or hyperextension of hip • Radiograph with blurred SI joint in advanced cases
Bursitis	• Inflammation of bursa (three around hip are trochanteric, iliopsoas, or ischiogluteal) • Caused by overuse or degenerative changes • Trochanteric (pain over greater trochanter, exacerbated by hip adduction) • Ischiogluteal (associated with sitting for long periods) • Radiograph unhelpful
Osteoarthritis	• Common, causing progressive restriction of motion in hip from synovitis, soft-tissue contractures, and loss of joint congruency • Pain in groin, buttock, anterior thigh or knee • Often with antalgic gain • Pain worse with weight bearing but may be present at rest • Examination with limited ROM and flexion contracture • Abduction and internal rotation are most restricted • Radiograph shows joint-space narrowing, cyst and osteophyte formation, and sclerotic changes in subchondral bone
Septic Arthritis	• Rare • Immunocompromised, renal failure, diabetes, intravenous drug users, those receiving corticosteroids or chemotherapy are at increased risk • High fever, exquisite pain, decreased motion • Radiograph shows widened joint space from effusion
Osteonecrosis	• Associated with femoral neck fractures and hip dislocations • Results of trauma from disruption of arterial supply to bone • Associated with showers of fat emboli • Nontraumatic risk factors (corticosteroid use, alcohol abuse, sickle cell disease, gout, Gaucher's disease, caisson disease, and hypercoagulable states) • MRI useful in early stages; advanced stages seen on plain radiograph
Contusions	• History of a direct blow to a specific area/bony prominence • Common in athletes of contact sports • Pt tenderness, bruising, hematoma common findings • Radiograph may show an associated avulsion fracture
Strains	• Injury to musculotendinous structures • Grade I: simple stretching of musculotendinous unit • Grade II: partial tear • Grade III: complete disruption
Athletic Pubalgia	• Chronic inguinal or pubic pain in athletes that worsens with exertion • Can be from hyperextension injury • MRI with nonspecific findings • Surgery often required for definitive resolution
Piriformis Syndrome	• Compression of the sciatic nerve as it exits the pelvis under the piriformis muscles, causing pain in sciatic distribution • Pain with hip flexion and internal rotation • Tenderness over piriformis tendon • Pain with resisted abduction and external rotation of thigh (Pace's sign)
Hamstring Syndrome	• Pain radiating from ischial tuberosity down the posterior aspect of thigh into popliteal fossa • Pain worse with hamstring stretch • Tenderness over ischial tuberosity • Pain with resisted leg extension
Stress Fracture	• From chronic repetitive motion • At risk: track and field, long-distance runners, military marchers • In femur: persistent groin pain with decrease ROM • In pelvis: inguinal pain, antalgic gain, full ROM

SI = sacroiliac; ROM = range of motion.

The differential diagnosis of hip pain includes contusions, strains, piriformis syndrome, hamstring syndrome, inflammatory disorders, bursitis (particularly of the trochanteric bursa), septic arthritis, osteoarthritis, and osteonecrosis (**Table 24**) (114). Contusions are generally the result of a direct blow to soft tissue on or around a bony prominence, most commonly occurring in football and hockey players. Strains are similarly benign injuries to soft tissue and are treated with symptomatic measures. Piriformis syndrome involves compression of the sciatic nerve as it travels under the piriformis muscles, exiting the pelvis. Pain is defined in the sciatic distribution and intensifies with hip flexion and internal rotation. MRI is sometimes necessary in patients with hip pain to detect inflammation around the sciatic nerve and is the first-line imaging test for suspected occult fracture, osteonecrosis, or muscle injury (115). Hamstring syndrome involves pain radiating from the ischial tuberosity down the posterior aspect of the thigh and into the popliteal fossa. Stretching activities, such as sprinting and hurdling, are frequent causes of this syndrome. Inflammatory conditions associated with hip pain include Reiter's syndrome (also known as reactive arthritis), psoriatic arthritis, ankylosing spondylitis, and inflammatory bowel disease. Pain in patients with inflammatory conditions can be reproduced by palpation directly over the sacroiliac joint, with evidence of sclerosis and a blurred joint space on radiography. Bursitis is common in patients with hip pain and is related to overuse or degenerative changes. Trochanteric bursitis can be confirmed in patients in whom hip adduction intensifies the pain or in those in whom the examination reveals pain and tenderness over the bursa. Local injection into the bursa with corticosteroids is highly effective and should be offered to patients with trochanteric bursitis when needed.

Most patients with chronic hip pain have degenerative arthritis, which is associated with other large-joint arthritis complaints. Treatment for degenerative arthritis includes analgesics, range-of-motion and strengthening exercises, and weight loss in patients who are obese. Corticosteroid injections may be used sparingly in patients with degenerative arthritis, but those with severe pain refractory to conservative management may benefit from total hip-replacement surgery. Osteonecrosis, or avascular necrosis of the femoral head in adults, is often associated with trauma, sickle cell disease, alcohol abuse, gout, corticosteroid use, and hypercoagulable states; it can also be idiopathic. Pain control is the mainstay of treatment in osteonecrosis, although there are several surgical options for treating this condition with proven benefit.

Knee Pain

Knee pain is present in up to 20% of the general population, accounts for over 1.9 million primary care outpatient visits annually, and is a source of considerable disability. Overall, 6% of primary care patients with physical complaints have knee pain, 17% of whom have pain for less than 3 days, and 46% of whom have pain for less than 1 month. Knee pain should be considered in terms of its chronicity (acute vs. chronic), location in the knee, and involvement of one or both knees. There are many possible differential diagnoses of knee pain. When knee pain is acute and monoarthritic, possible causes may include trauma, infection, and crys-

talline disease. Most chronic knee pain in the primary care setting is caused by osteoarthritis. Other causes of chronic knee pain include rheumatoid arthritis, spondyloarthropathy, meniscal tears, patellofemoral syndrome, and anserine bursitis. Anterior knee pain usually is caused by problems with the patella or the bursa around the patella. Deeper pain can be caused by osteoarthritis, rheumatoid arthritis, spondyloarthropathy, meniscal tears, infection, tears and sprains of the anterior or posterior cruciate ligaments, or crystalline disease (gout and pseudogout). Posterior knee pain may be due to a Baker's cyst, which is an outpocket of synovial fluid resulting from increased synovial pressure, usually caused by osteoarthritis. Pain in the medial part of the knee can be caused by pes anserine bursitis, medial meniscal tears, medial collateral ligament tears or sprains, or medial plica syndrome. Lateral knee pain occurs less commonly than medial knee pain but can be caused by lateral meniscal tears, lateral collateral ligament tears or sprains, or iliotibial band tendonitis.

The history of patients with knee pain can help pinpoint the underlying cause, particularly after trauma. With meniscal damage, patients describe a twisting injury with the foot in a weight-bearing position in which a popping or tearing sensation is often felt, followed by severe pain. Swelling occurs over several hours, in contrast to ligamentous injuries, in which swelling is immediate. Walking up and down stairs is difficult and squatting may be painful in patients with meniscal damage. Ligamentous damage usually occurs as a result of forceful stress or direct blows to the knee while the extremity is bearing weight. A valgus stress (that is, force applied to the lateral aspect of the knee) injures the medial collateral ligament; a varus stress (that is, force applied to the medial aspect of the knee) injures the lateral collateral ligament; hyperextension injures the posterior cruciate ligament; and excessive medial rotation with a planted foot stresses the anterior cruciate ligament. A popping or tearing sensation is also frequently reported in patients with ligamentous damage. For meniscal or ligamentous injuries, the physical examination is useful in establishing a diagnosis, with the likelihood of a tear less than 1% in patients with a negative examination; these patients require only clinical follow-up (**Table 25**) (116).

Specific maneuvers used in the evaluation of knee pain (**Figure 1**) include joint-line palpation and the McMurray maneuver for meniscal tears, and the anterior drawer sign and the Lachman and pivot tests for anterior cruciate ligament tears. Joint-line tenderness is assessed by palpating the joint line either medially or laterally; patients with meniscal tears find this maneuver to be painful. For the medial and lateral collateral ligaments, knee stability can be tested with varus or valgus stress at full extension and at 30 degrees.

The Ottawa knee rules are useful for deciding when to obtain a plain-film radiograph in patients with suspected fracture. Indications for obtaining radiographs include one or more of the following findings: age 55 years or older,

TABLE 25 Effect of Physical Examination and MRI Findings on the Likelihood of Knee Diagnoses*⁺

Knee Diagnosis	Pretest Probability	Post-Test Probability, if Positive		Post-Test Probability, if Negative	
		Physical Examination	*Magnetic Resonance Imaging*	*Physical Examination*	*Magnetic Resonance Imaging*
Anterior cruciate ligament tear	4	38	40	1	0.6
Posterior cruciate ligament tear	1	14	11	0.2	0.3
Medial meniscus	6	17	29	1	0.9
Lateral meniscus	6	41	55	0.8	1

* This table uses the pretest probability of the condition, based on the prevalence in primary care, and calculates the likelihood of having the problem with either a positive or a negative physical examination or magnetic resonance imaging result. ⁺Numbers represent percentages.

Reprinted with permission from Jackson, J. L. et. al. Ann Intern Med 2003;139:575-588.

Anterior Drawer Test

Lachman Test

Pivot Test

McMurray Test

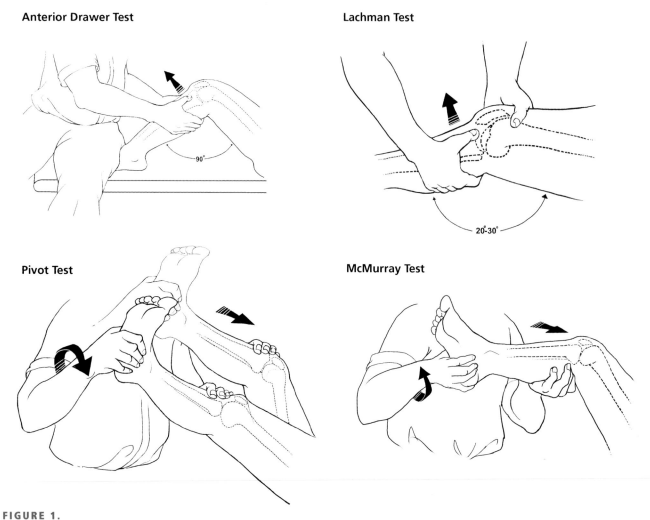

FIGURE 1.
Common maneuvers of the knee for assessing possible ligamentous and meniscal damage.

Reprinted with permission from Jackson JL, O'Malley PG, Kroenke K. Evaluation of acute knee pain in primary care. Ann Intern Med. 2003; 139:574-588.

TABLE 26 Common Causes of Foot Pain

Site	Diagnosis	Distinguishing Clinical Features
Posterior foot	Plantar fasciitis	Plantar pain when initiating walking, especially in the morning
	Calcaneal stress fracture	May follow excessive or repetitive weight-bearing exercise; ill-defined pain, worse with weight bearing
	Tarsal tunnel syndrome	Burning pain or numbness in heel, radiating to the sole and toes; aggravated by prolonged weight bearing, walking on hard surfaces; pain at night
	Achilles tendonitis	Pain with running, jumping; worse with dorsiflexion
	Achilles bursitis	Posterior calcaneal tenderness; caused by poorly fitting footwear
Anterior foot	Morton's neuroma	Forefoot pain and paresthesias, particularly in the third web space; aggravated by walking on hard surfaces, poorly fitting footwear; usually unilateral
	Hallux valgus	Deformities and pain of the first MTP joint with lateral deviation of the great toe
	Gout	Sudden onset of pain, redness, swelling of the first MTP joint (podagra). Exquisite tenderness

MTP = metatarsalphalangeal.

tenderness at the head of the fibula, isolated tenderness of the patella, and inability to flex to 90 degrees or inability to bear weight immediately and during evaluation. These rules are very sensitive, though not specific. In any patient, even in those who receive radiography, a fracture may still be missed. Patients whose symptoms do not improve need to return for re-evaluation and may be required to undergo repeated radiography to rule out fracture.

When the physical examination is suspicious for infection or crystalline disease, arthrocentesis is indicated. Features suggestive of infection or crystalline disease include pain, erythema, warmth, and effusions. Infection most commonly is manifested as disseminated gonococcal infection in young adults and either *Staphylococcus aureus* or *Streptococcus pneumoniae* in older patients. Patients with disseminated gonococcal infection typically present with a triad of tenosynovitis, vesiculopustular skin lesions, and polyarthralgias without purulent arthritis, or with purulent arthritis without skin lesions; analysis of the gram stain and culture of the synovial fluid are key in establishing the diagnosis. Although most infections are associated with leukocyte counts of 50,000 to 150,000 cells/μL, lower cell counts may be observed among immunocompromised patients and in those with infections caused by mycobacterial, some neisserial, and several gram-positive organisms. Other synovial fluid tests, such as protein, glucose, or lactose dehydrogenase, are not useful in establishing the diagnosis. Because nongonococcal bacterial arthritis can quickly destroy joints, these patients should receive empiric antibiotic therapy, with antibiotic choice based on the gram stain, until culture results become available. Patients with prosthetic joints are at highest risk for nongonococcal bacterial

arthritis in the first 3 months after placement of the joints, and most require removal of the prosthesis. Hip and shoulder infections often require surgical drainage, and early consultation in these cases is suggested. Patients who do not respond to antibiotics and in whom repeated aspirations show no decrease in leukocyte counts may require surgical intervention for other septic joints. Patients with crystalline diseases, such as gout (uric acid crystals) and pseudogout (calcium pyrophosphate crystals), often have findings suggestive of an infection. A diagnosis of crystalline disease can be established by synovial fluid analysis with a phase contrast microscope.

Osteoarthritis is the most common cause of chronic knee pain and can be diagnosed based on physical examination findings and medical history. Characteristic symptoms of this disease include pain with activity that is relieved by rest and morning stiffness that is relieved by activity. Other common findings include chronic effusion, crepitus and grating, restriction of motion, joint swelling, local tenderness, and bony deformity. The presence of bony enlargement of the knee or the presence of (all three) age older than 38 years, crepitus, and morning stiffness lasting less than 30 minutes is 89% sensitive and 88% specific for osteoarthritis. If a patient does not meet these clinical criteria, the likelihood that osteoarthritis is the cause of the knee pain is only 6%.

Foot and Ankle Pain

Foot symptoms (**Table 26**) account for nearly 1% of ambulatory care visits, and ankle sprains are among the most common injuries seen by primary care physicians. Hallux valgus (bunions) occurs when the great toe deviates toward the midline of the foot; pressure against footwear causes inflammation of the metatarsal head and bursa formation. The prevalence of hallux valgus is unknown, but women are affected more than men are, and ill-fitting footwear is a major cause. Orthoses and night splints are no more effective than no treatment for pain control of this condition or in preventing deterioration of the angle of deviation. Surgical procedures are performed when fitting footwear is difficult or in patients with impaired foot function or severe pain. Osteotomy leads to greater pain relief and functional improvement than conservative treatment in patients with hallux valgus; osteotomy may be more effective than arthroplasty in these patients, although data are limited (117).

Nerve-entrapment syndromes are another cause of foot pain. Morton's neuroma results from entrapment of interdigital nerves and causes forefoot pain and paresthesias, particularly in the third web spaces. Unilateral presentation is most common in patients with this condition, and women, usually in their fifth decade, are affected more often than are men. The plantar surface of the distal third and fourth metatarsals is usually tender in patients with nerve-entrapment syndromes, and compression can reproduce symptoms. The diagnosis of this syndrome is usually established clinically; although MRI may guide surgical interventions, routine imaging is not necessary. Broad-toed shoes, pronatory insoles, and corticosteroid injections are common treatments in patients with nerve-entrapment syndrome. Nerve excision and nerve transposition are offered to patients with refractory symptoms; however, a systematic review has found insufficient evidence to assess the effectiveness of these interventions (118).

Tarsal tunnel syndrome results from entrapment of the posterior tibial nerve under the medial flexor retinaculum, causing pain and paresthesias over the plantar and distal foot and toes. The syndrome can occur after traumatic injury, or, less commonly, from inflammatory conditions causing tenosynovitis. The differential diagnosis of tarsal tunnel syndrome includes peripheral neuropathy, reflex sympathetic dystrophy, sciatica, and compartment syndrome, although these conditions usually have other characteristic findings. The Tinel's test, performed by tapping the tibial nerve at the flexor retinaculum (posterior and inferior to the medial malleolus), may reproduce symptoms. The dorsiflexion-eversion test compresses the nerve by maximally everting and dorsiflexing the ankle while also maximally dorsiflexing the metatarsalphalangeal joints. The test had a sensitivity of 82% in patients undergoing decompression surgery and 100% specificity in normal control subjects (119). Plain-film radiography can detect bony abnormalities in patients with tarsal tunnel syndrome; MRI and electrodiagnostic testing are usually reserved for patients with refractory symptoms. Anti-inflammatory drugs, corticosteroid injections, shoe modifications, and orthotics are accepted conservative therapy in patients with tarsal tunnel syndrome, although little data support

these interventions. Outcomes of patients who undergo surgical decompression are variable, and controlled trials in these patients have not been reported.

Plantar fasciitis, the most common cause of inferior heel pain, is characterized by pain that worsens with walking, especially with the first steps in the morning or after resting, in addition to localized tenderness along the plantar fascia or the calcaneal insertion site. Obesity, prolonged standing, and repetitive microtrauma from running or dancing are risk factors for this condition. The differential diagnosis of plantar fasciitis includes calcaneal fractures, spondyloarthropathy, nerve-compression syndromes, and neuropathy. Plantar fasciitis is usually clinically diagnosed; radiographic bone spurs are neither specific nor sensitive findings in these patients. Imaging, including plain-film radiography, bone scans, ultrasonography, and MRI, is usually reserved for selected patients in whom the diagnosis of plantar fasciitis is uncertain or for evaluation of other causes of heel pain if conservative therapy is unsuccessful.

Symptoms of plantar fasciitis resolve in more than 80% of patients within 1 year. Conservative treatment is appropriate, although systematic reviews have found little evidence to guide clinical practice. A controlled trial showed that plantar fascial stretching exercises more effectively relieved pain than Achilles tendon stretches, although dropout rates in this study were substantial (120). Corticosteroid injections show short-term benefit compared with placebo in patients with plantar fasciitis. Trials assessing the benefit of extracorporeal shock wave therapy have equivocal results in these patients, although a recent controlled study of 293 patients reported significant pain reduction and increased activity at 3-month follow-up with treatment versus placebo (121). The benefits for orthotic devices, NSAIDs, avoidance of flat shoes and walking barefoot, and night splints are uncertain, although these are safe, inexpensive interventions. Plantar fasciotomy is reserved for the few patients with severe, persistent symptoms.

Lateral ankle ligament injuries resulting from inversion of the plantar-flexed foot are frequently encountered in primary care and emergency departments. Ankle sprains are classified according to clinical findings and functional loss. Most patients with grade I sprains, stretching of a ligament that causes mild pain and swelling but no joint instability or difficulty ambulating, do not seek medical care. Patients with grade II sprains have an incomplete ligament tear associated with moderate joint instability, pain, swelling, and difficulty ambulating. Those with grade III sprains have a complete ligament tear associated with more severe symptoms and instability and inability to ambulate. Fifteen percent of patients with sprains have complications involving fractures of the ankle or midfoot; however, decisions about routine radiography should be guided by the Ottawa ankle rules (**Figure 2**). These rules are based on a patient's ability to walk four steps and the presence of point tenderness in

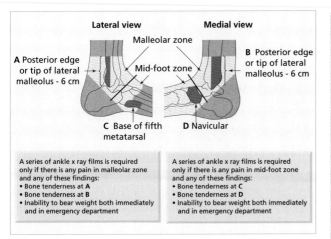

FIGURE 2.
Ottawa Ankle Rules.

Reprinted with permission from Bachman LM, Kolb MT, Steurer J, ter Riet G. Accuracy of Ottawa ankle rules to exclude fractures of the ankle and mid-foot: systematic review. BMJ 2003; 326:417.

malleolar and mid-foot zones. A systematic review has determined this instrument to be nearly 100% sensitive and able to reduce the number of unnecessary radiographs by 30% to 40% (122). Referral to an orthopedist is indicated in patients who have a significant (grade II or III) sprain or a fracture.

Functional treatment with an external support and early mobilization for acute lateral ankle ligament injuries can better relieve symptoms and decrease time away from work or sports compared with immobilization with braces or casts (123). Both semi-rigid and lace-up ankle supports are preferable to elastic bandages in the treatment of this type of injury. Although surgical repair is a consideration in patients with complete ligament tears, data from randomized trials are insufficient to determine the relative effectiveness of surgery versus conservative treatment for acute injuries. External ankle supports, including semi-rigid orthoses or air-cast braces, significantly reduce the risk of ligamentous injuries, particularly in patients with previous ankle sprains.

Fibromyalgia and Myofascial Pain

Fibromyalgia syndrome (FMS) and myofascial pain syndrome are prevalent in 2% to 4% of the U.S. adult general population and are eight times more likely to occur in women than in men. The central features of FMS are widespread musculoskeletal pain with localized tenderness unexplained by any other diagnosis, sleep disturbance, and fatigue. Myofascial pain syndrome is differentiated from FMS by the regional clustering of symptoms, particularly tender points, although it is unclear whether these are distinct entities. In 1990, The American College of Rheumatologists (ACR) published the most widely accepted (124) (**Table 27**) criteria for fibromyalgia, which consist of the presence of widespread pain for at least 3 months, and tenderness at 11 or more of 18 specific tender point sites on the four quadrants of the body (**Figure 3**).

TABLE 27 American College of Rheumatology 1990 Criteria for Fibromyalgia
Criterion 1. History of Widespread Pain
Definition: Pain in the right and left side of the body and above and below the waist and axial skeletal pain (cervical spine or anterior chest or thoracic spine or low back). In this definition, shoulder and buttock pain is considered as pain for each involved side. Low back pain is considered lower segment pain.
Criterion 2. Pain in 11 of 18 Tender Point Sites on Digital Palpation
Definition: Pain, on digital palpation, must be present in at least 11 of 18 specified tender point sites. Digital palpation should be performed with an approximate force of 4 kg. For a tender point to be considered "positive" for pain, the patient must state that the palpation was painful. "Tender" is not to be considered "painful."

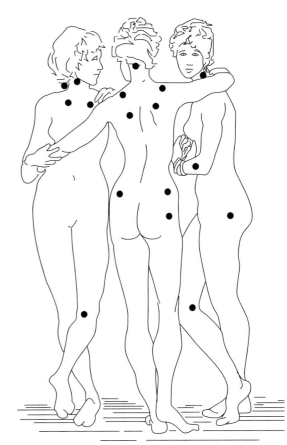

FIGURE 3.
Tender point locations for the 1990 classification criteria for fibromyalgia (The Three Graces, after Baron Jean-Baptiste Regnault, 1793, Louvre Museum, Paris).

In clinical practice, such tenderness is often found to be widespread and not limited to the points in question. Up to 25% of patients with systemic inflammatory conditions, such as

TABLE 28 Management Plan for Fibromyalgia

Focus on addressing factors that may prevent recovery, including stress and unhelpful coping behaviors, by implementing the following strategies.

1. Communicate a positive diagnosis, encourage self-management, be realistic

2. Provide relief for symptoms such as depression, pain, and sleep disturbance with agents such as antidepressants

3. Alter behavior to stabilize activity and retrain the body to function effectively (graded exercise, cognitive behavioral therapy)

4. Assist patients in managing the social and financial aspects of their illness and, when possible, remaining in or returning to employment

systemic lupus erythematosus and rheumatoid arthritis, meet the ACR criteria for fibromyalgia in the initial stages. Studies that have assessed the comorbidity of FMS with other symptom-defined syndromes have found high rates of chronic fatigue syndrome, migraine, irritable bowel syndrome, pelvic pain, and temporomandibular joint pain in patients with FMS. These patients also have an increased prevalence of lifetime and family history of major depression.

Factors associated with the development of fibromyalgia include female sex, age typically between 40 and 60 years, lower socioeconomic status, disability, and poor functional status. Some evidence suggests that patients are predisposed to develop FMS by some combination of genetics, previous experience, and, possibly, lack of social support. Many patients with FMS have experienced a precipitating accident, injury, or trauma. Physical inactivity or psychologic and behavioral factors may also be perpetuating factors in the development of FMS.

The following screening tests are appropriate in ruling out other medical conditions that may confound the diagnosis of FMS: serum thyroid-stimulating hormone assay (characterized by low levels in hyperthyroidism and high levels in hypothyroidism); erythrocyte sedimentation rate measurement (sensitive for polymyalgia rheumatica and any condition with systemic inflammation, such as rheumatologic conditions and chronic infections); complete blood count; basic serum chemistries; and withdrawal of potentially myopathic medications, particularly statins, with typical resolution of symptoms in 4 to 6 weeks of drug cessation. Sleep studies can be useful in excluding obstructive sleep apnea and narcolepsy in patients with suspected FMS. Depressive and anxiety disorders are appropriate for consideration in the differential diagnosis of FMS because of their treatment implications.

A common management strategy is to encourage and guide patients with FMS in self-management of their illness, advising them to be realistic about their expectations and avoid potentially harmful and expensive treatments (**Table 28**).

Although the causes of FMS remain unknown, it is typically thought to be caused by a combination of vulnerability and environmental stress likely to involve the brain and endocrine system, is potentially at least partially reversible, and is a disorder of bodily function rather than structure. Patients with this disorder may need to decrease the intensity and number of hours they work because of the stress associated with the illness and its symptoms. How to manage work demands, achieve a graded return to work, or plan an alternative career are important considerations in the management of these patients.

Most pharmacologic treatment studies in patients with FMS have focused on antidepressants, although many other agents have been advocated for use in treating this syndrome. Cyclobenzaprine (off-label use), a tricyclic agent chemically similar to amitriptyline but used as a muscle relaxant, has been shown to be efficacious in improving symptoms of fibromyalgia, especially pain and sleep disturbances. There are no data suggesting that NSAIDs (off-label use) are effective when used alone in the treatment of FMS, although they may be of some benefit in treating fibromyalgia when combined with amitriptyline (off-label use).

The mainstay of therapy in patients with FMS continues to be antidepressant drugs, which may be helpful for mood, pain, and sleep symptoms, but have limited effect on overall health outcomes. Patients who have pain and require nighttime sedation may be treated with tricyclic antidepressants, which have been shown to be effective in combination with selective serotonin reuptake inhibitors (SSRIs) (for example, fluoxetine [off-label use]). Higher doses of SSRIs than typically used for treating depression may be required to achieve a therapeutic response in some patients (125). The Food and Drug Administration has approved duloxetine as a new antidepressant drug for the treatment of FMS. This agent has been shown to be efficacious in alleviating most symptoms of fibromyalgia in patients with or without depression (126).

A rehabilitative outpatient program based on appropriately managed increases in activity, either as graded exercise therapy or as cognitive behavioral therapy (CBT), is the treatment of choice in this syndrome. Patient education, acupuncture, hypnosis, biofeedback, and mineral baths have all been shown to be efficacious in improving FMS symptoms (see also Reference 125) (**Table 29**).

FMS management focuses on maximizing functioning and quality of life, monitoring and treating comorbid depression and anxiety, and minimizing the risks for iatrogenic harm. This syndrome typically has a fluctuating-chronic course. The prognosis for patients who do not undergo rehabilitative therapy is for gradual improvement in most, but with few returning to premorbid functioning. Rehabilitative therapy improves outcomes, with 50% achieving partial or complete remission at 2 to 3 years after therapy. In general, poor outcome is predicted by longer illness duration, more

TABLE 29 Treatment of Fibromyalgia Syndrome

Pharmacologic Treatment

Strong Evidence for Efficacy

Amitriptyline: often helps sleep and overall well-being; dose, 25–50 mg at bedtime

Cyclobenzaprine: similar response and adverse effects; dose, 10–30 mg at bedtime

Modest Evidence for Efficacy

Tramadol: long-term efficacy and tolerability unknown; administered with or without acetaminophen; dose, 200–300 mg/d

SSRIs: Fluoxetine (only one carefully evaluated at this time): dose, 20–80 mg; may be used with tricyclic antidepressant given at bedtime; uncontrolled report of efficacy using sertraline

SNRIs: venlafaxine: one RCT ineffective, but two case reports found higher dose effective. Milnacipran: effective in single RCT. Duloxetine: effective in single RCT

Pregabalin: second-generation anticonvulsant; effective in single RCT

Weak Evidence for Efficacy

Growth hormone: modest improvement in subset of patients with FMS with low growth hormone levels at baseline

5-Hydroxytryptamine (serotonin): methodologic problems

Tropisetron: not commercially available

S-adenosyl-methionine: mixed results

No Evidence for Efficacy

Opioids, corticosteroids, NSAIDs, benzodiazepene and nonbenzodiazepene hypnotics, melatonin, calcitonin, thyroid hormone, guaifenesin, dehydroepiandrosterone, magnesium

Nonpharmacologic Treatment

Strong Evidence for Efficacy
(Wait-List or Flexibility Controls But Not Blinded Trials)

Cardiovascular exercise: efficacy not maintained if exercise stops

CBT: improvement often sustained for months

Patient education: group format using lectures, written materials, demonstrations; improvement sustained for 3 to 12 months

Multidisciplinary therapy, such as exercise and CBT or education and exercise

Moderate Evidence for Efficacy

Strength training, acupuncture, hypnotherapy, biofeedback, balneotherapy

Weak Evidence for Efficacy

Chiropractic, manual, and massage therapy; electrotherapy, ultrasonography

No Evidence for Efficacy

Tender (trigger) point injections, flexibility exercise

Reprinted with permission from Goldenberg D, et al. Management of fibromyalgia syndrome. JAMA. 2004;292(19):2388-95. Review.

CBT = cognitive behavioral therapy; RCT = randomized controlled trial; SSRI = selective serotonin reuptake inhibitor; SNRI = serotonin and norepinephrine reuptake inhibitor.

severe symptoms, older age, depression, and lack of social support. More severely ill patients attending specialist clinics have very poor prognoses for recovery.

KEY POINTS

- Most episodes of low back pain are benign and self-limited, with a serious underlying systemic disease or neurologic disorder present in less than 5% of patients.

- Spinal stenosis usually occurs in older adults and is characterized by neurogenic claudication exacerbated by walking and spinal extension but improved by sitting.

- Spinal infections are associated with fever, active urinary or skin infections, immunosuppression, immunodeficiency, injection drug use, or weight loss.

- A wide-based gait and abnormal Romberg test are highly specific findings for spinal stenosis.

- Maintaining normal activity improves pain control and functional status more than strict bed rest for acute low back pain, although not for sciatica.

- Tricyclic and tetracyclic antidepressants moderately reduce pain severity in patients with chronic low back pain but have an inconsistent effect on functional status.

- Bilateral radicular symptoms with or without involvement of the lower extremities should raise suspicion for cervical cord compression syndrome.

- In patients with acute cervical sprain or whiplash, immobilization is critical until radiography rules out a fracture, dislocation, or spinal cord injury.

- Patients with rotator cuff tendonitis have diffuse lateral shoulder pain that often interferes with sleep and is exacerbated by overhead reaching.

- Surgery may be necessary in patients with persistent severe rotator cuff pain despite conservative treatment, or in younger patients with large, acute tears.

- Treatment of DeQuervain's tenosynovitis includes splinting in the functional position, NSAIDs, and corticosteroid injection for persistent symptoms.

- Carpal tunnel syndrome (CTS) is characterized by neuropathic pain radiating into the thumb and index finger, which can be induced by either hyperextension or flexion of the wrist.

- Hip pain with fever may be suggestive of septic arthritis, psoas abscess, prostatitis, pelvic inflammatory disease, or urinary tract calculi or infection.

- Inflammatory conditions associated with hip pain include Reiter's syndrome (also known as reactive arthritis), psoriatic arthritis, ankylosing spondylitis, and inflammatory bowel disease.

- Patients with prosthetic joints are at highest risk for nongonococcal bacterial arthritis in the first 3 months after joint placement, with most infected patients requiring prosthesis removal.

- Osteotomy leads to greater pain relief and functional improvement than conservative treatment in patients with hallux valgus.

(continued)

- Plain-film radiography can detect bony abnormalities in patients with tarsal tunnel syndrome; MRI and electrodiagnostic testing are usually reserved for refractory symptoms.

- Plantar fasciitis is characterized by pain that worsens with walking, especially with the first steps in the morning or after resting, in addition to localized tenderness along the plantar fascia or the calcaneal insertion site.

- Corticosteroid injections provide short-term benefit to patients with plantar fasciitis compared with placebo.

- External ankle supports, including semi-rigid orthoses or air-cast braces, significantly reduce the risk of ligamentous injuries, particularly in patients with previous ankle sprains.

- Widespread pain for at least 3 months and tenderness at 11 or more of 18 specific tender point sites on the four quadrants of the body are criteria for fibromyalgia syndrome.

- Duloxetine is effective in alleviating most symptoms of fibromyalgia in patients with or without depression.

References

1. **Aaron LA, Buchwald D.** A review of the evidence for overlap among unexplained clinical conditions. Ann Intern Med. 2001;134:868-81. [PMID: 11346323]

2. **Kroenke K.** The interface between physical and psychological symptoms. Primary Care Companion. J Clin Psychiatry. 2003;5[suppl 7]:11-8. Available at: http://www.psychiatrist.com/pcc/pccpdf/v05s07/v05s0703.pdf. Accessed June 20, 2006.

3. **Khan AA, Khan A, Harezlak J, Tu W, Kroenke K.** Somatic symptoms in primary care: etiology and outcome. Psychosomatics. 2003;44:471-8. [PMID: 14597681]

4. **Jackson JL, Kroenke K.** The effect of unmet expectations among adults presenting with physical symptoms. Ann Intern Med. 2001;134:889-97. [PMID: 11346325]

5. **International Headache Society.** Classification and WHO ICD-10NA Codes. Cephalalgia. 2004;24(S1):138-49.

6. **Taylor FR.** Diagnosis and classification of headache. Prim Care. 2004;31:243-59, v. [PMID: 15172505]

7. **Dowson, A, Dahlof, C, Tepper, S, Newman, L.** Prevalence and diagnosis of migraine in a primary care setting. Cephalalgia. 2002; 22:590.

8. **Zwart JA, Dyb G, Hagen K, Svebak S, Holmen J.** Analgesic use: a predictor of chronic pain and medication overuse headache: the Head-HUNT Study. Neurology. 2003;61:160-4. [PMID: 12874392]

9. **Frediani F, Cannata AP, Magnoni A, Peccarisi C, Bussone G.** The patient with medication overuse: clinical management problems. Neurol Sci. 2003;24 Suppl 2:S108-11. [PMID: 12811605]

10. **Limmroth V, Katsarava Z.** Medication overuse headache. Curr Opin Neurol. 2004;17:301-6. [PMID: 15167065]

11. **Wenzel RG, Sarvis CA, Krause ML.** Over-the-counter drugs for acute migraine attacks: literature review and recommendations. Pharmacotherapy. 2003;23:494-505. [PMID: 12680479]

12. **Rains JC, Penzien DB, McCrory DC, Gray RN.** Behavioral headache treatment: history, review of the empirical literature, and methodological critique. Headache. 2005;45 Suppl 2:S92-109. [PMID: 15921506]

13. **Melchart D, Linde K, Fischer P, Berman B, White A, Vickers A, Allais G.** Acupuncture for idiopathic headache. Cochrane Database Syst Rev. 2001;(1):CD001218. [PMID: 11279710]

14. **Ernst E.** Manual therapies for pain control: chiropractic and massage. Clin J Pain. 2004 Jan-Feb;20(1):8-12. [PMID: 14668650]

15. **Linde K, Rossnagel K.** Propranolol for migraine prophylaxis. Cochrane Database Syst Rev. 2004;(2):CD003225. [PMID: 15106196]

16. **Silberstein SD.** Practice parameter: evidence-based guidelines for migraine headache (an evidence-based review): report of the Quality Standards Subcommittee of the American Academy of Neurology. Neurology. 2000;55:754-62. [PMID: 10993991]

17. **Moja PL, Cusi C, Sterzi RR, Canepari C.** Selective serotonin re-uptake inhibitors (SSRIs) for preventing migraine and tension-type headaches. Cochrane Database Syst Rev. 2005:CD002919. [PMID: 16034880]

18. **Schrader H, Stovner LJ, Helde G, Sand T, Bovim G.** Prophylactic treatment of migraine with angiotensin converting enzyme inhibitor (lisinopril): randomised, placebo controlled, crossover study. BMJ. 2001;322:19-22. [PMID: 11141144]

19. **Tronvik E, Stovner LJ, Helde G, Sand T, Bovim G.** Prophylactic treatment of migraine with an angiotensin II receptor blocker: a randomized controlled trial. JAMA. 2003;289:65-9. [PMID: 12503978]

20. **Johnson CD.** ABC of the upper gastrointestinal tract. Upper abdominal pain: Gall bladder. BMJ. 2001;323:1170-3. [PMID: 11711412]

21. **Srinivasan R, Greenbaum DS.** Chronic abdominal wall pain: a frequently overlooked problem. Practical approach to diagnosis and management. Am J Gastroenterol. 2002;97:824-30. [PMID: 12003414]

22. **Romagnuolo J, Bardou M, Rahme E, Joseph L, Reinhold C, Barkun AN.** Magnetic resonance cholangiopancreatography: a meta-analysis of test performance in suspected biliary disease. Ann Intern Med. 2003;139:547-57. [PMID: 14530225]

23. **Guthrie E, Thompson D.** Abdominal pain and functional gastrointestinal disorders. BMJ. 2002;325:701-3. [PMID: 12351366]

24. **Thomas SH, Silen W.** Effect on diagnostic efficiency of analgesia for undifferentiated abdominal pain. Br J Surg. 2003;90:5-9. [PMID: 12520567]

25. **Brandt LJ, Bjorkman D, Fennerty MB, Locke GR, Olden K, Peterson W, et al.** Systematic review on the management of irritable bowel syndrome in North America. Am J Gastroenterol. 2002;97:S7-26. [PMID: 12425586]

26. **Koloski NA, Talley NJ, Boyce PM.** Predictors of health care seeking for irritable bowel syndrome and nonulcer dyspepsia: a critical review of the literature on symptom and psychosocial factors. Am J Gastroenterol. 2001;96:1340-9. [PMID: 11374666]

27. **Whitehead WE, Palsson O, Jones KR.** Systematic review of the comorbidity of irritable bowel syndrome with other disorders: what are the causes and implications? Gastroenterology. 2002;122:1140-56. [PMID: 11910364]

28. **Lin HC.** Small intestinal bacterial overgrowth: a framework for understanding irritable bowel syndrome. JAMA. 2004;292:852-8. [PMID: 15316000]

29. **Gladman LM, Gorard DA.** General practitioner and hospital specialist attitudes to functional gastrointestinal disorders. Aliment Pharmacol Ther. 2003;17:651-4. [PMID: 12641513]

30. **Olden KW.** Diagnosis of irritable bowel syndrome. Gastroenterology. 2002;122:1701-14. [PMID: 12016433]

31. **Guilera M, Balboa A, Mearin F.** Bowel habit subtypes and temporal patterns in irritable bowel syndrome: systematic review. Am J Gastroenterol. 2005 May;100(5):1174-84. PMID: 15842596

32. **Holten KB.** Irritable bowel syndrome: minimize testing, let symptoms guide treatment. J Fam Pract. 2003;52:942-50. [PMID: 14653980]

33. **Patel SM, Stason WB, Legedza A, Ock SM, Kaptchuk TJ, Conboy L, et al.** The placebo effect in irritable bowel syndrome trials: a meta-analysis. Neurogastroenterol Motil. 2005;17:332-40. [PMID: 15916620]

34. **Hutton J.** Cognitive behaviour therapy for irritable bowel syndrome. Eur J Gastroenterol Hepatol. 2005;17:11-4. [PMID: 15647633]

35. **Lesbros-Pantoflickova D, Michetti P, Fried M, Beglinger C, Blum AL.** Meta-analysis: The treatment of irritable bowel syndrome. Aliment Pharmacol Ther. 2004;20:1253-69. [PMID: 15606387]

36. **Quartero AO, Meineche-Schmidt V, Muris J, Rubin G, de Wit N.** Bulking agents, antispasmodic and antidepressant medication for the treatment of irritable bowel syndrome. Cochrane Database Syst Rev. 2005:CD003460. [PMID: 15846668]

37. **Evans BW, Clark WK, Moore DJ, Whorwell PJ.** Tegaserod for the treatment of irritable bowel syndrome. Cochrane Database Syst Rev. 2004:CD003960. [PMID: 14974049]

38. **Cremonini F, Delgado-Aros S, Camilleri M.** Efficacy of alosetron in irritable bowel syndrome: a meta-analysis of randomized controlled trials. Neurogastroenterol Motil. 2003;15:79-86. [PMID: 12588472]

39. **Makris N, Barkun A, Crott R, Fallone CA.** Cost-effectiveness of alternative approaches in the management of dyspepsia. Int J Technol Assess Health Care. 2003;19:446-64. [PMID: 12962332]

40. **Moayyedi P, Deeks J, Talley NJ, Delaney B, Forman D.** An update of the Cochrane systematic review of *Helicobacter pylori* eradication therapy in nonulcer dyspepsia: resolving the discrepancy between systematic reviews. Am J Gastroenterol. 2003;98:2621-6. [PMID: 14687807]

41. **Soo S, Forman D, Delaney BC, Moayyedi P.** A systematic review of psychological therapies for nonulcer dyspepsia. Am J Gastroenterol. 2004;99:1817-22. [PMID: 15330925]

42. **Talley NJ.** Update on the role of drug therapy in non-ulcer dyspepsia. Rev Gastroenterol Disord. 2003;3:25-30. [PMID: 12684590]

43. **Kurata JH, Nogawa AN, Everhart JE.** A prospective study of dyspepsia in primary care. Dig Dis Sci. 2002;47:797-803. [PMID: 11991613]

44. **Manicourt DH, Brasseur JP, Boutsen Y, Depreseux G, Devogelaer JP.** Role of alendronate in therapy for posttraumatic complex regional pain syndrome type I of the lower extremity. Arthritis Rheum. 2004;50:3690-7. [PMID: 15529370]

45. **Ballantyne JC, Mao J.** Opioid therapy for chronic pain. N Engl J Med. 2003;349:1943-53. [PMID: 14614170]

46. **Brosseau L, Judd MG, Marchand S, Robinson VA, Tugwell P, Wells G, Yonge K.** Transcutaneous electrical nerve stimulation (TENS) for the treatment of rheumatoid arthritis in the hand. Cochrane Database Syst Rev. 2003;(3):CD004377. [12918009]

47. **Mailis-Gagnon A, Furlan AD, Sandoval JA, Taylor R.** Spinal cord stimulation for chronic pain. Cochrane Database Syst Rev. 2004:CD003783. [PMID: 15266501]

48. **Patterson DR, Jensen MP.** Hypnosis and clinical pain. Psychol Bull. 2003;129:495-521. [PMID: 12848218]

49. **Witt C, Brinkhaus B, Jena S, Linde K, Streng A, Wagenpfeil S, et al.** Acupuncture in patients with osteoarthritis of the knee: a randomised trial. Lancet. 2005;366:136-43. [PMID: 16005336]

50. **Widdicombe J, Kamath S.** Acute cough in the elderly: aetiology, diagnosis and therapy. Drugs Aging. 2004;21:243-58. [PMID: 15012170]

51. **Eccles R.** The powerful placebo in cough studies? Pulm Pharmacol Ther. 2002;15:303-8. [PMID: 12099783]

52. **Schroeder K, Fahey T.** Systematic review of randomised controlled trials of over the counter cough medicines for acute cough in adults. BMJ. 2002;324:329-31. [PMID: 11834560]

53. **Schroeder K, Fahey T.** Over-the-counter medications for acute cough in children and adults in ambulatory settings. Cochrane Database Syst Rev. 2004:CD001831. [PMID: 15495019]

54. **Smucny JJ, Flynn CA, Becker LA, Glazier RH.** Are beta2-agonists effective treatment for acute bronchitis or acute cough in patients without underlying pulmonary disease? A systematic review. J Fam Pract. 2001;50:945-51. [PMID: 11711010]

55. **Fukuda K, Straus SE, Hickie I, Sharpe MC, Dobbins JG, Komaroff A.** The chronic fatigue syndrome: a comprehensive approach to its definition and study. International Chronic Fatigue Syndrome Study Group. Ann Intern Med. 1994;121:953-9. [PMID: 7978722]

56. **Sullivan PF, Pedersen NL, Jacks A, Evengard B.** Chronic fatigue in a population sample: definitions and heterogeneity. Psychol Med. 2005;35:1337-48. [PMID: 16168156]

57. **Ross SD, Estok RP, Frame D, Stone LR, Ludensky V, Levine CB.** Disability and chronic fatigue syndrome: a focus on function. Arch Intern Med. 2004;164:1098-107. [PMID: 15159267]

58. **Darbishire L, Ridsdale L, Seed PT.** Distinguishing patients with chronic fatigue from those with chronic fatigue syndrome: a diagnostic study in UK primary care. Br J Gen Pract. 2003;53:441-5. [PMID: 12939888]

59. **Schmaling KB, Fiedelak JI, Katon WJ, Bader JO, Buchwald DS.** Prospective study of the prognosis of unexplained chronic fatigue in a clinic-based cohort. Psychosom Med. 2003;65:1047-54. [PMID: 14645784]

60. **Whiting P, Bagnall AM, Sowden AJ, Cornell JE, Mulrow CD, Ramirez G.** Interventions for the treatment and management of chronic fatigue syndrome: a systematic review. JAMA. 2001;286:1360-8. [PMID: 11560542]

61. **Sloane PD, Coeytaux RR, Beck RS, Dallara J.** Dizziness: state of the science. Ann Intern Med. 2001;134:823-32. [PMID: 11346317]

62. **Hanley K, O'Dowd T, Considine N.** A systematic review of vertigo in primary care. Br J Gen Pract. 2001;51:666-71. [PMID: 11510399]

63. **Parnes LS, Agrawal SK, Atlas J.** Diagnosis and management of benign paroxysmal positional vertigo (BPPV). CMAJ. 2003;169:681-93. [PMID: 14517129]

64. **Hoffman RM, Einstadter D, Kroenke K.** Evaluating dizziness. Am J Med. 1999;107:468-78. [PMID: 10569302]

65. **Colledge N, Lewis S, Mead G, Sellar R, Wardlaw J, Wilson J.** Magnetic resonance brain imaging in people with dizziness: a comparison with non-dizzy people. J Neurol Neurosurg Psychiatry. 2002;72:587-9. [PMID: 11971042]

66. **Yardley L, Donovan-Hall M, Smith HE, Walsh BM, Mullee M, Bronstein AM.** Effectiveness of primary care-based vestibular rehabilitation for chronic dizziness. Ann Intern Med. 2004;141:598-605. [PMID: 15492339]

67. Diagnostic and statistical manual of mental disorders. 4th ed. Washington, DC: American Psychiatric Association; 1994.

68. **Sateia MJ, Pigeon WR.** Identification and management of insomnia. Med Clin North Am. 2004;88:567-96, vii. [PMID: 15087205]

69. **Ringdahl EN, Pereira SL, Delzell JE Jr.** Treatment of primary insomnia. J Am Board Fam Pract. 2004;17:212-9. [PMID: 15226287]

70. **Krystal AD.** The changing perspective on chronic insomnia management. J Clin Psychiatry. 2004;65 Suppl 8:20-5. [PMID: 15153064]

71. **Silber MH.** Clinical practice. Chronic insomnia. N Engl J Med. 2005;353:803-10. [PMID: 16120860]

72. **Wang MY, Wang SY, Tsai PS.** Cognitive behavioural therapy for primary insomnia: a systematic review. J Adv Nurs. 2005;50:553-64. [PMID: 15882372]

73. **Zoorob RJ, Campbell JS.** Acute dyspnea in the office. Am Fam Physician. 2003;68:1803-10. [PMID: 14620600]

74. **Wang CS, FitzGerald JM, Schulzer M, Mak E, Ayas NT.** Does this dyspneic patient in the emergency department have congestive heart failure? JAMA. 2005;294:1944-56. [PMID: 16234501]

75. **Collins SP, Ronan-Bentle S, Storrow AB.** Diagnostic and prognostic usefulness of natriuretic peptides in emergency department patients with dyspnea. Ann Emerg Med. 2003;41:532-45. [PMID: 12658254]

76. **Knudsen CW, Omland T, Clopton P, Westheim A, Abraham WT, Storrow AB, et al.** Diagnostic value of B-Type natriuretic peptide and chest radiographic findings in patients with acute dyspnea. Am J Med. 2004;116:363-8. [PMID: 15006584]

77. **Morrison LK, Harrison A, Krishnaswamy P, Kazanegra R, Clopton P, Maisel A.** Utility of a rapid B-natriuretic peptide assay in differentiating congestive heart failure from lung disease in patients presenting with dyspnea. J Am Coll Cardiol. 2002;39:202-9. [PMID: 11788208]

78. **Milani RV, Lavie CJ, Mehra MR.** Cardiopulmonary exercise testing: how do we differentiate the cause of dyspnea? Circulation. 2004;110:e27-31. [PMID: 15277333]

79. **Kapoor WN.** Current evaluation and management of syncope. Circulation. 2002;106:1606-9. [PMID: 12270849]

80. **Benditt DG, van Dijk JG, Sutton R, Wieling W, Lin JC, Sakaguchi S, et al.** Syncope. Curr Probl Cardiol. 2004;29:152-229. [PMID: 15107784]

81. **Sarasin FP, Louis-Simonet M, Carballo D, Slama S, Rajeswaran A, Metzger JT, et al.** Prospective evaluation of patients with syncope: a population-based study. Am J Med. 2001;111:177-84. [PMID: 11530027]

82. **Grubb BP.** Clinical practice. Neurocardiogenic syncope. N Engl J Med. 2005;352:1004-10. [PMID: 15758011]

83. **Soteriades ES, Evans JC, Larson MG, Chen MH, Chen L, Benjamin EJ, et al.** Incidence and prognosis of syncope. N Engl J Med. 2002;347:878-85. [PMID: 12239256]

84. **Brignole M, Alboni P, Benditt DG, Bergfeldt L, Blanc JJ, Thomsen PE, et al.** Guidelines on management (diagnosis and treatment) of syncope-update 2004. Executive Summary. Eur Heart J. 2004;25:2054-72. [PMID: 15541843]

85. **Klinkman MS, Stevens D, Gorenflo DW.** Episodes of care for chest pain: a preliminary report from MIRNET. Michigan Research Network. J Fam Pract. 1994;38:345-52. [PMID: 8163958]

86. **Martina B, Bucheli B, Stotz M, Battegay E, Gyr N.** First clinical judgment by primary care physicians distinguishes well between nonorganic and organic causes of abdominal or chest pain. J Gen Intern Med. 1997;12:459-65. [PMID: 9276650]

87. **Patel H, Rosengren A, Ekman I.** Symptoms in acute coronary syndromes: does sex make a difference? Am Heart J. 2004;148:27-33. [PMID: 15215788]

88. **Wiest FC, Bryson CL, Burman M, McDonell MB, Henikoff JG, Fihn SD.** Suboptimal pharmacotherapeutic management of chronic stable angina in the primary care setting. Am J Med. 2004;117:234-41. [PMID: 15308432]

89. **Bugiardini R, Bairey Merz CN.** Angina with "normal" coronary arteries: a changing philosophy. JAMA. 2005;293:477-84. [PMID: 15671433]

90. **Wang WH, Huang JQ, Zheng GF, Wong WM, Lam SK, Karlberg J, et al.** Is proton pump inhibitor testing an effective approach to diagnose gastroesophageal reflux disease in patients with noncardiac chest pain?: a meta-analysis. Arch Intern Med. 2005;165:1222-8. [PMID: 15956000]

91. **Deyo RA.** Diagnostic evaluation of LBP: reaching a specific diagnosis is often impossible. Arch Intern Med. 2002;162:1444-7; discussion 1447-8. [PMID: 12090877]

92. **Deyo RA, Weinstein JN.** Low back pain. N Engl J Med. 2001;344:363-70. [PMID: 11172169]

93. **Wadell G, McCulloch JA, Kummel E, Venner RM.** Nonorganic physical signs in low-back pain. Spine. 1980 Mar-Apr;5(2):117-25. [PMID: 6446157]

94. **Jarvik JG, Deyo RA.** Diagnostic evaluation of low back pain with emphasis on imaging. Ann Intern Med. 2002;137:586-97. [PMID: 12353946]

95. **Jarvik JG, Hollingworth W, Martin B, Emerson SS, Gray DT, Overman S, et al.** Rapid magnetic resonance imaging vs radiographs for patients with low back pain: a randomized controlled trial. JAMA. 2003;289:2810-8. [PMID: 12783911]

96. **Cherkin DC, Sherman KJ, Deyo RA, Shekelle PG.** A review of the evidence for the effectiveness, safety, and cost of acupuncture, massage therapy, and spinal manipulation for back pain. Ann Intern Med. 2003;138:898-906. [PMID: 12779300]

97. **Staiger TO, Gaster B, Sullivan MD, Deyo RA.** Systematic review of antidepressants in the treatment of chronic low back pain. Spine. 2003;28:2540-5. [PMID: 14624092]

98. **Salerno SM, Browning R, Jackson JL.** The effect of antidepressant treatment on chronic back pain: a meta-analysis. Arch Intern Med. 2002;162:19-24. [PMID: 11784215]

99. **Gibson JN, Grant IC, Waddell G.** The Cochrane review of surgery for lumbar disc prolapse and degenerative lumbar spondylosis. Spine. 1999;24:1820-32. [PMID: 10488513]

100. **Devereaux MW.** Neck pain. Prim Care. 2004;31:19-31. [PMID: 15110156]

101. **Hoffman JR, Mower WR, Wolfson AB, Todd KH, Zucker MI.** Validity of a set of clinical criteria to rule out injury to the cervical spine in patients with blunt trauma. National Emergency X-Radiography Utilization Study Group. N Engl J Med. 2000;343:94-9. [PMID: 10891516]

102. **Figgitt DP, Noble S.** Botulinum toxin B: a review of its therapeutic potential in the management of cervical dystonia. Drugs. 2002;62:705-22. [PMID: 11893235]

103. **Kay TM, Gross A, Goldsmith C, Santaguida PL, Hoving J, Bronfort G, et al.** Exercises for mechanical neck disorders. Cochrane Database Syst Rev. 2005:CD004250. [PMID: 16034925]

104. **Gross AR, Hoving JL, Haines TA, Goldsmith CH, Kay T, Aker P, et al.** Manipulation and mobilisation for mechanical neck disorders. Cochrane Database Syst Rev. 2004:CD004249. [PMID: 14974063]

105. **Buchbinder R, Green S, Youd JM.** Corticosteroid injections for shoulder pain. Cochrane Database Syst Rev. 2003:CD004016. [PMID: 12535501]

106. **Green S, Buchbinder R, Hetrick S.** Physiotherapy interventions for shoulder pain. Cochrane Database Syst Rev. 2003;(2):CD004258. Review. PMID: 12804509

107. **Hay EM, Thomas E, Paterson SM, Dziedzic K, Croft PR.** A pragmatic randomised controlled trial of local corticosteroid injection and physiotherapy for the treatment of new episodes of unilateral shoulder pain in primary care. Ann Rheum Dis. 2003;62:394-9. [PMID: 12695148]

108. **Gerdesmeyer L, Wagenpfeil S, Haake M, Maier M, Loew M, Wortler K, et al.** Extracorporeal shock wave therapy for the treatment of chronic calcifying tendonitis of the rotator cuff: a randomized controlled trial. JAMA. 2003;290:2573-80. [PMID: 14625334]

109. **Buchbinder R, Hoving JL, Green S, Hall S, Forbes A, Nash P.** Short course prednisolone for adhesive capsulitis (frozen shoulder or stiff painful shoulder): a randomised, double blind, placebo controlled trial. Ann Rheum Dis. 2004;63:1460-9. [PMID: 15479896]

110. **Ly-Pen D, Andreu JL, de Blas G, Sanchez-Olaso A, Millan I.** Surgical decompression versus local steroid injection in carpal tunnel syndrome: a one-year, prospective, randomized, open, controlled clinical trial. Arthritis Rheum. 2005;52:612-9. [PMID: 15692981]

111. **Gerritsen AA, de Krom MC, Struijs MA, Scholten RJ, de Vet HC, Bouter LM.** Conservative treatment options for carpal tunnel syndrome: a systematic review of randomised controlled trials. J Neurol. 2002;249:272-80. [PMID: 11993525]

112. Gerritsen AA, de Vet HC, Scholten RJ, Bertelsmann FW, de Krom MC, Bouter LM. Splinting vs surgery in the treatment of carpal tunnel syndrome: a randomized controlled trial. JAMA. 2002;288:1245-51. [PMID: 12215131]

113. Katz JN, Simmons BP. Clinical practice. Carpal tunnel syndrome. N Engl J Med. 2002;346:1807-12. [PMID: 12050342]

114. DeAngelis NA, Busconi BD. Assessment and differential diagnosis of the painful hip. Clin Orthop Relat Res. 2003:11-8. [PMID: 12578995]

115. Newberg AH, Newman JS. Imaging the painful hip. Clin Orthop Relat Res. 2003:19-28. [PMID: 12578996]

116. Jackson JL, O'Malley PG, Kroenke K. Evaluation of acute knee pain in primary care. Ann Intern Med. 2003;139:575-88. [PMID: 14530229]

117. Ferrari J, Higgins JP, Prior TD. Interventions for treating hallux valgus (abductovalgus) and bunions. Cochrane Database Syst Rev. 2004:CD000964. [PMID: 14973960]

118. Thomson CE, Gibson JN, Martin D. Interventions for the treatment of Morton's neuroma. Cochrane Database Syst Rev. 2004:CD003118. [PMID: 15266472]

119. Kinoshita M, Okuda R, Morikawa J, Jotoku T, Abe M. The dorsiflexion-eversion test for diagnosis of tarsal tunnel syndrome. J Bone Joint Surg Am. 2001;83-A:1835-9. [PMID: 11741063]

120. DiGiovanni BF, Nawoczenski DA, Lintal ME, Moore EA, Murray JC, Wilding GE, et al. Tissue-specific plantar fascia-stretching exercise enhances outcomes in patients with chronic heel pain. A prospective, randomized study. J Bone Joint Surg Am. 2003;85-A:1270-7. [PMID: 12851352]

121. Ogden JA, Alvarez RG, Levitt RL, Johnson JE, Marlow ME. Electrohydraulic high-energy shock-wave treatment for chronic plantar fasciitis. J Bone Joint Surg Am. 2004;86-A:2216-28. [PMID: 15466731]

122. Bachmann LM, Kolb E, Koller MT, Steurer J, ter Riet G. Accuracy of Ottawa ankle rules to exclude fractures of the ankle and mid-foot: systematic review. BMJ. 2003;326:417. [PMID: 12595378]

123. Kerkhoffs GM, Rowe BH, Assendelft WJ, Kelly K, Struijs PA, van Dijk CN. Immobilisation and functional treatment for acute lateral ankle ligament injuries in adults. Cochrane Database Syst Rev. 2002:CD003762. [PMID: 12137710]

124. Wolfe F, Smythe HA, Yunus MB, Bennett RM, Bombardier C, Goldenberg DL, et al. The American College of Rheumatology 1990 Criteria for the Classification of Fibromyalgia. Report of the Multicenter Criteria Committee. Arthritis Rheum. 1990;33:160-72. [PMID: 2306288]

125. Goldenberg DL, Burckhardt C, Crofford L. Management of fibromyalgia syndrome. JAMA. 2004;292:2388-95. [PMID: 15547167]

126. Arnold LM, Lu Y, Crofford LJ, Wohlreich M, Detke MJ, Iyengar S, et al. A double-blind, multicenter trial comparing duloxetine with placebo in the treatment of fibromyalgia patients with or without major depressive disorder. Arthritis Rheum. 2004;50:2974-84. [PMID: 15457467]

HYPERLIPIDEMIA

Although all patients should receive hypercholesterolemia screening, the recommendation for initial screening age varies by organization. The Adult Treatment Panel (ATP III) of the National Cholesterol Education Program (NCEP) recommends obtaining a fasting (9 to 12 hours) serum lipid profile consisting of total cholesterol, low-density lipoprotein (LDL) cholesterol, high-density lipoprotein (HDL) cholesterol, and triglycerides beginning at age 20

TABLE 30 Classification of Total, LDL, and HDL Cholesterol and Triglycerides

LDL cholesterol (mg/dL)	
<100	Optimal
100–129	Near optimal/above optimal
130-159	Borderline high
160-189	High
≥190	Very high
Total cholesterol (mg/dL)	
<200	Desirable
200-239	Borderline high
≥240	High
HDL cholesterol (mg/dL)	
<40	Low
≥60	High
Serum Triglycerides (mg/dL)	
<150	Normal
150-199	Borderline high
200-499	High
≥500	Very high

Adapted from National Cholesterol Education Program: Third Report of the Expert Panel on Detection, Evaluation, and Treatment of High Blood Cholesterol in Adults (Adult Treatment Panel III) Executive Summary: accessed at http://www.nhlbi.nih.gov/guidelines/cholesterol/atp_iii.htm

LDL = low-density lipoprotein; HDL = high-density lipoprotein.

years, with repeated testing every 5 years for patients in whom values are acceptable (1). The United States Preventive Services Task Force (USPSTF) recommended in 2001 that women aged 45 years and older and men aged 35 years and older undergo screening, with a total and HDL cholesterol nonfasting measurement repeated every 5 years (2). If total cholesterol in a nonfasting sample is >200 mg/dL or HDL is <40 mg/dL, then a fasting panel should be obtained. The USPSTF recommends that cholesterol screening begin at age 20 years in patients with a history of multiple cardiovascular risk factors, diabetes mellitus, or family history of either elevated cholesterol levels or premature cardiovascular disease (younger than age 50 years in men or 60 years in women). A separate measurement of LDL particle size has gained popularity since research has indicated that small, dense, LDL particles may contribute to coronary artery disease (CAD). Because these particles are often present when patients have other high-risk characteristics, including high serum triglyceride levels and low HDL cholesterol levels, diabetes, and the metabolic syndrome, LDL subclass measurement does not add additional information to typical measurements of cholesterol values (3). The ATP III and the USPSTF do not recommend measurement of LDL particle size for screening purposes.

The ATP III has established a classification of acceptable cholesterol levels (**Table 30**) and a step-wise approach to the

TABLE 31 Evaluation and Management of Cholesterol

Step	Action	Key features or Cross-Referenced Table
1	Determine cholesterol levels	See Table 30
2	Identify presence of CAD or CAD equivalent	CAD: myocardial infarction, unstable angina, coronary artery procedures, or evidence of myocardial ischemia
		CAD-equivalent: diabetes mellitus, symptomatic carotid artery disease, peripheral artery disease, and abdominal aortic aneurysm
3	Determine presence of risk factors other than LDL	See Table 33
4	Calculate 10-year risk of CAD (only for patients without CAD or equivalent and >2 risk factors)	Go to http://www.nhlbi.nih.gov/guidelines/cholesterol/risk_tbl.htm
5	Determine risk category	See Table 32
6	Initiate therapeutic lifestyle changes if indicated	Dietary changes (see Table 35) with weight reduction and increased physical activity
7	Add drug therapy if indicated	See Table 36
8	Identify and treat metabolic syndrome	Identification (see Table 34)
		Treatment: reduce underlying obesity and physical inactivity, treatment of other CAD risk factors
9	Treat elevated triglycerides	Encourage increased physical activity and weight loss. Use fibrates or a nicotinic acid if drug treatment indicated

Adapted from National Cholesterol Education Program: ATP III Guidelines At-A-Glance Quick Desk Reference. Accessed at: http://www.nhlbi.nih.gov/guidelines/cholesterol/atglance.pdf

CAD = coronary artery disease; LDL = low-density lipoprotein.

TABLE 32 ATP III LDL Goals for Therapeutic Lifestyle Changes (TLC) and Drug Therapy

Risk Category	LDL goal	Initiate TLC	Consider Drug Therapy
High risk: CAD, CAD equivalents, 10-year risk >20%	<100 mg/dL (optional goal: <70 mg/dL)	≥100 mg/dL	≥100 mg/dL (<100 mg/dL: consider drug options)
Moderately high risk: 2+ risk factors with 10-year risk 10% to 20%	<130 mg/dL	≥130 mg/dL	≥130 mg/dL (100 to 129 mg/dL: consider drug options)
Moderate risk: 2+ risk factors with 10-year risk <10%	<130 mg/dL	≥130 mg/dL	≥160 mg/dL
Lower risk: 0 to 1 risk factor	<160 mg/dL	≥160 mg/dL	≥190 mg/dL (160 to 189 mg/dL: LDL-lowering drug optional)

Adapted from Grundy SM, Cleeman JI, Bairey CN, Brewer Jr. HB, Clark LT, Hunninghake DB, Pasternak RC, Smith Jr. SC, Stone NJ for the Coordinating Committee of the National Cholesterol Education Program. Implications of recent clinical trials for the National Cholesterol Education Program Adult Treatment Panel III Guidelines. Circulation. 2004;110:227-239.

LDL = low-density lipoprotein; CAD = coronary artery disease.

evaluation and management of cholesterol (**Table 31**). Studies published since the last executive summary of the NCEP show that reducing LDL cholesterol to very low levels benefits patients at high risk for CAD, and the ATP III has modified its previous recommendations for some LDL goals for patients at high and moderately high risk for CAD (**Table 32**) (4).

For patients with high cholesterol levels, the ATP III recommends either therapeutic lifestyle changes, medications to reduce high LDL cholesterol levels, or both, depending on the risk for CAD (see Table 32). High-risk patients include those with a history of CAD (myocardial infarction, unstable angina, coronary artery procedures, or evidence of myocardial ischemia) or risk-equivalent conditions, including diabetes, symptomatic carotid artery disease, peripheral artery disease, and abdominal aortic aneurysm. Additionally, this high-risk category includes any patient with a 10-year risk >20% based on the Framingham risk table (http://www.nhlbi.nih.gov/guidelines/cholesterol/risk_tbl.htm). Moderately high-risk patients include those with two or more CAD risk factors (**Table 33**) and a 10-year risk for CAD of 10% to 20% based on the Framingham risk table.

The ATP III recommends an LDL goal of <70 mg/dL in patients at the very highest risk for CAD, including those with cardiovascular disease plus 1) multiple major risk factors

TABLE 33 Major Risk Factors (Exclusive of LDL Cholesterol) That Modify LDL Goals

Cigarette smoking
Hypertension (blood pressure ≥140/90 mm Hg or taking antihypertensive medication)
Low HDL cholesterol (<40 mg/dL)*
Family history of premature CAD (male first-degree relative age <55 y; female first-degree relative age <65 y)
Age (men ≥45 y; women ≥55 y)

Data are from the National Cholesterol Education Program: Third Report of the Expert Panel on Detection, Evaluation, and Treatment of High Blood Cholesterol in Adults (Adult Treatment Panel III) Executive Summary. Accessed at http://www.nhlbi.nih.gov/guidelines/cholesterol/atp_iii.htm

*HDL cholesterol ≥60 mg/dL constitutes as a "negative" risk factor. This removes one risk factor from the total count

HDL = high-density lipoprotein. CAD = coronary artery disease.

Table 34 Criteria for Metabolic Syndrome

Any Three of the Following

Risk Factor	*Defining Level*
Abdominal obesity	Waist circumference
Men	>102 cm (>40 in)
Women	>88 cm (>35 in)
Triglycerides	≥150 mg/dL
HDL cholesterol	
Men	<40 mg/dL
Women	<50 mg/dL
Blood pressure	≥130/≥85 mm Hg
Fasting glucose	≥110 mg/dL

Adapted from National Cholesterol Education Program: Third Report of the Expert Panel on Detection, Evaluation, and Treatment of High Blood Cholesterol in Adults (Adult Treatment Panel III) Executive Summary: accessed at http://www.nhlbi.nih.gov/guidelines/cholesterol/atp_iii.htm.

TABLE 35 Nutrient Composition of the Therapeutic Lifestyle Change Diet

Nutrient	Recommended Intake
Saturated fat	Less than 7% of total calories
Polyunsaturated fat	Up to 10% of total calories
Monounsaturated fat	Up to 20% of total calories
Total fat	25% to 35% of total calories
Cholesterol	Less than 200 mg/d
Carbohydrate	50% to 60% of total calories
Fiber	20 to 30 g/d
Protein	Approximately 15% of total calories
Plant stanols/sterols	2 g/d
Total calories	Balance intake and expenditure to avoid weight gain

Adapted from National Cholesterol Education Program: Third Report of the Expert Panel on Detection, Evaluation, and Treatment of High Blood Cholesterol in Adults (Adult Treatment Panel III) Executive Summary: accessed at http://www.nhlbi.nih.gov/guidelines/cholesterol/atp_iii.htm

including diabetes, 2) severe and poorly controlled risk factors including cigarette smoking, 3) multiple risk factors for the metabolic syndrome (**Table 34**), or 4) patients with acute coronary syndromes. Further clinical trials to more clearly define whether LDL levels should be uniformly decreased to <70 mg/dL in all high-risk patients are ongoing, because no trials clearly show clinical benefit for sustaining this value in patients with stable CAD.

Therapeutic lifestyle changes are appropriate for any persons with lifestyle-related risk factors for CAD, such as obesity, physical inactivity, elevated triglyceride levels, low HDL levels, or metabolic syndrome (see Table 34). Therapeutic lifestyle changes include 1) dietary modifications as outlined in **Table 35**, 2) weight reduction, and 3) increased physical activity. High amounts of vegetables, fruits, legumes, and whole grains as part of the low-fat diet reduce LDL and total cholesterol levels (5). The addition of plant sterols/stanols enhance fecal elimination of cholesterol and can produce a 10% to 15% reduction in total and LDL cholesterol (6, 7).

Plant sterols/stanols in small amounts are available naturally in fruits, vegetables, seeds, and legumes and can be added to spreads extracted from pine needles or soy. Examples of products with plant sterols/stanols added include *Benecol*® and *Take Control*® spreads that are used instead of margarine. Maximal dietary therapy as indicated in Table 35 can lower LDL cholesterol by as much as 25% to 30%. Lipid panels in patients adopting therapeutic lifestyle changes should be rechecked after 6 weeks of initiation of this therapy, with intensification of therapeutic lifestyle changes or the addition of medication recommended, depending on risk.

Patients who are at high risk or moderately high risk for CAD should receive medication in addition to therapeutic lifestyle changes if cholesterol values are above goal. In other risk categories, it is recommended that medication be added to therapeutic lifestyle changes after 3 months if needed. In all patients in whom lipid-lowering treatment is used, the lipid panel should be rechecked after 6 weeks of therapy. In the past, the ATP III has not been explicit about how much the LDL level should be lowered below a recommended goal. For every 1% reduction in LDL, there is an approximate 1% reduction in CAD risk. The ATP III therefore recommends initiating statin therapy at standard doses (**Table 36**) adequate to lower LDL levels by 30% to 40%, allowing reduction of CAD events by approximately the same percentage, instead of using the minimal dose of medication to only achieve the goal LDL reduction. The ATP III notes that a 30% to 40% reduction is not the main objective of therapy, but rather a guideline for treatment.

Table 36 illustrates the range of doses available for cholesterol-lowering medications. Elevated LDL levels are best treated with statins. If standard doses of statins are not enough to lower LDL cholesterol values below goal, the dose

TABLE 36 Drugs affecting lipoprotein metabolism

Drug Class	Agent	Daily Dose	Standard Dose (mg/d) (LDL ↓30-40%)*	Lipoprotein Reductions Across Dose Range (%)	Side Effects	Contraindications
HMG CoA reductase inhibitors (statins)	Lovastatin Pravastatin Simvastatin Fluvastatin Atorvastatin Rosuvastatin	20-80 mg 20-40 mg 20-80 mg 20-80 mg 10-80 mg 5-40 mg	40 40 20-40 40-80 10 10	LDL: ↓18-55 HDL: ↑5-15 TG: ↓7-30	Myopathy Increased liver enzymes	Absolute: active or chronic liver disease Relative: concomitant use of certain drugs†
Cholesterol absorption inhibitor	Ezetimibe	10 mg		LDL: ↓14-18 HDL: ↑1-3 TG: ↓2	Headache GI distress	Absolute: Severe hepatic disease, Concomitant use of fibric acid derivatives Relative: renal impairment or mild hepatic disease
Bile acid sequestrants	Cholestyramine Colestipol Colesevelam	4-16 g 5-20 g 2.6-3.8 g		LDL: ↓15-30 HDL: ↑3-5 TG: no change	GI distress Constipation Decreased absorption of other drugs	Absolute: dysbetalipoproteinemia, TG >400 mg/dL Relative: TG >200 mg/dL
Nicotinic acid	Immediate release Extended release Sustained release	1.5-3 g 1-2 g 1-2 g		LDL: ↓5-25 HDL: ↑15-35 TG: ↓20-50	Flushing Hyperglycemia Hyperuricemia Upper GI distress Hepatotoxicity	Absolute: chronic liver disease, severe gout Relative: diabetes, hyperuricemia, peptic ulcer disease
Fibric acids	Gemfibrozil Fenofibrate Clofibrate	600 mg BID 200 mg 1000 mg BID		LDL: ↓5-20 HDL: ↑10-20 TG: ↓20-50	Dyspepsia Gallstones Myopathy	Absolute: Severe renal or hepatic disease
Omega-3 fatty acids (fish oils)		3-12 g/d		LDL: HDL: TG: ↓ 20-50	Interference with platelet function Dyspepsia Taste perversion Eructation	Sensitivity or allergy to fish

*Applies to research completed with statins only

†Cyclosporine, macrolide antibiotics, various anti-fungal drugs, cytochrome P-450 inhibitors

Adapted from National Cholesterol Education Program: Third Report of the Expert Panel on Detection, Evaluation, and Treatment of High Blood Cholesterol in Adults (Adult Treatment Panel III) Executive Summary: http://www.nhlbi.nih.gov/guidelines/cholesterol/atp_iii.htm; and Bruckert E. New advances in lipid-modifying therapies for reducing cardiovascular risk. Cardiology. 2002;97:59-66; and The Medical Letter, Inc. Treatment Guidelines from The Medical Letter: Drugs for Lipids. 2005;3:15-22.

HDL = high-density lipoprotein; LDL = low-density lipoprotein; TG = triglyceride; BID = twice daily; GI = gastrointestinal.

of statin may be increased, or a second agent can be added (see Table 36), such as ezetimibe, bile acid sequestrants, or nicotinic acid. The combination of a fibric acid derivative with a statin should be avoided, if possible, because of the increased risk for myopathy this combination confers.

The mechanism of action of statins is to inhibit the rate-limiting step in cholesterol biosynthesis and stimulation of LDL receptor activity in hepatocytes. Statins additionally decrease levels of the inflammatory marker C-reactive protein, improve endothelial function, reduce plasma viscosity, and decrease platelet aggregation and thrombin formation. Studies of statins have shown reduced clinical endpoints for low-risk (absence of CAD) and higher-risk patients. All statins, except pravastatin, are metabolized through the cytochrome P-450 system. Because statins have varied

effects on this system, fluvastatin and rosuvastatin portend a somewhat lower risk for drug interactions than the other statins, as does pravastatin.

Common dose-related statin-induced muscle symptoms include 1% to 5% focal or diffuse myalgia and serum creatine kinase (CK) elevations that are less than 10 times the upper limit of normal. Serum CK levels may rise after exercise, and statins appear to increase this effect. Muscle weakness can also occur, but the frequency of this symptom is unknown. Myopathy, a serum CK level more than 10 times the upper limit of normal, occurs in about 0.1% to 0.5% of patients treated with statins in clinical trials (8). Rhabdomyolysis occurs at a rate of 0.44 per 10,000 person-years of therapy with atorvastatin, pravastatin, or simvastatin, and is dose-dependent (9). If any one of these statins is combined with a fibrate, the rate of rhabdomyolysis occurrence increases to 5.98 per 10,000 person-years, whereas the rate of rhabdomyolysis occurrence in patients taking a fibrate alone is 5.34 per 10,000 person-years (see also Reference 9). The potential risk factors for the occurrence of rhabdomyolysis include older age, female sex, low BMI, hypothyroidism, diabetes mellitus, and impaired renal or hepatic function. Some medications other than fibrates also increase the risk for statin-associated myopathy, including cyclosporine, macrolide antibiotics, various antifungal drugs, and cytochrome P-450 inhibitors (see also Reference 8). Serum CK levels should be measured before patients begin taking statins and again on development of muscle pain (10). The ATP III does not specifically provide recommendations on CK testing in patients taking statins. Statin therapy should be discontinued in patients with a serum CK 3 to 10 times the upper limit of normal. Some patients in whom myalgia develops from one statin may be able to tolerate another statin (see also Reference 10).

In 1% to 2 % of patients, an increase in aminotransferase liver enzymes of more than three times normal can occur. A baseline liver enzyme measurement should be taken before patients begin statin therapy, then 3 months after initiation of the statin therapy, and then annually (see also Reference 10). The ATP III does not specifically provide recommendations on frequency of liver enzyme evaluation. Patients in whom elevated liver enzyme levels develop may be able to tolerate another statin or a lower dose of the same statin (see also Reference 10).

Ezetimibe inhibits intestinal absorption of cholesterol and plant sterols. Because of reduced cholesterol absorption, hepatic LDL receptor activity increases, and more LDL is cleared from the plasma. Most of the cholesterol within the intestinal lumen is from the bile; therefore, a patient maintaining a zero-cholesterol diet can benefit from ezetimibe, which can be used as monotherapy for patients who cannot tolerate statins, or in combination with statins. This drug seems to be well tolerated and has minimal effects on the cytochrome P-450 system. No trials have evaluated clinical endpoints for patients taking this medication, and future studies may more clearly show the long-term risks and benefits of this treatment.

The bile acid sequestrants cholestyramine, colestipol, and colesevelam are anion-exchange resins. These drugs speed clearance of LDL from plasma by increasing LDL receptor activity and are useful in combination with statins or nicotinic acid. Because this group of agents acts within the intestine, it is relatively safe. Bile acid sequestrants stimulate very-low-density lipoprotein (VLDL) secretion and might worsen hypertriglyceridemia, which is a relative contraindication to their use.

Nicotinic acid is a B vitamin, and in doses much higher than needed for vitamin replacement, it has anticholesterol properties and reduces the concentration of lipoprotein (a), an atherogenic lipoprotein. Nicotinic acid reduces the secretion of VLDL by the liver. Patients who take aspirin 30 minutes before taking nicotinic acid experience decreased flushing, which is a major limiting side effect of this drug.

Fibric acid derivatives (fenofibrate, gemfibrozil, and clofibrate) increase lipoprotein lipase activity, reduce synthesis of aproprotein C-III (an inhibitor of lipoprotein lipase), and increase synthesis of the major HDL lipoproteins (apoprotein A-I and aproprotein A-II). Because of the increased lipoprotein lipase activity in patients who take fibric acid derivatives, VLDL and remnant lipoproteins are cleared more readily.

Fish oils are unsaturated omega-3 fatty acids present in cold water fish and sold in capsules. Taken regularly, the oil can reduce hepatic triglyceride production and increase clearance of serum triglycerides. Over long courses of treatment, they may also increase HDL levels. Large doses may interfere with platelet function.

Modification of other risk factors beyond LDL can also help reduce the risk for CAD. The metabolic syndrome represents a constellation of lipid and nonlipid risk factors of metabolic origin, closely linked to insulin resistance, with 22% of Americans qualifying for this syndrome in the 2001 Third National Nutrition and Health Examination Survey (11). The ATP III recommends that the diagnosis of metabolic syndrome be established in patients with three or more risk factors (see Table 34) for this syndrome. Excessive body fat (especially abdominal obesity) and physical inactivity promote the development of insulin resistance, but there is also a genetic predisposition to this syndrome. The risk factors for metabolic syndrome enhance risk for CAD at any given LDL cholesterol level. Management of the metabolic syndrome includes reduction of underlying causes (obesity and physical inactivity) and treatment of risk factors (hypertension, elevated triglycerides, and low HDL levels).

Although the primary goal of treatment in CAD risk reduction is to decrease cholesterol levels, elevated triglyceride levels are also an independent risk factor for CAD. Table 30 illustrates the ATP III classification of serum triglyceride levels. The ATP III recommends the non-HDL cholesterol level (total cholesterol minus HDL) as a secondary target of therapy in patients at high risk for CAD with high triglyceride levels (>200 mg/dL), with the target level for non-HDL cholesterol 30 mg/dL higher than the goal LDL cholesterol. All patients with borderline high triglyceride levels (150 to 199 mg/dL) should be advised to lose weight and increase physical activity. Patients with high triglyceride levels (200 to 499 mg/dL) may need drug therapy (see Table 36) consisting of intensification of LDL-lowering medication or the addition of nicotinic acid or a fibrate. The ATP III does not specifically recommend the use of fish oils to decrease triglyceride levels. The initial goal for patients with very high triglyceride levels (>500 mg/dL), before treating LDL, is prevention of pancreatitis by maintaining very-low-fat diets (<15% of calorie intake) and beginning a program of weight reduction and increased physical activity, and use of a nicotinic acid or fibrate.

Low HDL cholesterol (<40 mg/dL), also an independent risk factor for CAD, may be caused by factors associated with insulin resistance, cigarette smoking, very-high-carbohydrate diets, and certain drugs (β-blockers, anabolic corticosteroids, and progestational agents). The evidence is insufficient to suggest a specific goal for raising HDL levels, but the primary target in patients with low HDL levels is to ensure that the LDL level is at or below goal. If the LDL goal is on target, then weight reduction and physical activity is recommended. When low HDL cholesterol levels are associated with high triglyceride levels, the focus of treatment should be on decreasing non-HDL cholesterol. If the triglyceride level is <200 mg/dL, treatment for isolated low HDL cholesterol levels is mostly reserved for persons with CAD or CAD risk-equivalent problems. Specific medications that increase HDL levels include nicotinic acid and the fibric acid class (see Table 36). Further treatment of low HDL cholesterol levels is currently investigational. A preliminary study of a synthetic HDL infusion resulted in a reduction of coronary artery atherosclerotic lesions, but further study of clinical endpoints is needed to determine whether this is a feasible treatment (12).

KEY POINTS

- Women aged 45 years and older and men aged 35 years and older should receive cholesterol screening, with repeated screening every 5 years.

- Cholesterol screening is recommended beginning at age 20 years in patients with a history of multiple cardiovascular risk factors, diabetes mellitus, or family history of either elevated cholesterol levels or premature cardiovascular disease.

- For patients with high cholesterol levels, therapeutic lifestyle changes, medications to reduce high serum low density lipoprotein (LDL) cholesterol levels, or both are recommended, depending on coronary artery disease (CAD) risk factors.

- An LDL goal of <70 mg/dL is recommended in patients at the very highest risk for CAD.

- The addition of plant sterols/stanols enhances fecal elimination of cholesterol and can produce a 10% to 15% reduction in total and LDL cholesterol.

- Studies of statins have shown reduced clinical endpoints for low-risk and higher-risk patients.

- Serum creatine kinase (CK) levels should be measured before patients begin taking statins and again on development of muscle pain.

- Statin therapy should be discontinued in patients with a serum CK level that is 3 to 10 times the upper limit of normal.

- A baseline liver enzyme measurement should be taken before patients begin statin therapy, then 3 months after initiation of therapy, and then annually.

- The risk factors for metabolic syndrome enhance risk for CAD at any given LDL cholesterol level.

References

1. **National Cholesterol Education Program.** Third report of the expert panel on detection, evaluation, and treatment of high blood cholesterol in adults (Adult Treatment Panel III) executive summary [National Heart Blood, and Lung Web site]. NIH Publication No. 01-3670. May 2001. Available at: http://www.nhlbi.nih.gov/guidelines/cholesterol/atp_iii.htm. Accessed September 7, 2005.

2. **United States Preventive Services Task Force.** Screening for lipid disorders in adults [Agency for Healthcare Research and Quality Web site]. March 2001. Available at: http://www.ahrq.gov/clinic/uspstf/uspschol.htm. Accessed September 7, 2005.

3. **Sacks FM, Campos H.** Clinical review 163: Cardiovascular endocrinology: Low-density lipoprotein size and cardiovascular disease: a reappraisal. J Clin Endocrinol Metab. 2003;88:4525-32. [PMID: 14557416]

4. **Grundy SM, Cleeman JI, Merz CN, Brewer HB Jr, Clark LT, Hunninghake DB, et al.** Implications of recent clinical trials for the National Cholesterol Education Program Adult Treatment Panel III guidelines. Circulation. 2004;110:227-39. [PMID: 15249516]

5. **Gardner CD, Coulston A, Chatterjee L, Rigby A, Spiller G, Farquhar JW.** The effect of a plant-based diet on plasma lipids in hypercholesterolemic adults: a randomized trial. Ann Intern Med. 2005;142:725-33. [PMID: 15867404]

6. **Cleghorn CL, Skeaff CM, Mann J, Chisholm A.** Plant sterol-enriched spread enhances the cholesterol-lowering potential of a fat-reduced diet. Eur J Clin Nutr. 2003;57:170-6. [PMID: 12548313]

7. **Miettinen TA, Gylling H.** Plant stanol and sterol esters in prevention of cardiovascular diseases. Ann Med. 2004;36:126-34. [PMID: 15119832]

8. **Thompson PD, Clarkson P, Karas RH.** Statin-associated myopathy. JAMA. 2003;289:1681-90. [PMID: 12672737]

9. **Graham DJ, Staffa JA, Shatin D, Andrade SE, Schech SD, La Grenade L, et al.** Incidence of hospitalized rhabdomyolysis in patients treated with lipid-lowering drugs. JAMA. 2004;292:2585-90. [PMID: 15572716]

10. Drugs for lipids. Treat Guidel Med Lett. 2005 Mar;3(31):15-22. [PMID: 15726011]

11. **Ford ES, Giles WH, Dietz WH.** Prevalence of the metabolic syndrome among US adults: findings from the third National Health and Nutrition Examination Survey. JAMA. 2002;287:356-9. [PMID: 11790215]

12. **Nissen SE, Tsunoda T, Tuzcu EM, Schoenhagen P, Cooper CJ, Yasin M, et al.** Effect of recombinant ApoA-I Milano on coronary atherosclerosis in patients with acute coronary syndromes: a randomized controlled trial. JAMA. 2003;290:2292-300. [PMID: 14600188]

OBESITY

Epidemiology and Definition of Obesity

Obesity is a problem of increasing magnitude in the industrialized countries including the United States, where its prevalence in adults has increased from 13% to 31% over the past 4 decades (1, 2). Obesity rates in the United States are also rising among children and adolescents. The World Health Organization defines obesity as a BMI of ≥30. Obesity is further stratified into three classes: 1) class I has a BMI of 30 to 34.9, class II has a BMI of 35 to 39.9, and class III has a BMI of ≥40. Persons with a BMI between 25 and 29.9 are defined as overweight.

The BMI is calculated by weight in pounds, divided by height in inches squared, multiplied by 703; or as weight in kilograms, divided by height in meters squared. The National Institute of Health provides a BMI calculator at www.nhlbisupport.com/bmi and a table at www.nhlbi.nih.gov/guidelines/obesity/bmi_tbl.htm. The BMI is an appropriate screening measure because it is easy to calculate and has been determined to be reliable and valid in identifying adults at risk for increased morbidity and mortality because of being overweight or obese.

Risk Factors for Obesity

Risk factors for obesity include increasing age, female sex, and African American, Hispanic American, and Native American ethnicity/race. Among immigrant subgroups, the number of years of residence in the United States is positively associated with higher BMI after 10 years of residency (3).

Obesity is associated with increased total mortality and increased risk for chronic conditions, including coronary artery disease, stroke, type 2 diabetes mellitus, heart failure, dyslipidemia, hypertension, reproductive and gastrointestinal cancer, gallstones, fatty liver disease, osteoarthritis, and sleep apnea. The pattern of fat deposition is a prognostic factor in patients who are obese, with increased cardiovascular risk in persons with central or visceral fat accumulation, especially among the elderly. Waist circumference can be used as a measure of central adiposity. A circumference of >102 cm (40 in) in men and >88 cm (35 in) in women indicates central adiposity. The thresholds for central adiposity are not reliable for persons with a BMI of >35. The number of deaths attributable to obesity (BMI >30) was reported to have decreased over the past decade in a recent analysis (BMI >25 and <30) of data from the National Health and Nutrition Examination Survey (4). However, temporal trends in the attributable mortality due to obesity are controversial and reflect the complexity of statistical analyses used to determine attributable risk.

Screening and Primary Prevention of Obesity

Primary prevention of obesity is recommended through the promotion of healthy lifestyles. The U.S. Preventive Services Task Force (USPSTF) recommends that clinicians screen all adult patients for obesity and offer high-intensity counseling and behavioral interventions to encourage sustainable weight loss for obese adults. A high-intensity intervention is defined as more than one (group or individual) person-to-person session per month for at least 3 months. This recommendation is a level B recommendation, reflecting fair evidence that this intervention will improve health outcomes and provide more benefit than risks to obese persons. However, the USPSTF found insufficient evidence to recommend for or against the use of counseling of any intensity or behavioral interventions to promote sustained weight loss in adults who are overweight, but not obese (BMI >25 but <30). The most effective interventions for overweight adults combine nutrition education and diet and exercise counseling with behavioral strategies to help patients acquire skills and the support needed to change eating patterns and to become physically active.

There are differing recommendations defining what is an adequate amount of physical activity. In 1995, the Centers for Disease Control and Prevention and the American College of Sports Medicine (CDC/ACSM) recommended that adults should have at least 30 minutes a day, most if not all days of a week, of moderate-intensity physical activity. The American Heart Association issued similar recommendations. Conversely, the Institute of Medicine (IOM) Committee on Dietary References Intakes report from 2002 recommended 60 minutes of daily moderate-intensity physical activity, stating that 30 minutes/day of such activity may not be sufficient to maintain body weight in adults in the BMI range of 18.5 to 25.

Diagnosis and Evaluation of Obesity

A diagnosis of obesity is established by using weight and height measurements to determine BMI. A BMI of ≥30 meets the WHO criteria for obesity. The clinical evaluation of an obese patient should include history and physical examination to screen for comorbid disease (**Table 37**), with a chronologic history of weight gain to elicit a precipitating cause for the obesity, such as daily stressors. Family history may suggest a genetic predisposition to obesity, and medication history can help identify drugs that may contribute to weight gain, such as corticosteroids, antidepressants (tricyclic antidepressants), antipsychotic agents (phenothiazines and butyrophenones), anticonvulsants (valproate and carbamazepine), lithium, and antidiabetic agents (insulin, sulfonylurea, and thiazolidinediones). Additional key aspects to the clinical history are dietary history, level of activity or exercise, history of eating disorders, and history of depression. The differential diagnosis for obesity includes the endocrine disorders of Cushing's disease, polycystic ovary disease, and hypothyroidism.

During the physical examination, the BMI, waist circumference, and blood pressure should be determined, and any signs of Cushing's disease, polycystic ovary disease, hypothyroidism, and cardiovascular disease should be identified. Baseline laboratory studies should include a biochemical profile, fasting plasma glucose and serum lipid profile, and serum thyroid-stimulating hormone measurement. The metabolic syndrome, characterized by abdominal obesity combined with other coronary artery disease risk factors, is a consideration in patients who are obese (see Hyperlipidemia section).

TABLE 37 Key Factors in the Evaluation of Obesity

Screening and Prevention	Clinical Evaluation for Comorbid Disease	Physical Examination and Laboratory Studies	Treatment Options
Monitor BMI in all patients as a screen for obesity	Coronary heart disease	BMI	Dietary and exercise counseling and behavior modification
	Type 2 DM	Biochemical profile	
A BMI ≥30 meets WHO criteria for obesity	Sleep apnea	Fasting glucose	Pharmacologic therapy
	Osteoarthritis	Lipid profile	Surgical therapy
Nutritional education, diet, and exercise	Gallbladder disease	TSH	
	Stress incontinence		
	Metabolic syndrome		

BMI = body mass index; WHO = World Health Organization; DM = diabetes mellitus; TSH = thyroid-stimulating hormone.

Treatment of Obesity

The management of patients who are obese includes dietary counseling and behavioral modification, pharmacologic intervention, or surgical intervention. The WHO has defined successful management of patients who are obese as a 5% to 15% reduction in initial weight. Caloric restriction has been successful in short-term weight loss, but less so over the long-term. Patients who receive counseling on low-calorie diets (1000 to 1200 kcal/d) achieve reduced body weight by an average of 8% over 3 to 12 months. Very-low-calorie diets result in greater initial weight loss but results are similar to standard calorie-restricted diets beyond 1 year. Low-fat diets have been no more effective in helping patients achieve long-term weight loss than calorie-restricted diets (5, 6). Low-carbohydrate diets are typically defined as <60 g/day of carbohydrates, with the lowest carbohydrate diet consisting of <20g/day of carbohydrates. A meta-analysis of the efficacy and safety of low-carbohydrate diets found insufficient evidence to recommend for or against the use of these diets. Low-carbohydrate diets have not been adequately evaluated for use longer than 90 days in persons 53 years of age or older or in those with hyperlipidemia, hypertension, or diabetes.

Patients who received counseling on physical activity achieved weight loss of 2% to 3% of initial weight and reduced abdominal fat (7). A systematic review of major commercial weight loss programs concluded that only one large randomized controlled trial of Weight Watchers provided evidence to support the efficacy of these interventions. The Weight Watchers study reported a loss of 3.2% of initial weight at 2 years (8).

Pharmacologic Therapy

A recent meta-analysis found that sibutramine, orlistat, phentermine, bupropion (off-label use), topiramate (off-label), and probably diethylpropion and fluoxetine (off-label use) were effective in promoting modest weight loss (3 to 5 kg [6.62 to 11 lb]) when given with diet recommendations. Sibutramine and orlistat are the most-studied drugs for weight loss (9). Sibutramine is a nonadrenergic agent and a selective serotonin reuptake inhibitor. The most common adverse effects of this drug are related to increased adrenergic activity and include dry mouth, headache, insomnia, and constipation. Sibutramine can cause a dose-related increase in blood pressure and is not recommended for persons with poorly controlled hypertension. Sibutramine has also been associated with an increased pulse rate. Patients with cardiac arrhythmias, congestive heart failure, coronary artery disease, or a history of stroke should undergo a risk–benefit assessment before taking sibutramine. Orlistat is an inhibitor of pancreatic/intestinal lipase and increases fecal fat loss. This effect is dose related and reaches a plateau with a dosage of 400 to 600 mg/day. Side effects of orlistat are related to malabsorption of fat in the gastrointestinal tract and include steatorrhea, bloating, and oily discharge. Fecal incontinence and malabsorption of fat-soluble vitamins (vitamins A, D, E, and K) have also been reported. Sibutramine and orlistat are approved for persons with a BMI of ≥30 or for persons with a BMI of ≥27 with other cardiovascular risk factors, such as hypertension, diabetes, or dyslipidemia. A meta-analysis of sibutramine reported a mean difference in weight loss of 4.45 kg (95% CI, 3.62 to 5.29) at 12 months compared with placebo groups. In patients who took sibutramine, heart rate was increased by about 4 beats/min. A meta-analysis of orlistat found a mean difference in weight loss of 2.89 kg (95% CI, 2.27–3.51) at 12 months compared with placebo groups. In patients who took orlistat, gastrointestinal side effects, including diarrhea, flatulence, bloating, abdominal pain, and dyspepsia, were noted. Sibutramine and orlistat are Food and Drug Administration approved for long-term use and maintenance of weight loss.

Surgical Therapy

In 1991, the National Institutes of Health established guidelines for the surgical therapy of morbid obesity, defined as a BMI of ≥40, or ≥35 in the presence of comorbidities. Surgical therapy for obesity is called bariatric surgery. Categories of bariatric surgery include gastric binding, gastric bypass (principally Roux-en-Y), gastroplasty, and biliopancreatic diversion or duodenal switch. The two meta-analyses of bariatric surgery report that surgery is more effective than nonsurgical treatment for weight loss and control of some comorbid conditions for persons with a BMI of ≥40. One meta-analysis of bariatric surgery reported a mean excess weight loss of 61.2% (95% CI, 58.1 to 64.4), combining the experience from all bariatric procedures. Surgical mortality within 30 days was 0.1% in patients who underwent gastric-binding procedures, 0.5% in those who underwent gastric bypass, and 1.1% in those who underwent biliopancreatic diversion or duodenal switch. Early postoperative complications of bariatric surgery include anastomotic leaks, wound infections, dehiscence, ileus, cardiopulmonary failure, pulmonary embolism, pneumonia, and myocardial infarction. In addition, rapid postoperative weight loss is associated with cholelithiasis from cholesterol stones. Other complications included incisional hernias, which are common and are usually repaired 12 to 18 months after surgery; B_{12} deficiency; anemia; depression; cholecystitis; and gastritis. Significant rates of resolution or improvement of comorbidities in patients who underwent bariatric surgery were also reported; diabetes was completely resolved in 76.8%, hyperlipidemia was improved in 70%, hypertension was resolved in 61.7%, and obstructive sleep apnea was resolved in 85.7% (10).

A second meta-analysis reported a 20- to 30-kg (44- to 66-lb) weight loss that was maintained for up to 10 years in patients with a BMI of ≥40 who underwent bariatric surgery. The benefit for persons with a BMI of 35 to 39 was suggested but not conclusively demonstrated. The overall mortality in patients who underwent bariatric surgery was <1%, with adverse events occurring in 20% of cases. Outcomes were improved in patients whose surgeons had performed more procedures. Based on this evidence, the American College of Physicians recommends surgery as a treatment option for patients with a BMI of ≥40 who failed an exercise and diet program with or without drug therapy and who have obesity-related chronic conditions. A physician–patient discussion of surgical options should include the long-term side effects of bariatric surgery or possible need for re-operation, gall bladder disease, and malabsorption. Another recommendation is for patients who are obese and considering bariatric surgery to be referred to high-volume centers experienced in performing this type of procedure. Studies of quality of life after bariatric surgery indicate that patients experience social and economic benefits from the significant weight loss (11).

KEY POINTS

- The pattern of fat deposition is a prognostic factor in patients who are obese, with increased cardiovascular risk in persons with central or visceral fat accumulation, especially among the elderly.

- All adult patients should receive obesity screening and be offered high-intensity counseling and behavioral interventions to encourage sustainable weight loss.

- Patients who receive counseling on low-calorie diets (1000 to 1200 kcal/day) achieve reduced body weight by an average of 8% over 3 to 12 months.

- Very-low-calorie diets result in greater initial weight loss but similar results beyond 1 year.

- Low-fat diets have been no more effective in helping patients achieve long-term weight loss than calorie-restricted diets.

- A systematic review found that participants of the Weight Watchers study reported a loss of 3.2% of initial weight at 2 years.

- Bariatric surgery is more effective than nonsurgical treatment for weight loss and control of some comorbid conditions in persons with a BMI of ≥40.

References

1. Screening for obesity in adults: recommendations and rationale. Ann Intern Med. 2003;139:930-2. [PMID: 14644896]

2. **McTigue KM, Harris R, Hemphill B, Lux L, Sutton S, Bunton AJ, et al.** Screening and interventions for obesity in adults: summary of the evidence for the U.S. Preventive Services Task Force. Ann Intern Med. 2003 Dec 2;139(11):933-49. [PMID: 14644897]

3. **Goel MS, McCarthy EP, Phillips RS, Wee CC.** Obesity among US immigrant subgroups by duration of residence. JAMA. 2004;292:2860-7. [PMID: 15598917]

4. **Flegal KM, Graubard BI, Williamson DF, Gail MH.** Excess deaths associated with underweight, overweight, and obesity. JAMA. 2005;293:1861-7. [PMID: 15840860]

5. **Labib M.** ACP Best Practice No 168. The investigation and management of obesity. J Clin Pathol. 2003;56:17-25. [PMID: 12499427]

6. **Pirozzo S, Summerbell C, Cameron C, Glasziou P.** Advice on low-fat diets for obesity. Cochrane Database Syst Rev. 2002;(2):CD003640. [PMID: 12076496]

7. **Bravata DM, Sanders L, Huang J, Krumholz HM, Olkin I, Gardner CD, et al.** Efficacy and safety of low-carbohydrate diets: a systematic review. JAMA. 2003 Apr 9;289(14):1837-50 Review. [PMID: 12684364]

8. **Tsai AG, Wadden TA.** Systematic review: an evaluation of major commercial weight loss programs in the United States. Ann Intern Med. 2005;142:56-66. [PMID: 15630109]

9. **Li Z, Maglione M, Tu W, Mojica W, Arterburn D, Shugarman LR, et al.** Meta-analysis: pharmacologic treatment of obesity. Ann Intern Med. 2005;142:532-46. [PMID: 15809465]

10. **Maggard MA, Shugarman LR, Suttorp M, Maglione M, Sugerman HJ, Sugarman HJ, et al.** Meta-analysis: surgical treatment of obesity. Ann Intern Med. 2005;142:547-59. [PMID: 15809466]

11. **Snow V, Barry P, Fitterman N, Qaseem A, Weiss K.** Pharmacologic and surgical management of obesity in primary care: a clinical practice guideline from the American College of Physicians. Ann Intern Med. 2005;142:525-31. [PMID: 15809464]

GENITOURINARY AND RENAL DISORDERS

RECENT ADVANCE

- **Transurethral microwave therapy in benign prostatic hyperplasia**

TABLE 38 Common Sexual Dysfunctions by Gender	
Men	Decreased libido
	Anorgasmia
	Premature ejaculation
	Erectile dysfunction
	Performance anxiety
	Sex not pleasurable
Women	Decreased libido
	Anorgasmia
	Dyspareunia
	Performance anxiety
	Trouble lubricating
	Sex not pleasurable

Sexual Dysfunction

Sexual dysfunction is a common problem (**Table 38**) that can adversely affect quality of life and signal the presence of serious medical or psychosocial problems. Male sexual dysfunction is categorized by decreased libido (lack of interest in sexual activity), erectile dysfunction, ejaculatory disorders, and anatomical abnormalities. Female sexual dysfunction is characterized by decreased libido, arousal disorders, orgasmic disorders, or pain with intercourse. Among adults aged 40 to 80 years sampled for the Global Study of Sexual Attitudes and Behaviors, women (39%) were more likely than men (28%) were to report sexual dysfunction (1). Men most commonly reported erectile dysfunction and early ejaculation, whereas women most frequently reported lack of sexual interest, inability to reach orgasm, and difficulty lubricating. Sexual dysfunction was relatively uncommon before age 50 years in a study of male health professionals; the prevalence of erectile dysfunction then increased substantially with age. Healthy 75- to 79-year-old men had a relative risk for erectile dysfunction of 6.1 (95% CI, 5.0 to 7.4) compared with 55- to 59-year-old men. Obesity, inactivity, smoking, alcohol consumption, and chronic medical conditions are also associated with erectile dysfunction (2).

Sexual dysfunction occurs at a younger age in women, although problems with lubrication are most prevalent at midlife. Poor health, history of a sexually transmitted disease, emotional problems, urinary tract symptoms, sexual trauma, and deteriorating socioeconomic status are associated with sexual dysfunction in women.

Although psychogenic causes for sexual dysfunction are common, endocrine abnormalities, medications, and medical conditions account for most cases. Testosterone deficiency, hyperprolactinemia, and thyroid disorders can cause erectile dysfunction; testosterone deficiency can also decrease libido. Diminished estrogen levels in women can lead to vaginal epithelial atrophy, insufficient lubrication, and dyspareunia, whereas hyperprolactinemia and thyroid disorders can decrease libido. Autonomic neuropathy, especially complicating diabetes, Parkinson's disease, or multiple sclerosis, can cause retrograde ejaculation and erectile dysfunction and inhibit arousal and orgasm. Vascular insufficiency, resulting from atherosclerosis or diabetes, can impair arousal by preventing genital vasocongestion. Erectile dysfunction may be the initial manifestation of atherosclerotic vascular disease. Assessment of cardiovascular risk is indicated in men with erectile dysfunction. Numerous medications cause sexual dysfunction, most notably antihypertensive drugs (thiazide diuretics, calcium channel blockers, ACE inhibitors, and sympathetic blockers), lipid-lowering agents, anticholinergics, antiandrogens, narcotics, and antidepressants. Tobacco, alcohol, marijuana, amphetamines, cocaine, and heroin can decrease libido and inhibit orgasm.

A sexual history should encompass sexual interest, activity, and function. When a patient describes a history of sexual dysfunction, the symptoms and onset, duration, and severity should be ascertained. Further history should focus on determining whether the problem is organic and associated with medical illnesses, habits, medications, or substance abuse, or psychologic. Rapid onset of sexual dysfunction suggests psychogenic causes or medication effects, whereas a more gradual onset suggests the presence of medical illnesses. Decreased libido suggests hormonal deficiencies, psychogenic causes, or medication effects.

Pertinent physical findings in men with sexual dysfunction include evidence of a penile plaque (Peyronie's disease), testicular abnormalities, gynecomastia, visual field defects, neuropathy, and vascular insufficiency. Nocturnal penile tumescence detected using a home monitoring device suggests a psychogenic cause, although hypogonadal men may also have some nocturnal erectile function. Routine laboratory studies may identify underlying chronic diseases, and measurement of total serum testosterone, prolactin, and thyroid levels helps to identify the most prevalent hormonal causes for erectile dysfunction. When total testosterone levels are in the low-normal range, measuring bioavailable (free) testosterone levels helps to establish a diagnosis of hypogonadism in the setting of conditions such as obesity, liver disease, or old age that affect sex hormone–binding serum globulin levels. Measurement of serum follicle-stimulating hormone and luteinizing hormone levels can determine whether a low testosterone level indicates primary or secondary hypogonadism.

Women with sexual dysfunction should be evaluated for endocrine, neurologic, and vascular disorders and undergo a detailed gynecologic examination of the external and internal genitalia. Serum hormone studies may be indicated in women

TABLE 39 Treatment Options for Erectile Dysfunction

Treatment	Benefits/Use	Risks/Limitations
Phosphodiesterase type-5 inhibitors Sildenafil (25 to 100 mg) Vardenafil (2.5 to 20 mg) Tadalafil (2.5 to 20 mg)	Oral, safe, easy to use. Taken 1 h before intercourse. Duration of action longer with tadalafil (36 h) than sildenafil or vardenafil (both 4 h)	Cannot use with nitrates; headache, flushing, dyspepsia, blue-tinged vision (sildenafil only). Cannot use vardenafil or tadalafil with α-blockers. Associated with vision loss from nonarteritic ischemic optic neuritis
Yohimbine (5.4 mg three times/d)	Oral, used for psychogenic erectile dysfunction	Anxiety, insomnia; may increase blood pressure
Testosterone Injection (100 mg weekly 200 to 300 mg every 2 to three wk) Transdermal patch 5 to 10 mg/d	Intramuscular injection or transdermal patch. Can increase libido	Erythrocytosis, skin reactions (with patch), may exacerbate lower urinary tract symptoms, uncertain or risk for prostate cancer (requires monitoring)
Trazodone (50 to 100 mg)	Oral, used for psychogenic erectile dysfunction, depression	Priapism, dizziness, lethargy
Intraurethral suppository Alprostadil	Relatively noninvasive	Limited efficacy, burning sensation
Penile injection therapy Alprostadil Phentolamine Papaverine	Most effective nonsurgical option, rapid onset	Invasive, risk of priapism and fibrosis. Initial trial dose should be administered under healthcare provider supervision
Vacuum device	Noninvasive	Mechanical, cumbersome
Penile prosthesis	Effective, simple	Invasive, risk of mechanical failure, infection

Data are from Morgentaler A. JAMA 2004;291(24):2994-3003.

with sexual dysfunction, particularly to evaluate for thyroid disorders, ovarian failure, hyperprolactinemia, and congenital disorders.

Most clinical trials of sexual dysfunction have studied erectile dysfunction (**Table 39**). Initial treatments of this disorder include psychosexual therapy or counseling, lifestyle modifications, medication adjustments, oral erectogenic agents, and vacuum constriction devices. Other therapies for erectile dysfunction include androgen replacement, intraurethral or intrapenile erectogenic drugs, and penile prostheses.

The oral agents sildenafil, vardenafil, and tadalafil facilitate erection by selectively inhibiting the metabolism of cyclic guanosine monophosphate by phosphodiesterase type 5 (PDE-5) in the corpora cavernosa. This inhibition enhances nitrous oxide–mediated penile smooth-muscle relaxation, leading to penile engorgement. The PDE-5 inhibitors do not enhance libido or normal erectile function. A systematic review of 27 trials demonstrated a significantly higher overall percentage of successful sexual intercourse attempts in patients who took sildenafil versus placebo (57% vs. 21%), but this drug was less effective (24%) following radical prostatectomy (3). Although sildenafil did not increase the risk for cardiovascular events, concomitant use of PDE-5 inhibitors with nitrates is contraindicated because of case reports of sudden death in patients who took this combination. Sildenafil improved erectile function in men with major depression that was in remission and sexual dysfunction associated with selective serotonin reuptake inhibitors (4). A systematic review of

six trials also suggested that the antidepressant trazodone might provide benefit to men with psychogenic erectile dysfunction (5).

Intracavernous injection and transurethral administration of prostaglandin E1 administered immediately before intercourse significantly increases the chance of having at least one successful attempt at intercourse compared with placebo in patients with sexual dysfunction. A randomized trial of lifestyle modifications showed that losing weight and increasing physical activity benefited approximately 30% of obese men with erectile dysfunction (6).

Psychotherapy and behavioral therapy have been the primary treatment in patients with premature ejaculation. Selective serotonin reuptake inhibitors and topical anesthetics can delay ejaculation with minimal side effects, but they have not received approval from the Food and Drug Administration (FDA) for this indication.

Depending on the cause, treatments for female sexual dysfunction include psychosexual therapy or counseling, lifestyle modifications, genitourinary surgery, medication adjustments, and pharmacotherapy. Evidence for sildenafil in treating arousal disorders in younger women is inconclusive, and the manufacturer is not seeking regulatory approval for this indication. A systematic review found only six placebo-controlled trials of pharmacotherapy for female sexual dysfunction in postmenopausal women (7). Estrogen replacement therapy alone and in combination with testosterone shows short-term improvement in libido and vaginal lubrication in women with sexual dysfunction; however, oral estrogen is associated with an increased risk for cardiovascular disease, breast cancer and endometrial cancer, and venous thromboembolism. Although androgen replacement therapy can increase sexual desire and activity, adverse effects are common, and androgen monotherapy has not received FDA approval for treatment of female sexual dysfunction.

KEY POINTS

- Obesity, inactivity, smoking, alcohol consumption, and chronic medical conditions are associated with erectile dysfunction.

- Poor health, history of a sexually transmitted disease, emotional problems, urinary tract symptoms, sexual trauma, and deteriorating socioeconomic status are associated with sexual dysfunction in women.

- A significantly higher overall percentage of successful sexual intercourse attempts was reported in men who took sildenafil versus placebo, but sildenafil was less effective after radical prostatectomy.

- Concomitant use of phosphodiesterase type-5 inhibitors with nitrates is contraindicated because of case reports of sudden death after treatment with this combination.

- Sildenafil improved erectile function in men with major depression that was in remission in addition to selective serotonin reuptake inhibitor–associated sexual dysfunction.

- Intracavernous injection and transurethral administration of prostaglandin E1 administered immediately before intercourse significantly increases the chance of having at least one successful attempt at intercourse compared with placebo in men with erectile dysfunction.

- Losing weight and increasing physical activity benefited approximately 30% of obese men with erectile dysfunction.

Urinary Incontinence

Normal bladder filling and emptying require accommodation of increased bladder volumes at a low intravesicular pressure, a bladder outlet that is closed at rest and remains closed during increased abdominal pressure, and the absence of involuntary bladder contractions. Age-related physiologic changes leading to incontinence are decline in bladder capacity, decrease in urethral closing pressure, uninhibited detrusor contractions, loss of elasticity of the bladder tissue, increased prostate size with outlet obstruction in men, and pelvic muscle laxity in women. Urinary incontinence is categorized by symptoms and physiology (**Table 40**).

Urinary incontinence is a common problem, especially in the elderly population. Estimates of prevalence are 10% to 35% in community-dwelling adults and 50% to 70% in the nursing home population. Risk factors for urinary incontinence

include female sex (with this disorder occurring twice as commonly in women as in men), increasing age, recurrent urinary tract infections, obesity, constipation, and other bowel problems. Incontinence is also more common in patients with diabetes, stroke, hypertension, cognitive impairment, Parkinson's disease, arthritis, back problems, and hearing or visual impairment than in those without these problems. In women, parity, vaginal mode of delivery, hysterectomy in women 60 years of age or older, cystocele, and uterine prolapse are additional risk factors for urinary incontinence (8), whereas benign prostatic hyperplasia and radical prostatectomy for prostate cancer are risk factors for urinary incontinence in men (9). Several medications are associated with incontinence (**Table 41**). Although urge incontinence is more common among young women than young men, the gap narrows as age increases, especially after age 75 years.

Patients are reluctant to mention symptoms of incontinence with their physician. The basic clinical evaluation of patients with such symptoms includes a detailed history and physical examination, urinalysis, and serum creatinine and plasma glucose measurement. Having patients with urinary incontinence record in a diary the frequency, timing, and amount of voiding for 24 to 72 hours before the examination visit is helpful. The history helps to determine the category of incontinence as urge incontinence, stress incontinence, or overflow incontinence. Total incontinence refers to continuous loss of urine with minimal activity. Functional incontinence refers to that caused by mental or physical activities that impede normal voiding or the ability to get to the toilet. Mixed incontinence is characterized by symptoms of both urge and stress incontinence. Postsurgical incontinence refers to incontinence occurring in men after they have undergone radical prostatectomy.

The clinical evaluation of patients with incontinence should focus on neurologic disease and functional status. A rectal examination is useful in identifying fecal impaction, rectal masses, and sphincter tone. In men, a genitourinary examination to evaluate the prostate gland for hyperplasia or a mass is appropriate, as is evaluation of the urethra. In women, a pelvic examination is indicated to identify signs of atrophic vaginitis, pelvic prolapse, cystocele, or rectocele. Reversible conditions associated with incontinence are summarized by the mnemonic DIAPPERS (*d*elirium, *i*nfection of the urinary tract [symptomatic], *a*trophic urethritis/vaginitis, *p*harmaceuticals, *p*sychologic disorders [especially depression], *e*xcessive urine output [associated with heart failure or hyperglycemia], *r*estricted mobility, and *s*tool impaction) (10).

A Cochrane systematic review found insufficient evidence to determine whether management based on urodynamic findings leads to better outcomes in patients with urinary incontinence when compared with standard management based on history and clinical examination (11). Therefore, urodynamic testing is usually reserved for patients who do not

TABLE 40 Types of Urinary Incontinence

Type	Characteristics	Pathophysiology	Treatment
Urge incontinence, overactive bladder dysfunction	Daytime voiding Frequency Nocturia Bothersome urgency	Involuntary contraction of the bladder Decreased control of the detrusor muscle Decreased competence of the urethral sphincter in men	Biofeedback Bladder training Anticholinergics Oxybutynin Tolterodine
Stress incontinence	Involuntary release of urine secondary to effort or exertion, such as from sneezing, coughing, or physical exertion	Pelvic muscle laxity, nerve injury, or urologic surgery Poor intrinsic sphincter function	Pelvic floor muscle training for women (Kegel) Biofeedback Electrical stimulation Open retropubic colposuspension Suburethral sling procedure
Overflow	Associated with over-distension of the bladder	Underactive detrusor muscle or outlet obstruction	Pelvic floor muscle training with biofeedback in early postprostatectomy period External penile clamp

Note: Tricyclic antidepressants are an off-label treatment for urge incontinence. α-Adrenergic agonist midodrine is an off-label treatment for stress incontinence.

TABLE 41 Medications Associated with Urinary Incontinence

Type of Medication	Potential Effects on Continence
Diuretics	Polyuria, frequency, urgency
Anticholinergics	Urinary retention, overflow
Psychotropics Antidepressants Antipsychotics	Anticholinergic actions, sedation Anticholinergic actions, sedation, rigidity, immobility
Sedatives/Hypnotics	Sedation, delirium, immobility, muscle relaxation
Narcotic analgesics	Urinary retention, fecal impaction, sedation, delirium
α-Adrenergic blockers	Urethral relaxation
α-Adrenergic agonists	Urinary retention
β-Adrenergic agonists	Urinary retention
Calcium channel blockers	Urinary retention
Alcohol	Polyuria, frequency, urgency, sedation, delirium, immobility

Adapted from Merkel I. Urinary Incontinence in the Elderly. Southern Medical Journal 2001;94:952-957.

respond to urinary incontinence therapy based on the initial clinical evaluation.

Treatment of urinary incontinence consists of behavioral, pharmacologic, and surgical approaches, depending on type of incontinence (see Table 40). Treatments have been more widely studied in female than in male patients with this complaint.

Pelvic-floor muscle training, or Kegel exercise, involves repeated voluntary pelvic-floor muscle contractions and can be performed with or without the use of biofeedback techniques.

Recent Cochrane systematic reviews have found pelvic-floor muscle training to be effective treatment for women with stress or mixed incontinence compared with no treatment or placebo (12). Other nonpharmacologic approaches that have demonstrated some benefit in clinical trials compared with usual care are electrical stimulation, vaginal cones, bladder training, or prompted voiding. Electrical stimulation works through stimulation of the sacral posterior roots, reducing urge incontinence. The treatment usually is administered daily for a period of months.

The first-line pharmacologic intervention for urge and mixed incontinence consists of anticholinergic medications, which act by blocking parasympathetic signals to the detrusor muscle and inhibiting involuntary bladder contractions (13). Tolterodine tartrate is associated with fewer anticholinergic side effects than oxybutynin because of uroselectivity. Transdermal oxybutynin has fewer cholinergic side effects than oral oxybutynin. A 2- to 4-week trial of this drug is recommended before assessing the degree of benefit. A Cochrane systematic review of anticholinergic drugs for urge incontinence found that anticholinergic medications resulted in better subjective cure and improvement rates (RR 1.41, 95% CI 1.29 to 1.54) compared with placebo (14). The most common side effect of anticholinergic agents is dry mouth. Central nervous system side effects include drowsiness, hallucinations, cognitive impairment, and delirium. Elderly patients have a higher potential for adverse central nervous system effects from anticholinergic medications than do younger patients (15). Doxepin, a tricyclic antidepressant, has been studied in women with detrusor instability or urinary incontinence. Although shown effective in some studies, this drug has not received approval from the Food and Drug Administration (FDA) for the treatment of incontinence. Doxepin results in subjective improvement compared with placebo (OR 23.80, 95% CI 3.99 to 141.97), but not in objective improvement in bladder stability; side effects include electrocardiographic abnormalities, cardiac arrhythmias, and hypertension. α-Adrenergic agonists and serotonin and norepinephrine agonists are being evaluated for the treatment of stress incontinence but are not currently FDA approved for this indication. A recent Cochrane systematic review found only limited evidence to suggest that adrenergic agonist drugs are better than placebo in treating incontinence (16). Potential adverse effects of these agents include palpitations, cardiac arrhythmias, hypertension, and insomnia.

Surgical procedures for stress incontinence are designed to correct urethral closure problems and improve support of the urethrovesical junction. Procedures include open retropubic colposuspension, bladder-neck needle suspension, anterior vaginal repair, laparoscopic retropubic colposuspension, suburethral sling procedure, and periurethral injections. Adverse outcomes may include perioperative complications, new urgency and urge incontinence, voiding difficulties, recurrent or new pelvic prolapse, and the need for repeated surgery.

KEY POINTS

- **Parity, vaginal mode of delivery, hysterectomy at $\geq$60 years, cystocele, and uterine prolapse are risk factors for urinary incontinence in women, whereas benign prostatic hyperplasia and radical prostatectomy for prostate cancer are risk factors for urinary incontinence in men.**
- **Pelvic-floor muscle training was effective treatment for women with stress or mixed incontinence compared with no treatment or placebo.**
- **Anticholinergic medications were found to be better than placebo in rates of subjective cure or improvement in patients with urge incontinence.**

Benign Prostatic Hyperplasia

Benign prostatic hyperplasia (BPH) is a nonmalignant enlargement of the prostate gland that becomes increasingly prevalent with age. Histologic changes of hyperplasia are found in more than 50% of men in their 50s and in nearly 90% of men in their 80s. More than 30% of men 65 years and older have lower urinary tract symptoms caused by BPH. By age 80 years, an estimated one in four men will have undergone treatment to relieve BPH symptoms.

The symptoms of BPH involve a dynamic component (smooth-muscle contraction in the prostate, prostate capsule, and bladder neck) and a fixed component (enlarged prostate compressing the urethra). BPH leads to irritative (urgency, frequency, and nocturia) and obstructive (decreased stream, intermittency, incomplete emptying, and straining) symptoms. The differential diagnoses for these symptoms include urethral stricture, bladder-neck contracture, urinary tract

infection, carcinoma of the prostate or bladder, bladder calculi, diabetes mellitus, and neurogenic bladder.

The diagnosis of BPH is established primarily by medical history and digital rectal examination. Urinalysis is recommended to identify other causes of lower urinary tract symptoms. Although BPH is not a risk factor for prostate cancer, American Urologic Association guidelines recommend offering prostate-specific antigen (PSA) testing to men for whom a prostate cancer diagnosis or an elevated PSA value would change BPH management (17). Optional tests for evaluating BPH include measurement of serum creatinine level and urine cytology, and measurements of urinary flow rate and postvoid residual urine volume. Cystoscopy, transrectal ultrasonography, and upper urinary tract imaging are not routinely recommended.

When a diagnosis of BPH has been established, the AUA symptom index (**Table 42**), which ranges from 0 to 35 points, quantifies symptom severity. Symptom scores <8 are considered mild; 8 to 19, moderate; and >19, severe. Transurethral resection of the prostate (TURP), the goldstandard treatment for BPH, is recommended in patients with refractory urinary retention, persistent gross hematuria, recurrent urinary tract infections, bladder stones, or renal insufficiency clearly attributable to BPH. In the absence of these indications, medical management is appropriate, although watchful waiting is reasonable in men with mild symptoms.

The two major BPH drug classes are α-adrenergic blockers (terazosin, tamsulosin, doxazosin, alfuzosin, and prazosin), which relax smooth muscle in the bladder neck and prostate, and the 5-α reductase inhibitors (finasteride and dutasteride), which reduce the size of the prostate gland. Short-term studies have shown α-adrenergic blockers superior to finasteride in reducing urinary symptoms and improving urinary flow, although meta-analyses have shown both drugs to be superior to placebo (18). The Medical Therapy of Prostate Symptoms study found that long-term doxazosin plus finasteride therapy reduced the risk for overall clinical progression of BPH, including symptom worsening, acute urinary retention, renal insufficiency, recurrent urinary tract infections, urinary incontinence, and the need for invasive therapy, more than either drug when used alone (19). Both drugs were more effective than placebo, although doxazosin alone did not reduce the risk for urinary retention or the need for invasive therapy. However, adverse outcomes in patients taking these drugs were uncommon, and monotherapy with the quicker-acting α-adrenergic blockers is still appropriate. Adding finasteride to the therapeutic regimen is reasonable in men with progressive symptoms or in those with a prostate volume >40 mL. Because doxazosin monotherapy was less cardioprotective than other antihypertensive agents in the ALLHAT study (20), α-blockers should be used cautiously as a single agent in men with hypertension and BPH. Herbal preparations often are

TABLE 42 AUA Symptom Index*

	Not at all	Less than 1 time in 5	Less than half the time	About half the time	More than half the time	Almost always
Over the past month, how often have you had a sensation of not emptying your bladder completely after you finish urinating?	0	1	2	3	4	5
Over the past month, how often have you had to urinate again less than 2 hours after you finished urinating?	0	1	2	3	4	5
Over the past month, how often have you stopped and started again several times when you urinated?	0	1	2	3	4	5
Over the past month, how often have you found it difficult to postpone urination?	0	1	2	3	4	5
Over the past month, how often have you had a weak urinary stream?	0	1	2	3	4	5
Over the past month, how often have you had to push or strain to begin urination?	0	1	2	3	4	5
Over the past month, how many times did you most typically get up to urinate from the time you went to bed at night until the time you got up in the morning?	0	1	2	3	4	5

Reprinted with permission from Barry MJ, et al. J Urol 1992; 148:1549-57.

*Note: Symptom classification based on cumulative score: mild (0 to 7), moderate (8 to 19), severe (20 to 35). AUA = American Urologic Association.

used for treating symptoms of prostatism. Meta-analyses have shown symptom and urinary flow improvement with the use of *Pygeum africanum* but only symptom improvement with *Serenoa repens* (saw palmetto extract), β-sitosterol, and cernitin. However, a recent study found no evidence that saw palmetto improved symptoms or urinary flow (21). No herbal preparation reduced prostate volume. The long-term safety and effectiveness of these preparations in preventing BPH complications are unknown. Men with symptomatic BPH should avoid antihistamine and anticholinergic drugs that can impair bladder function and sympathomimetic drugs that can increase outflow resistance. Finasteride can reduce PSA levels by 50%; therefore, biopsy referral thresholds should be adjusted accordingly in men undergoing prostate cancer screening. Although TURP significantly improves symptom scores and peak urinary flow compared with watchful waiting, this procedure requires hospitalization and can be complicated by infection, blood loss requiring transfusion, retrograde ejaculation, and severe hyponatremia. Minimally invasive outpatient surgical procedures have been developed to reduce complications and hospital length-of-stay in patients with BPH. Laser prostatectomy (22) and transurethral microwave thermotherapy (23) are outpatient procedures that significantly improve urinary symptoms and peak urinary flow, although less effectively than TURP. Minimally invasive treatments result in fewer transfusions and strictures than TURP, but higher re-operation rates in patients with BPH.

- Offering prostate-specific antigen (PSA) testing is recommended only in men for whom a prostate cancer diagnosis or an elevated PSA value would change benign prostatic hyperplasia (BPH) management.

- Transurethral resection of the prostate is recommended in patients with refractory urinary retention, persistent gross hematuria, recurrent urinary tract infections, bladder stones, or renal insufficiency clearly attributable to BPH.

- Short-term studies have shown α-adrenergic blockers superior to finasteride in reducing urinary symptoms and improving urinary flow in BPH, although meta-analyses have shown both drugs to be superior to placebo.

- Long-term doxazosin plus finasteride reduced the risk for overall clinical progression of BPH, including symptom worsening, acute urinary retention, renal insufficiency, recurrent urinary tract infections, urinary incontinence, and the need for invasive therapy, more than either drug when used alone.

- In men with BPH, adding finasteride to the therapeutic regimen is reasonable for progressive symptoms or in men with a prostate volume >40 mL.

- α-Blockers should be used cautiously as a single agent in men with hypertension and BPH.

- Meta-analyses have shown symptom and urinary flow improvement with *Pygeum africanum* but only symptom improvement with *Serenoa repens*, β-sitosterol, and cernitin in patients with BPH.

- Because finasteride can reduce PSA levels by 50%, biopsy referral thresholds should be adjusted accordingly in men undergoing prostate cancer screening.

Testicular and Scrotal Abnormalities

Conditions that affect the scrotum and testicle range from the extremely benign to medical emergencies that require immediate surgical correction. In patients with acute testicular pain, the most important condition to rule out immediately is torsion of the testicle. Early identification of this problem with prompt surgical attention prevents the need for orchidectomy. Patients with torsion of the testicle usually have acute onset of testicular pain in one testis that makes walking uncomfortable. This condition is frequently associated with abdominal pain, nausea, and vomiting. On examination, there is evidence of inflammation on one side; the affected testicle is tender to touch, hot, and swollen. Testicular pain can occur at any age but occurs most commonly in males between ages 15 and 30 years. If the testicle is found to be viable during surgery once untwisted, further episodes can be prevented with bilateral orchidopexy. In the presence of vascular compromise, an orchidectomy may be indicated in patients with torsion of the testicle.

Epididymitis is the other main consideration among the differential diagnoses in this clinical scenario; however, patients with epididymitis tend to be older than 30 years and have symptoms of urinary tract infection and a more gradual onset of pain than those with torsion of the testicle.

The examination of patients with a mass in the groin or scrotum should focus on whether the mass 1) is cystic or solid (that is, whether it transilluminates); 2) has a superior edge that can be appreciated by palpating above it; and 3) is separate from the testicle. Epididymal cysts, which are separate from the testis and are cystic, are a benign condition occurring in adult men (24). The treatment of this condition is removal of the cyst only in symptomatic patients. Hydroceles and varicoceles occur within the testicle and are cystic. Hydroceles occur frequently in young men and are treated with aspiration or removal only when they are large and symptomatic. Patients with varicoceles, which are characterized by a "bag of worms" consistency, require only reassurance. Epididymoorchitis is generally a solid mass that is separate from the testicle, with clear tenderness just at the superior pole. Common causes of this condition include *Escherichia coli*, mumps, gonococcal infection, or tuberculosis. First-catch urine samples and inspection for urethral discharge are helpful in establishing the diagnosis. Inguinal hernias may also extend into the scrotum. It is difficult to palpate above the lesion in patients with inguinal hernias, because it extends superiorly into the canal.

A painless testicular mass that is solid on examination is highly suspicious for testicular cancer, the most common cancer in young men (25). Testicular cancer affects almost 9000 men in the United States annually and has slowly increased in incidence in the past 40 years. This disease affects whites four to five times more often than blacks, and occurs most frequently in men between the ages of 20 and 40 years. The main risk factor for testicular cancer is a history of cryptorchidism; however, a newly identified association of seminomas with HIV has been reported in patients with testicular cancer. The evaluation of a suspicious mass should include ultrasonography with serum β-human chorionic gonadotropin, α-fetoprotein, and lactate dehydrogenase measurement. Chest radiography and abdominal CT scan are essential components of staging in patients with confirmed malignancy. Seminomas and the more aggressive nonseminomas identified at early stages have an almost 95% cure rate in patients with testicular cancer.

References

1. **Nicolosi A, Laumann EO, Glasser DB, Moreira ED Jr, Paik A, Gingell C, et al.** Sexual behavior and sexual dysfunctions after age 40: the global study of sexual attitudes and behaviors. Urology. 2004;64:991-7. [PMID: 15533492]

2. **Bacon CG, Mittleman MA, Kawachi I, Giovannucci E, Glasser DB, Rimm EB.** Sexual function in men older than 50 years of age: results from the health professionals follow-up study. Ann Intern Med. 2003;139:161-8. [PMID: 12899583]

3. **Fink HA, Mac Donald R, Rutks IR, Nelson DB, Wilt TJ.** Sildenafil for male erectile dysfunction: a systematic review and meta-analysis. Arch Intern Med. 2002;162:1349-60. [PMID: 12076233]

4. **Nurnberg HG, Hensley PL, Gelenberg AJ, Fava M, Lauriello J, Paine S.** Treatment of antidepressant-associated sexual dysfunction with sildenafil: a randomized controlled trial. JAMA. 2003;289:56-64. [PMID: 12503977]

5. **Fink HA, MacDonald R, Rutks IR, Wilt TJ.** Trazodone for erectile dysfunction: a systematic review and meta-analysis. BJU Int. 2003;92:441-6. [PMID: 12930437]

6. **Esposito K, Giugliano F, Di Palo C, Giugliano G, Marfella R, D'Andrea F, et al.** Effect of lifestyle changes on erectile dysfunction in obese men: a randomized controlled trial. JAMA. 2004;291:2978-84. [PMID: 15213209]

7. **Modelska K, Cummings S.** Female sexual dysfunction in postmenopausal women: systematic review of placebo-controlled trials. Am J Obstet Gynecol. 2003;188:286-93. [PMID: 12548231]

8. **Holroyd-Leduc JM, Straus SE.** Management of urinary incontinence in women: scientific review. JAMA. 2004;291:986-95. [PMID: 14982915]

9. **Moore KN, Gray M.** Urinary incontinence in men: Current status and future directions. Nurs Res. 2004 Nov-Dec;53(6 Suppl):S36-41. [PMID: 15586146]

10. **Vapnek JM.** Urinary incontinence. Screening and treatment of urinary dysfunction. Geriatrics. 2001;56:25-9; quiz 32. [PMID: 11641859]

11. **Hunter KF, Moore KN, Cody DJ, Glazener CM.** Conservative management for postprostatectomy urinary incontinence. Cochrane Database Syst Rev. 2004;(2):CD001843. [PMID: 15106164]

12. **Hay-Smith EJ, Dumoulin C.** Pelvic floor muscle training versus no treatment, or inactive control treatments, for urinary incontinence in women. Cochrane Database Syst Rev. 2006 Jan 25;(1):CD005654. Review. [PMID: 16437536]

13. **Haeusler G, Leitich H, van Trotsenburg M, Kaider A, Tempfer CB.** Drug therapy of urinary urge incontinence: a systematic review. Obstet Gynecol. 2002 Nov;100(5 Pt 1):1003-16. Review. [PMID: 12423868]

14. **Hay-Smith J, Herbison P, Ellis G, Morris A.** Which anticholinergic drug for overactive bladder symptoms in adults. Cochrane Database Syst Rev. 2005 Jul 20;(3):CD005429. Review. [PMID 16034974]

15. **Scheife R, Takeda M.** Central nervous system safety of anticholinergic drugs for the treatment of overactive bladder in the elderly. Clin Ther. 2005;27:144-53. [PMID: 15811477]

16. **Alhasso A, Glazener CMA, Pickard R, N'Dow J.** Adrenergic drugs for urinary incontinence in adults. Cochrane Database Syst Rev. 2005 Jul 20;(3):CD001842. [PMID: 16034867]

17. AUA guideline on management of benign prostatic hyperplasia (2003). Chapter 1: Diagnosis and treatment recommendations. J Urol. 2003;170:530-47. [PMID: 12853821]

18. **Wilt TJ, Howe W, MacDonald R.** Terazosin for treating symptomatic benign prostatic obstruction: a systematic review of efficacy and adverse effects. BJU Int. 2002;89:214-25. [PMID: 11856101]

19. **McConnell JD, Roehrborn CG, Bautista OM, Andriole GL Jr, Dixon CM, Kusek JW, et al.** The long-term effect of doxazosin, finasteride, and combination therapy on the clinical progression of benign prostatic hyperplasia. N Engl J Med. 2003;349:2387-98. [PMID: 14681504]

20. Major cardiovascular events in hypertensive patients randomized to doxazosin vs chlorthalidone: the antihypertensive and lipid-lowering treatment to prevent heart attack trial (ALLHAT). ALLHAT Collaborative Research Group. JAMA. 2000;283:1967-75. [PMID: 10789664]

21. **Bent S, Kane C, Shinohora K, Neuhas J, Hudes ES, Goldberg H, et al.** Saw palmetto for benign prostatic hyperplasia. N Engl J Med. 2006;354:557-66. [PMID: 16467543]

22. **Hoffman RM, MacDonald R, Slaton JW, Wilt TJ.** Laser prostatectomy versus transurethral resection for treating benign prostatic obstruction: a systematic review. J Urol. 2003;169:210-5. [PMID: 12478138]

23. **Hoffman RM, MacDonald R, Monga M, Wilt TJ.** Transurethral microwave thermotherapy vs transurethral resection for treating benign prostatic hyperplasia: a systematic review. BJU Int. 2004;94:1031-6. [PMID: 15541122]

24. **Rubenstein RA, Dogra VS, Seftel AD, Resnick MI.** Benign intrascrotal lesions. J Urol. 2004;171:1765-72. [PMID: 15076274]

25. **MacVicar GR, Pienta KJ.** Testicular cancer. Curr Opin Oncol. 2004;16:253-6. [PMID: 15069322]

VASCULAR DISORDERS

Chronic Venous Insufficiency and Lymphedema

Edema is the abnormal accumulation of fluid in extravascular interstitial space, resulting from alterations in capillary hemodynamics, including increased hydrostatic pressure, decreased oncotic pressure, or increased capillary permeability, and renal retention of sodium and water. Causes of lower-extremity edema include congestive heart failure, constrictive pericarditis, restrictive cardiomyopathy, nephrotic syndrome, hypoproteinemia, cirrhosis, pregnancy, chronic venous insufficiency, deep venous thrombosis, lymphedema, cellulitis, Baker's cyst, thyroid disease, and medication effects.

Chronic venous insufficiency results from persistent venous hypertension caused by venous incompetence or occlusion. Manifestations of chronic venous insufficiency include edema, skin hyperpigmentation, stasis dermatitis, varicose veins (distended and tortuous superficial leg veins), lipodermatosclerosis (fibrosing panniculitis of the subcutaneous tissue), cellulitis, and ulceration (**Table 43**). Venous diseases are among the most commonly encountered chronic conditions. The estimated prevalence of chronic venous insufficiency ranges widely, from <1% to 17% in men and <1% to 40% in women, depending on the diagnostic criteria and geographic location. The estimated prevalence of varicose veins is 25% to 30% in women and 10% to 20% in men, whereas the lifetime risk of venous ulcers is approximately 1%. Ulcer prevalance is higher among women and increases with age. The strongest risk factor for venous insufficiency is a history of deep venous thrombosis or phlebitis; leg injury, age, and obesity also increase the risk for this condition.

Clinical examination is usually sufficient for establishing a diagnosis of chronic venous insufficiency. Duplex ultrasonography can accurately detect venous incompetence (in patients considering invasive procedures) and deep vein thrombosis, as well as popliteal cysts, hematomas, aneurysms, and soft-tissue masses. Ankle-brachial index measurements help establish whether patients have coexisting arterial disease, although these measurements are unreliable in patients with diabetes mellitus who have vascular calcification.

Varicose veins, which can occur in the absence of chronic venous insufficiency, are cosmetically distressing and cause aching pain, limb heaviness, itching, cramping, and edema. Uncommon complications of varicose veins include thrombophlebitis, venous ulceration, and variceal rupture. Initial treatment of this disorder includes leg elevation, weight loss, and graduated compression stockings, although serious complications may be an indication for surgical procedures (for example, ligation, stripping, or avulsion). Injection sclerotherapy or surgery is a consideration in patients who do not respond to conservative treatment for varicose veins. A systematic review found no controlled trials comparing sclerotherapy with observation and only a single controlled trial comparing sclerotherapy with graduated compression stockings (1). Sclerotherapy more effectively improved varicose vein symptoms and cosmetic appearance in pregnancy compared with graduated compression stockings. Another systematic review of nine controlled trials comparing sclerotherapy with surgery in patients with varicose veins found insufficient evidence to recommend a treatment (2). Although sclerotherapy was less expensive, resulted in fewer complications, and was more effective than surgery in the first post-therapy year, long-term outcomes favored surgery in patients with varicose veins.

Venous ulcers, typically located on the medial ankle, can require protracted therapy. Leg elevation and compression therapy are standard initial interventions in patients with venous ulcers. Compression heals approximately 70% to 80% of venous ulcers within 3 to 6 months. A systematic review found that compression bandages were more effective than no compression in healing ulcers, with multilayered, elastic, high compression (30 to 40 mm Hg at the ankle) more effective than single-layered, low compression (3). The benefits of

Category	Clinical signs
Class 0	No visible or palpable signs of venous disease
Class 1	Telangiectasias, reticular veins, malleolar flares
Class 2	Varicose veins
Class 3	Edema without skin changes
Class 4	Skin changes due to venous disease (hyperpigmentation, stasis, lipodermatosclerosis)
Class 5	Venous skin changes with healed ulceration
Class 6	Venous skin changes with active ulceration

TABLE 43 Classification and Grading of Chronic Venous Disease

Reprinted with permission from Porter J. J Vasc Surgery 1995;21:635

intermittent pneumatic compression in the treatment of venous ulcers are uncertain. Compression is contraindicated in patients with arterial insufficiency.

Effective adjunctive medications for healing ulcers include aspirin; horse chestnut seed extract, which induces prostaglandins-mediated vasoconstriction; and pentoxifylline. Short-term diuretic therapy may be appropriate in patients with severe edema, but volume depletion can occur in these patients because edema from venous insufficiency is poorly mobilized.

The 12-month recurrence rate for venous ulcers ranges from 26% to 69%. A randomized trial of superficial venous surgery to correct reflux in combination with multilayered, high-compression bandages reported similar healing rates when compared with compression alone (65% for each treatment), but 12-month recurrence rates were significantly lower in the surgical group (12% vs. 28%) (4). Although compression stockings are often used to prevent recurrent ulcerations, there are no published comparisons of patients who have used compression stockings with those who have not. Recurrence rates may be lower in patients who use higher-pressure versus lower-pressure compression stockings.

Below-knee elastic compression stockings reduced the 2-year incidence of post-thrombotic syndrome in patients after a first episode of symptomatic proximal deep venous thrombosis by approximately 50% compared with a control group (5).

Alterations in lymphatic transport can lead to lymphedema. Primary lymphedema is caused by congenital abnormalities in the lymphatic system that occur early in life as familial or sporadic disease, at puberty (lymphedema praecox), or in adulthood (lymphedema tarda). Secondary lymphedema results from an acquired reduction in lymphatic flow. Worldwide, the most common cause of secondary lymphedema is the parasitic infection lymphatic filariasis, but in Western populations, malignancy due to tumor compression, lymph node dissection, and/or radiation; trauma; and cellulitis are more prevalent causes of lymphedema (6). Lower-extremity lymphedema, which complicates 10% to 49% of pelvic and genital cancer treatments, initially may be characterized by unilateral or bilateral aching leg pain, heaviness, and pitting edema. Early in its course, lymphedema may be confused with chronic venous insufficiency, myxedema, or lipedema. Advanced lymphedema is recognized by the characteristic nonpitting "peau d'orange" edema resulting from progressive fibrosis of cutaneous and subcutaneous tissue and by hyperkeratosis and papillomatosis. The dorsum of the foot is most commonly affected, and the toes appear blunted in patients with advanced lymphedema. When the clinical diagnosis is uncertain, the gold-standard diagnostic procedure in patients with suspected lymphedema is radionuclide lymphoscintigraphy. CT and MRI also help to establish the diagnosis of lymphedema and can also identify anatomic abnormalities (see also Reference 6).

Lymphedema requires lifelong treatment to reduce edema, including leg elevation, use of gradient pressure stockings and inelastic bandages, and massage therapy, thermal therapy, and external pneumatic compression (see also Reference 6). No drugs effectively treat lymphedema, and diuretics should be avoided because they poorly mobilize lymphedematous fluid and deplete intravascular volume. Chronic lymphedema predisposes patients to recurrent cellulitis; meticulous skin care and prompt antibiotics can reduce infectious complications. Surgical interventions for patients with lymphedema include debulking and excisional and bypass procedures; none has been rigorously evaluated, and complications can lead to poor functional and cosmetic outcomes.

KEY POINTS

- Compression heals approximately 70% to 80% of venous ulcers within 3 to 6 months.

- The 12-month recurrence rate for venous ulcers ranges from 26% to 69%.

- Below-knee elastic compression stockings reduced the 2-year incidence of post-thrombotic syndrome in patients after a first episode of symptomatic proximal deep venous thrombosis by approximately 50% compared with a control group.

- The gold-standard diagnostic procedure in patients with suspected lymphedema is radionuclide lymphoscintigraphy.

- No drugs effectively treat lymphedema, and diuretics should be avoided in these patients because they poorly mobilize lymphedematous fluid and deplete intravascular volume.

References

1. Tisi PV, Beverley CA. Injection sclerotherapy for varicose veins. Cochrane Database Syst Rev. 2002:CD001732. [PMID: 11869605]

2. Rigby KA, Palfreyman SJ, Beverley C, Michaels JA. Surgery versus sclerotherapy for the treatment of varicose veins. Cochrane Database Syst Rev. 2004:CD004980. [PMID: 15495134]

3. Cullum N, Nelson EA, Fletcher AW, Sheldon TA. Compression for venous leg ulcers. Cochrane Database Syst Rev. 2001:CD000265. [PMID: 11405957]

4. Barwell JR, Davies CE, Deacon J, Harvey K, Minor J, Sassano A, et al. Comparison of surgery and compression with compression alone in chronic venous ulceration (ESCHAR study): randomised controlled trial. Lancet. 2004;363:1854-9. [PMID: 15183623]

5. Prandoni P, Lensing AW, Prins MH, Frulla M, Marchiori A, Bernardi E, et al. Below-knee elastic compression stockings to prevent the post-thrombotic syndrome: a randomized, controlled trial. Ann Intern Med. 2004;141:249-56. [PMID: 15313740]

6. Tiwari A, Cheng KS, Button M, Myint F, Hamilton G. Differential diagnosis, investigation, and current treatment of lower limb lymphedema. Arch Surg. 2003;138:152-61. [PMID: 12578410]

DERMATOLOGIC DISORDERS

RECENT ADVANCES

- Methicillin-resistant *Staphylococcus aureus* in community-acquired disease

- Tacrolimus and pimecrolimus safety concerns

Pruritis

Pruritis is a sensation of itch and pain transmitted by unmyelinated C fibers, whose receptors are assumed to be in the dermis and epidermis. A broad array of substances can induce pruritis, including histamine, serotonin, papain, opioids, neuropeptides, and certain products of eosinophils and platelets. Many of these compounds act through effects on mast-cell degranulators and the release of histamine. Pruritis may be indicative of various dermatologic diseases or psychiatric and systemic conditions (Table 44) (1).

The two most common dermatalogic causes of pruritis are dermatitis, including contact dermatitis, and xerosis (dry skin). Frequent bathing, poor chronic hydration, and dry winter weather exacerbate dry skin and the accompanying itch. The treatment of xerosis should include advice about using a humidifier in dry weather conditions, avoiding excess bathing and scrubbing of skin, use of moisturizing soaps, and routine use of moisturizers and occlusives. Moisturizers, including mineral oil, coconut oil, lactate, and urea, are all effective at supplying water to the skin (2). Occlusives with petrolatum help to reduce water loss from skin and are appropriate for use in combination with moisturizers.

Precipitating factors for contact dermatitis include new soaps, herbal supplements, or other medications. Environmental factors, such as fleas and mites from pets, or a change in environment (for example, different sheets or carpets), may also

TABLE 44 Evaluation of Itch Without Obvious Cause

History

Periodicity
  Day or night, intermittent or continuous

Nature
  Burning, pricking, insects crawling

Location
  Scapula/subscapula in nostalgia paresthetica (a localized itch in the scapular area, presumably neuropathic)
  Palms of hand and soles of feet (cholestasis)

Provoking factors
  Activity/exercise, cold, sunlight, water

Medications
  Opioids, hypersensitivity reactions

Atopic history
  Subclinical eczema

Travel history
  Parasitic infections

Examination

Dry skin

Scabies

Icteric conjunctiva

Weight loss

Change in mental status

Laboratory

Complete blood count
  If anemic, plasma iron, total iron-binding capacity, ferritin

Erythrocyte sedimentation rate

Plasma creatinine

Biochemical liver tests
  Total/direct bilirubin, alkaline phosphatase, gammaglutamyl transpeptidase, aspartate aminotransferase, alanine aminotransferase, fasting total plasma bile acids

Thyroid function

T4 and thyroid-stimulating hormone

Fasting plasma glucose

Fecal analysis for ova and parasites

polycythemia vera, lymphoma, psychiatric illness, HIV, hepatitis C infection, multiple sclerosis, cholestasis of pregnancy, and some types of cancer. Pruritis is the presenting symptom in 50% of all patients with polycythemia vera; in up to 85% of patients with end-stage renal disease who are receiving dialysis; in 30% of those with Hodgkin's lymphoma; and in 100% of those with T-cell lymphoma (Sezary syndrome). Laboratory studies in patients who have itch without obvious cause might include a complete blood count; measurement of erythrocyte sedimentation rate, serum creatinine, serum thyroid-stimulating hormone, and plasma glucose; and liver chemistry tests.

Nonpharmacologic treatment of pruritis includes recommending that patients wear lightweight clothing to keep cool, achieving an ambient environment that is not too dry, and avoiding hot showers and baths (4). Patients with pruritis should be encouraged to keep their nails very short to avoid skin damage from scratching. Drug treatment includes topical agents and systemic medications. Topical antipruritic agents are the most helpful for treating localized itchy rashes and insect bites. Effective compounds for topical relief of itching include menthol and phenol, calamine lotion, topical H_1-receptor antagonist antihistamines, capsaicin, and local anesthetics. Systemic antihistamines are the drug of choice for pruritis, especially for patients with histamine-mediated itch. H_2-receptor antagonists can also be helpful, particularly for patients with urticaria. Doxepin, a tricyclic antidepressant, is also a potent H_1- and H_2-receptor antagonist that provides relief to some patients with pruritis. The itch from epidural opioids and chronic cholestasis has been effectively treated by intravenous ondansetron. Paroxetine and mirtazapine have also been used successfully in some patients with pruritis, although the effect is short-lived, diminishing after 4 to 6 weeks of therapy. Some HIV-positive patients with itch have had benefit from indomethacin (5).

KEY POINTS

- Systemic disease may be responsible for itch without obvious cause based on evidence from retrospective clinical studies.

- Laboratory studies in patients who have itch without obvious cause include a complete blood count; measurement of erythrocyte sedimentation rate, serum creatinine, serum thyroid-stimulating hormone, and plasma glucose levels; and liver chemistry tests.

- Systemic antihistamines are the drug of choice for patients with pruritis, especially for those with histamine-mediated itch.

Urticaria

Urticaria, also known as hives, is a common skin finding that arises from a recurrent, but transient, cutaneous swelling with sudden erythema caused by vascular extravasation (**Figure 4**).

cause pruritis. The distribution of localized pruritis and any excoriations found on examination may be helpful in establishing the diagnosis.

Pruritis without obvious cause requires prompt further investigation (see Table 44). Systemic disease was present in 10% to 50% of such patients based on four retrospective clinical studies of generalized pruritis, and in 22% as reported in a recent retrospective analysis. (3). Underlying conditions of pruritis include hypo- and hyperthyroidism, diabetes mellitus, uremia, obstructive biliary disease, iron-deficiency anemia,

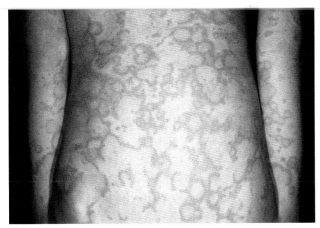

FIGURE 4.
Annular lesions of urticaria.

This condition can signify a completely benign, almost evanescent nuisance, or a severe, life-threatening form of urticaria called "angioedema," a sudden, temporary edema of a localized area of skin or mucosa, usually the lips, face, hands, feet, penis, or scrotum. The hallmark of urticaria is the rapid appearance of the weal, a superficial itchy, sometimes painful, swelling of the skin. Weals can be multiple or isolated and usually involve the trunk and extremities, sparing the palms and soles. Those involving the skin around the mouth are considered an emergency, requiring careful observation and investigation for airway obstruction. Concomitant angioedema and urticaria occur in 40% of patients, with another 40% having hives alone, and 20% having angioedema but no urticaria (6).

The clinical classification of urticaria depends on symptom duration and precipitating factors (**Table 45**). Acute urticaria is generally related to environmental allergens, including drugs, foods, and, occasionally, inhalants. Penicillin, aspirin, NSAIDs, contrast dyes, and sulfonamides are the most common drug-related causes of acute urticaria. Other common exposures that precipitate acute urticaria are latex, nuts, fish, eggs, and chocolate. With a careful history, the source of this acute skin finding usually can be identified. When chronic urticaria occurs, patient diaries are often helpful in determining the cause. An individual weal in acute urticaria typically lasts from 2 to 24 hours. It will not last more than 24 hours (7).

Physical urticaria represents 15% to 20% of all patients with chronic urticaria and is considered an IgE-mediated reaction to a host of known physical causes, such as cold, heat, elevated body temperature, pressure, vibration, ultraviolet rays, and even water on the skin. The weals of physical urticaria disappear within an hour except in patients with delayed-pressure urticaria, which take longer to develop and to fade. Angioedema without weals should raise suspicion for a C1 esterase inhibitor deficiency. The evaluation of these patients should focus on family history and the presence of abdominal pain. A complete blood count with differential is recommended in patients who are refractory to antihistamines to identify the presence of eosinophilia, an elevated ery-

TABLE 45 Clinical Classification of Urticaria and Angioedema
Ordinary Urticaria
Acute: up to 6 wk of continuous activity
Chronic: 6 wk or more of continuous activity
Episodic: intermittent
Physical Urticaria
Reproducibly induced by the same physical stimulus
Aquagenic urticaria
Cholinergic urticaria
Cold urticaria
Delayed pressure urticaria
Dermographism
Localized heat urticaria
Solar urticaria
Vibratory angioedema
Angioedema Without Weals
Contact Urticaria
Induced by biologic or chemical skin contact
Urticarial Vasculitis
Defined by vasculitis on skin biopsy

throcyte sedimentation rate possibly indicative of urticarial vasculitis, and serum thyroid-stimulating hormone measurement to identify possible thyroid dysfunction. Any weal persisting for more than 24 hours is suspicious for vasculitis and requires lesion biopsy for histologic confirmation. If biopsy results are positive for this disease, serum complement levels should also be measured (8).

Antihistamines (H_1-receptor antagonists) are the preferred treatment in patients with urticaria, demonstrating undisputed efficacy and safety. Patients should be offered the choice of at least two different H_1-receptor antagonists, because individual responses and tolerance to these drugs vary substantially. Frequently, antihistamine doses higher than the manufacturers' licensed recommended dose are required in the treatment of urticaria, with strong benefits of increased dosage outweighing the potential risks (9). Adding an H_2 antagonist to the treatment regimen can improve control of symptoms in some patients with urticaria. Combination medications with nonsedating daytime antihistamines and sedating antihistamines at night may help some patients. All antihistamines should be avoided during pregnancy, especially in the first and last trimesters. Clemastine, dexchlorpheniramine, and diphenhydramine are sedating antihistamines that are officially labeled category B drugs by the Food and Drug Administration, with only cetirizine and loratidine qualifying as nonsedating options. Epinephrine can be a life-saving agent in patients with anaphylaxis and severe laryngeal angioedema. Inhaled racemic epinephrine can also be helpful in this setting. Epinephrine is not considered effective for angioedema caused by C1 esterase inhibitory deficiency.

In patients with severe chronic urticaria, experimental therapies, such as cyclosporine, plasmapheresis, and intravenous immunoglobulin, have been used. The few studies on these agents in this setting have been small, uncontrolled, and unconfirmed. In general, only 25% of these patients experience long-term improvement. Systemic and topical corticosteroids have not been routinely beneficial in patients with severe chronic urticaria.

In the rare case of urticaria from C1 esterase inhibitory deficiency, treatment includes anabolic steroids, such as stanozolol and danazol.

KEY POINTS

- Penicillin, aspirin, NSAIDs, contrast dyes, and sulfonamides are the most common drug-related causes of acute urticaria.

- Antihistamines are the preferred treatment in patients with urticaria, demonstrating undisputed efficacy and safety.

- Frequently, antihistamine doses higher than the manufacturers' licensed recommended dose are required in patients with urticaria, with strong benefits of increased dosage outweighing the potential risks.

- Epinephrine can be a life-saving agent in patients with anaphylaxis and severe laryngeal angioedema.

Acne

There are four physiologic factors involved in acne vulgaris: 1) androgen-mediated stimulation of sebaceous gland activity; 2) abnormal keratinization leading to follicular plugging (that is, comedo formation); 3) proliferation of the bacterium *Propionibacterium acnes* in the follicle; and 4) inflammation.

Acne is almost universal at the age of puberty, although its severity and persistence into adulthood is variable. Genetic factors may contribute to the severity of acne, and family history is a risk factor for this condition. Evidence suggests that acne is exacerbated by emotional stress. There are no proven correlations between dirt or diet and acne.

Acne is a clinical diagnosis, based on the presentation of typical skin lesions. The evaluation of acne includes assessment of severity, possible exacerbating factors, and the potential for associated endocrine disease processes. Acne is classified by severity and type as comedonal-only acne, mild-to-moderate inflammatory acne, moderate-to-severe inflammatory acne, and severe papulnodular inflammatory acne (**Figure 5**). In patients with acne, a microcomedo may develop into visible open comedos ("blackheads") or closed comedones ("whiteheads"). Subsequent inflammatory papules, pustules, or nodules may develop. Nodulocystic acne consists of pustular lesions >0.5 cm.

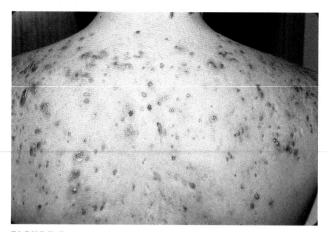

FIGURE 5.
Patient with severe acne vulgaris on the back.

Pustules and cysts are considered to be inflammatory acne. Acne lesions most commonly develop in areas that have a high concentration of sebaceous glands, including the face, neck, chest, upper arms, and back. Exacerbating factors for acne include mechanical obstructions, such as clothing, or medications, including anabolic steroids (for example, danazol and testosterone), corticosteroids, isoniazid, lithium, and dilantin. Endocrine causes of acne include diseases that lead to increased androgen exposure, including Cushing's disease, polycystic ovary syndrome, and congenital adrenal hyperplasia. The differential diagnosis of acne includes rosacea, perioral dermatitis, bacterial folliculitis, and drug-induced acneiform eruptions. The presence of comedones confirms the diagnosis of acne. Laboratory evaluation in patients with acne is required only in women who have a rapid onset of hyperandrogenism and virilization; the presence of an androgen-secreting ovarian or adrenal tumor can be ruled out in these patients when serum testosterone and dehydroepiandrosterone (DHEA)-S levels are normal. Women with acne and irregular menses, hirsutism, or obesity should be evaluated for polycystic ovary syndrome (10).

The approach to treatment of acne is dictated by its severity. Most acne treatment regimens require continuation of therapy for 6 to 8 weeks before efficacy is determined. For comedonal-only acne, topical retinoids are the mainstay of treatment. These agents are derivatives of vitamin A and prevent comedone formation by normalizing desquamation of follicular epithelium. Creams and lower-concentration formulations of retinoids are less irritating but may take longer to produce a response than gels and higher-concentration formulations. For mild-to-moderate–severity inflammatory acne (papules and pustules), topical antibiotics are the treatment of choice. Topical retinoids combined with topical antibiotics or benzoyl peroxide are more effective than topical antibiotics alone in these patients. For moderate-to-severe inflammatory acne, oral antibiotics are the treatment of choice, primarily the tetracyclines. Antibiotic-resistant strains of *P. acnes* have increased over the past few decades, are associated with treatment failures, and occur most commonly with the use of erythromycin and least commonly with the use of minocycline. Recommendations for reducing antibiotic resistance include using combined topical therapy, such as topical antibiotics, retinoids, and benzoyl peroxide, and avoidance of long-term use of topical or oral antibiotics (11).

Oral isotretinoin is indicated in patients with severe papulonodular acne, in those who have not responded to treatment, or in those with scarring or relapsing acne. A rare adverse effect of isotreninoin is acne fulminans, which requires treatment with systemic corticosteroids. Isotretinoin is a proven teratogen, and treatment in women of reproductive years requires documentation of contraception use and periodic pregnancy testing. It is strongly recommended that two negative pregnancy tests be obtained 1 week before oral isotretinoin therapy is initiated and monthly pregnancy tests be performed once therapy has begun. It is preferable that two methods of contraception be used, and contraception must be continued for at least 6 weeks after treatent is completed. Physicians in the United States must note on the prescription that patients meet the qualifications for isotretinoin therapy and have provided informed consent to use this treatment. Several oral contraceptives have Food and Drug Administration approval for treating acne in women, and androgen receptor blockers are an off-label-use treatment for acne in women (**Table 46**).

KEY POINTS

- **The presence of comedones confirms the diagnosis of acne.**
- **Laboratory evaluation in patients with acne is required only in women who have a rapid onset of hyperandrogenism and virilization to rule out polycystic ovary syndrome.**
- **For comedonal-only acne, topical retinoids are the mainstay of treatment.**
- **For mild-to-moderate–severity inflammatory acne, topical antibiotics are the treatment of choice.**
- **For moderate-to-severe inflammatory acne, oral antibiotics are the treatment of choice.**
- **Oral isotretinoin is indicated in patients with severe papulonodular acne, in those who have not responded to treatment, or in those with scarring or relapsing acne.**
- **Isotretinoin is a proven teratogen, and treatment in women of reproductive years requires documentation of contraception use and periodic pregnancy testing.**

Atopic Dermatitis

Atopic dermatitis, also known as atopic eczema, is a chronic inflammatory condition of the skin, often associated with other atopic diseases, including hay fever and asthma. Areas most affected include the creases of the skin and the hands.

The type of lesion in atopic dermatitis varies from vesicles (nonpustular fluid collections) to lichenification (thickening of the skin) on a background of poorly demarcated redness, with dry skin as an often-associated finding. An outbreak of skin lesions begins with itchy skin; patients often have a lower threshold for itching and response to irritants than those without this disorder. Factors that worsen the condition include allergens, irritants, climate/seasonal changes, infection, repeated washing/drying of skin, certain foods, and stress. Bath and shower oils advertised for treatment of dry skin can worsen atopic dermatitis (12).

The differential diagnosis for atopic dermatitis includes seborrheic dermatitis, contact dermatitis, dyshidrotic dermatitis (involving the palms and soles), nummular dermatitis (involving the trunk and lower extremities), and drug reactions. Emollients are an important first-line treatment for this condition in reducing dry skin. They work through various mechanisms, including by trapping water in the skin (petrolatum), introducing water into the skin (aqueous cream), or increasing the water-holding capacity of the skin (urea) (13). The patient can choose the emollient that works the best, because one type is not better than another type. Emollients may reduce the need for topical corticosteroids or augment the effect that corticosteroids have on the skin (see also Reference 13). Other treatments for atopic dermatitis include avoiding triggers, such as low humidity, perspiration, and heat; limiting bathing and washing, or applying emollients immediately after bathing; using 100% cotton clothing; avoiding fabric softeners; and using stress-management techniques. Pharmacologic treatments for atopic dermatitis are outlined in **Table 47**.

As indicated in Table 47, tacrolimus and pimecrolimus are indicated in patients with at least moderate dermatitis who are not responsive to or tolerant of topical corticosteroids. In March 2005, the Food and Drug Administration released an alert stating that a potential connection existed between the use of these medications and lymphomas and skin cancers based on case reports and studies in animals; therefore, these medications should be used only for short-term and intermittent treatment (14).

KEY POINTS

- **The differential diagnosis for atopic dermatitis includes seborrheic dermatitis, contact dermatitis, dyshidrotic dermatitis (involving the palms and soles), nummular dermatitis (involving the trunk and lower extremities), and drug reactions.**
- **Emollients are an important first-line treatment for atopic dermatitis.**
- **Tacrolimus and pimecrolimus have been associated with lymphomas and skin cancers in case reports and animal studies and should be used for short-term and intermittent treatment only.**

TABLE 46 Medications for Acne

Medication	Form or Dose	Indication	Adverse Effects/Notes
Retinoids Tretinoin Adapalene Tazarotene	Topical	Comedones only	Reduce the number of comedones and inflammatory lesions from 40% to 70% Irritation that occurs early in therapy Adapalene is less likely to cause skin irritation and is better tolerated than tretinoin or tazarotene Topical tretinoin is not teratogenic May be combined with topical antibiotics
Tetracycline Doxycycline Minocycline Erythromycin	250 mg BID to QID orally 50 to 100 mg/day to BID orally 50 to 100 mg/d to BID 150 mg BID to QID orally	Moderate to severe inflammatory acne	Adverse effects of oral tetracycline are gastrointestinal tract dyspepsia, vaginal candidiasis in women, photosensitivity Doxycycline causes gastrointestinal symptoms and photosensitivity Adverse effects of minocycline include vertigo, dizziness, ataxia, and, rarely, a bluish discoloration. Has also been associated with drug-induced lupus, autoimmune hepatitis, and a hypersensitivity syndrome
Isotretinoin	0.5 to 1 mg/kg/d	Severe nodular acne and acne unresponsive to other therapy	Used as a single therapy except in women who are on oral contraceptives Most common adverse effects are cheilitis, teratogenicity, hypertriglyceridemia, elevated liver chemistry values, and elevated cholesterol Proven teratogen. Use necessitates contraception during and 6 weeks after therapy, baseline and monthly pregnancy tests. Prescription must identify the above and patient must sign consent
Oral contraceptives (OCs)	Ethinyl estradiol and norethindrone	Women with acne	Contraindications to OCs include smoking, migraine headaches with aura, and hypertension Can be used with other standard therapies as listed in this table

Note: For women with acne, androgen receptor blockers (flutamide and spironolactone) are an off-label medication.

BID = twice daily; QID = four times daily.

Contact Dermatitis

Contact dermatitis is the result of an irritant (80%) or allergic reaction. In irritant dermatitis, any substance that damages the outer skin layer can cause skin irritation and result in either mild dryness and erythema or an eczematous reaction that is erythematous, scaly, or vesicular; repeated lip licking is an example of irritant contact dermatitis. Allergic contact dermatitis develops when the repeated, direct contact of the offending substance causes a type-IV hypersensitivity reaction that develops over 10 to 14 days. Re-exposure to the antigen then causes an eczematous reaction within 12 to 48 hours. The most common cause of allergic contact dermatitis is urushiol, a plant resin found in poison oak, poison ivy, and poison sumac, and only a few exposures can cause the reaction. Contrary to popular belief, vesicles from active lesions do not cause spread of the dermatitis. Other common, but less-potent, sensitizers include nickel from jewelry, formaldehyde from clothes and nail polish, preservatives in skin products, fragrances, topical medications (including topical corticosteroids, neomycin, bacitracin, and benzocaine), and latex. The shape and location of the rash can help identify the offending substance in patients with contact dermatitis, but allergens may spread to other sites by inadvertent contact, such as in eyelid dermatitis caused by nail polish. The scalp, palms, and soles are often resistant to allergic contact dermatitis. A combination of sun exposure and allergens spread through the air, such as ragweed, can cause a rash on the face and exposed areas of the skin.

Treatment of allergic contact dermatitis includes minimizing the use of topical products; avoiding treatments with common skin sensitizers, such as paraben, lanolin, and fragrance; and, if topical corticosteroids are needed, use of topical ointments instead of creams. Pimecrolimus and tacrolimus are costly alternatives (off-label uses), and topical tacrolimus has been shown to help reduce nickel-induced allergic dermatitis (15). In March 2005, the Food and Drug Administration released an alert stating that a potential connection existed between the use of these medications and lymphomas and skin cancers based on case reports and studies in animals; therefore, the use of these medications is recommended for short-term and intermittent treatment only (see also Reference 14). Specific treatment for poison ivy dermatitis has not been well studied, but clinical experience shows that cold compresses and cool baths with or without colloidal oatmeal can be helpful. High-potency topical corticosteroids do not penetrate blisters but reduce erythema in patients with poison ivy dermatitis; low-potency corticosteroids are of limited benefit in these patients. Pimecrolimus was not found to be efficacious in the treatment of poison ivy dermatitis when compared with a placebo cream

TABLE 47 Treatment of Atopic Dermatitis

Intervention	Use	Recommendations	Anticipated Benefits	Potential Harms	Comments
Topical corticosteroids	First-line treatment after emollients; moderate-to-severe dermatitis	Use lowest effective potency; use only mild preparations on face, neck, intertriginous areas; once daily is probably aseffective as twice daily	Reduced itching and improvements in sleep and the appearance of the skin	Short-term: stinging on application (for potentpreparations); long-term: skin changes, systemic effects	Optimal methods of use are unclear
Topical tacrolimus and pimecrolimus	Second-line treatment; moderate-to-severe dermatitis unrespon-sive to or intolerant of topical steroids	Use twice daily until symptoms resolve, then intermittently	Reduced itching and improvements in sleep and the appearance of the skin	Stinging and burning on application (tacrolimus, 43%; pimecrolimus, 17%). Potential skin cancer and lymphoma risk	Studies have shown reduced need for topical corticosteroids and less flares of dermatitis†; fairly costly
Oral antihistamines	Adjunctive therapy	Unclear	Possible reduced itching and improved sleep	Drowsiness	Unclear benefit
Refined coal tar	Mild-to-moderate dermatitis	Twice daily	Reduced itching, redness, and lichenification	Itching and stinging (17%); odor; staining clothes and skin	Data limited
Topical doxepin	Adjunctive	Thin layer 3 to 4 times/d (maximum 12 g/d)	Reduced itching (short-term)	Drowsiness, stinging, and burning	Evidence of short-term (24- to 48-h) relief
Oral corticosteroids	Severe flare	Intermittent use only	Reduced itching, skin redness, infiltration, oozing		No randomized trials; optimal dose unknown; can use prednisolone 0.5 mg/kg, tapered over 2 to 3 wk, with specialist support

Adapted from Williams HC. Atopic dermatitis. NEJM. 2005;352:2314-24.

†Data from Luger TA, Lahfa M, Folster-Holst R, et al. Long-term safety and tolerability of pimecrolimus cream 1% and topical corticosteroids in adults with moderate to severe atopic dermati-tis. J Dermatolog Treat. 2004 Jun;15(3):169-78; and Meurer M, Folster-Holst R, Wozel G, et al. for the CASM-DE-01 study group. Pimecrolimus cream in the long-term management of atopic dermatitis in adults: a six-month study. Dermatology. 2002;205(3):271-7.

(16). Patients with severe poison ivy dermatitis can be treated with oral prednisone (maximum 60 mg/day), with a tapered dose administered over 2 to 3 weeks.

KEY POINTS

- **The most common cause of allergic contact dermatitis is urushiol, a plant resin found in poison oak, poison ivy, and poison sumac, and only a few exposures are needed to cause the reaction.**

- **Treatment of allergic contact dermatitis includes mini-mizing the use of topical products, avoiding treat-ments with common skin sensitizers, and using topical ointments versus creams.**

Psoriasis

Psoriasis is thought to have a primary T-lymphocytic–based immunopathogenesis. Histologically, psoriasis is character-ized by marked keratinocyte hyperproliferation, a dense inflammatory infiltrate consisting of T-cells and neutrophils, and vascular dilatation and proliferation.

Psoriasis is a common disorder, affecting 2% to 3% of the U.S. population. The median age of onset is 28 years, with a biphasic distribution of age of onset. Evidence suggests a genetic predisposition to psoriasis. Psoriasis is more common in the northern latitudes and in those with a family history of this disorder. In the United States, this disease is less common among blacks than in the remainder of the population (17, 18).

The diagnosis of psoriasis is established primarily based on clinical presentation. The differential diagnosis includes seborrhoeic dermatitis, lichen simplex chronicus, tinea cor-poris, lichen planus, and subacute cutaneous lupus erythe-matosus. The most common form of psoriasis is plaque pso-riasis, occurring in more than 80% of cases. The skin lesions of this disorder are sharply demarcated erythematous plaques (**Figure 6**) covered by silvery-white scales that affect the scalp and extensor surfaces (elbows and knees) as well as nails. Inverse psoriasis is characterized by the presence of lesions in

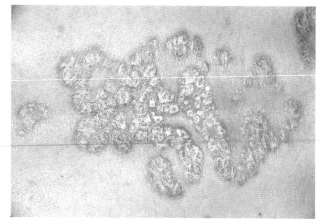

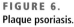

FIGURE 6.
Plaque psoriasis.

flexural sites, such as the axillae and antecubital fossae. Guttate psoriasis is manifested by the sudden development of erythematous scaling papules on the trunk and extremities, usually affecting children and young adults, and often developing after infection with β-hemolytic streptococcus (**Figure 7**). Erythrodermic psoriasis is characterized by generalized inflammation, erythema, and widespread scaling of the skin, affecting up to 100% of the body surface. Generalized pustular psoriasis of von Zumbusch is characterized by sterile pustules over large portions of the trunk. Erythrodermic psoriasis and generalized pustular psoriasis are rare and severe variants of psoriasis in which the skin can lose its protective function, causing susceptibility to infection and sepsis. Patients receiving systemic corticosteroids or cyclosporine are at risk for acute erythrodermic or pustular flares with sudden cessation of medication. An inflammatory, seronegative spondlyoarthropathy, psoriatic arthritis, can occur in up to 25% of patients with psoriatic skin lesions (**Figure 8**). Inflammatory bowel disease—ulcerative colitis and Crohn's disease—occurs more commonly in patients with psoriasis (19).

Patients with mild or limited psoriasis are treated with mid- to high-potency topical corticosteroids, topical vitamin D_3 analogues (calcipotriol or tacalcitol), and a topical retinoid (tazarotene). Topical corticosteroids are the most commonly used treatment in the United States. Therapy should be initiated with a medium-strength agent (classes 3, 4, and 5). Low-potency agents (classes 6 and 7) are used for the face, groin, and axillary areas. High-potency agents (classes 1 and 2) are used for treatment of thick, chronic plaques. Adverse effects of topical corticosteroids include cutaneous atrophy, telangiectasias, and striae. Vitamin D analogues are less effective than topical corticosteroids in the treatment of psoriasis and cause local irritation, but they are not associated with cutaneous atrophy and may be used in conjunction with topical corticosteroids. Topical retinoids can cause local irritation. For moderate-to-severe psoriasis, phototherapy and/or systemic medications may be helpful.

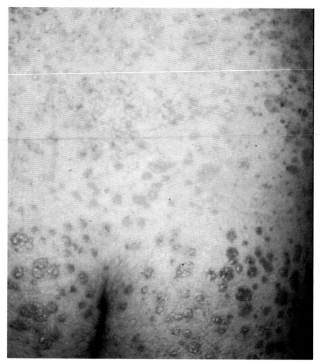

FIGURE 7.
Guttate psoriasis characterized by numerous erythematous scaling papules.

Reprinted from The Lancet, Vol. 361. Lebwohl M. Psoriasis. Lancet 2003;361:1197-204. Copyright © 2003, reprinted with permission from Elsevier.

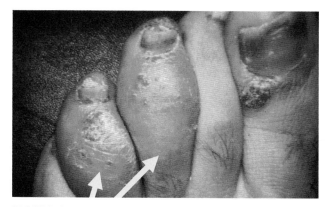

FIGURE 8.
Small joint polyarthritis with typical psoriac skin lesions and nail pitting.

©1972–2004 American College of Rheumatology Clinical Slide Collection. Used with permission.

Systemic therapies include those that target keratinocyte function, are immunosuppressive, or are immune-response modifiers (**Table 48**). Traditional phototherapy includes broad-band and narrow-band ultraviolet B (UVB) therapy; narrow-band UVB therapy has been found to be more effective than broad-band UVB therapy. Photochemotherapy (PUVA) involves ingestion of oral psoralen followed by irradiation with ultraviolet A. PUVA is highly effective in the

TABLE 48 Options for Psoriasis Treatment

Mild or Limited Disease

Topical Corticosteroids
Low potency
  Desonide
  Alclometasone dipropionate
Medium potency
  Triamcinolone acetonide
  Hydrocortisone valerate
  Fluticasone propionate
  Halcinonide
High potency
  Halobetasol propionate
  Betamethasone dipropionate

Topical Vitamin D Analogues
Calcipotriol
Calcitriol
Tacalcitol

Topical Retinoids
Tazarotene

Moderate to Severe Disease

Targeting Keratinocyte Functions
Methotrexate
Acitretin (retinoid)

Phototherapy
Broadband UVB
Narrowband UVB
Photochemotherapy (PUVA)

Climatotherapy
Sunlight
Exposure to long-wave UVB rays

Immunosuppressive Therapy
Fumarates
Cyclosporin

Immune Response Modifiers
Alefacept
Efalizumab
Etanercept

UVB = ultraviolet B; PUVA = psoralen followed by ultraviolet A radiation therapy.

treatment of psoriasis but is associated with squamous cell carcinoma. A number of systemic oral therapies are available for patients with psoriasis. Methotrexate is highly effective in these patients but is associated with the short-term side effects of nausea, aphthous stomatitis, and bone marrow toxicity and the long-term side effects of hepatic fibrosis. Systemic retinoids are moderately effective in treating psoriasis and are associated with mucocutaneous side effects; they are also teratogenic, and their use is limited in women of childbearing age.

Cyclosporin is effective in the treatment of psoriasis, but long-term use of this drug is associated with nephrotoxicity. Newer biologically targeted treatments of psoriasis in the category of immune response modifiers have also received Food and Drug Administration approval (see Table 48).

Psoriasis has a chronic and fluctuating course. Factors that can exacerbate this disease include infection, particularly streptococcal infections of the upper respiratory tract; injury to the skin; and medication (lithium and β-blockers). Psoriasis may have an adverse effect on quality of life.

KEY POINT

- Patients with mild or limited psoriasis are treated with mid- to high-potency topical corticosteroids, topical vitamin D_3 analogues, and a topical retinoid.

Papulosquamous Disorders

Patients are evaluated for four common papulosquamous disorders in primary care settings: 1) pityriasis versicolor (also called tinea versicolor), 2) seborrheic dermatitis, 3) rosacea, and 4) lichen planus. The lipophilic yeasts of the *Malassezia* species are associated with the skin disorders of pityriasis versicolor and seborrheic dermatitis. Rosacea is a chronic skin condition of unknown origin. Lichen planus is an inflammatory mucocutaneous condition caused by a cell-mediated immune response.

Pityriasis versicolor is a chronic, benign skin condition, characterized by scaly, hypo- or hyperpigmented macules, primarily affecting lipid-rich areas of the body, including the upper trunk, neck, or upper arms (20). The lesions may coalesce to cover large areas of the body surface. The condition is usually asymptomatic, and the primary concerns are cosmetic. It affects primarily young adults and occurs more frequently in the tropics and in the summer months. Options for treatment include the keratolytic agents selenium sulfide and propylene glycol and topical and oral antifungal agents, such as ketoconazole, itraconazole, and fluconazole. Itraconazole is the most costly of these treatments. Treatment is usually effective, but discolored areas can persist for months. Itraconazole is also effective in prophylactic treatment of pityriasis versicolor.

Seborrheic dermatitis is a chronic, benign skin condition, characterized by red, flaking patches located most commonly on the scalp, nasolabial folds, eyebrows, ears, and chest. It affects 1% to 3% of the adult population in the United States. Some experts consider dandruff to be a severe form of scalp seborrheic dermatitis.

Seborrheic dermatitis is more common in men, in patients with HIV or AIDS, or in those whose health is otherwise immunocompromised than in those without these characteristics. It has a bimodal distribution and most commonly occurs in adolescents, young adults, and in patients older than 50 years. Exacerbations are more frequent and severe in the winter. Options for treatment of seborrheic dermatitis include topical agents with keratolytic activity (selenium sulfide and propylene glycol), topical corticosteroids for short-term use, topical antifungal agents, and oral antifungal agents. Topical agents are considered first-line therapy for patients with seborrheic dermatitis. Classes of antifungal agents used for the treatment of this disorder include the azoles (ketoconazole and itraconazole) and allylamines (terbinafine). A newer class of topical medications, the noncorticosteroid topical immunomodulators tacrolimus and pimecrolimus, are off-label treatments for seborrheic dermatitis, but these agents are associated with safety concerns (see Contact Dermatitis section for discussion of these agents). Long-term prophylaxis may be required with the use of topical or oral antifungal therapy.

Rosacea is a common chronic, benign skin condition affecting the face and characterized by flushing, redness, papules, pustules, and dilated blood vessels (**Figure 9**). Ocular changes, usually manifested as nonspecific symptoms such as burning of the eyes, are present in 50% of patients. Rosacea is more common in women, those with a family history of this condition, and in whites of Celtic origin (21). The typical age of onset of this condition is between 30 and 50 years. The diagnosis of rosacea is established clinically, and its course is chronic, with flares and relapses. Heat, sunlight, ingestion of hot liquids, alcohol ingestion, and hot/spicy foods can precipitate flares of rosacea. The four subtypes of this disease are erythematotelangiectatic (flushing), papulopustular, phymatous, and ocular. The goals of treatment are to modify exacerbating factors, decrease facial erythema, reduce the number of papules, and maintain remission. Nonpharmacologic treatment includes protection from ultraviolet light with sunscreen and sun-avoidance strategies. In milder disease, topical therapy is used. A recent Cochrane review found evidence that topical metronidazole and azelaic acid cream in addition to oral metronidazole and tetracycline are effective treatments in patients with rosacea (22). In mild disease, topical therapy is used. In moderate-to-severe disease, a combination of topical therapy and oral antibiotics (tetracyclines or erythromycin) is indicated. Among the topical agents that have received approval from the Food and Drug Administration for treatment of rosacea are metronidazole 0.75%, sulfacetamide 10%/sulfur 5%, and azelaic acid 15% gel. Light-based therapies have also received Food and Drug Administration approval for rosacea treatment. Agents under investigation for treatment of this disorder include the nonsteroidal immunomodulators tacrolimus and pimecronlimus, topical retinoid therapy, and subantimicrobial doses of doxycyline. Retinoid therapy is appropriate for phymatous changes in the early stages of this disease; however, dermatosurgical intervention is the only effective treatment for advanced rosacea.

Patients with lichen planus typically have violaceous polygonal flat-topped papules and plaques (**Figure 10**); pruritis in these patients may be severe. Most cases of lichen planus are idiopathic, but some may be caused by medications, such as gold, antimalarial agents, penicillamine, thiazide diuretics, β-blockers, nonsteroidal anti-inflammatory drugs, quinidine, and ACE inhibitors. Lichen planus occurs most commonly in women and blacks. The usual age of onset is between 30 and 50 years. A skin biopsy can establish the diagnosis of lichen planus. Patients with oral lichen planus have a 50-fold increased risk for oral cancer. Treatment options for this disorder include topical steroids, antihistamines, corticosteroids, cyclosporine, PUVA (photochemotherapy involving ingestion of oral psoralen followed by irradiation with ultraviolet A), systemic corticosteroids, systemic retinoids, and interferon alfa 2a or 2b. An evidence-based analysis of lichen planus treatment concluded that the retinoid acitretin is first-line therapy in patients with cutaneous lichen planus, and topical corticosteroids are first-line therapy in patients with mucosal erosive lichen planus (23).

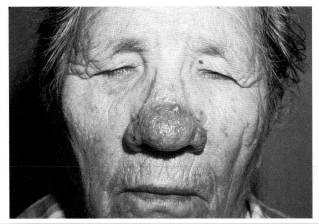

FIGURE 9.
Patient with rosacea, with involvement of the nose and central face and characterized by hyperplastic sebaceous glands, erythema, and pustules. The enlargement of the nose is termed rhinophyma.

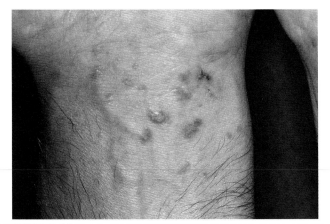

FIGURE 10.
Lichen planus, consisting of purple, polygonal papules on glabrous skin.

- Pityriasis versicolor is characterized by scaly, hypo- or hyperpigmented macules, primarily affecting lipid-rich areas of the body, including the upper trunk, neck, or upper arms.
- Seborrheic dermatitis is characterized by red, flaking patches, located most commonly on the scalp, nasolabial folds, eyebrows, ears, and chest.
- Rosacea affects the face and is characterized by flushing, redness, papules, pustules, and dilated blood vessels; it is more common in whites of Celtic origin.
- Flares of rosacea can be precipitated by heat, sunlight, ingestion of hot liquids, alcohol ingestion, and hot/spicy foods.
- Patients with lichen planus typically have violaceous polygonal flat-topped papules, plaques and pruritis.
- A skin biopsy is indicated to establish the diagnosis of lichen planus.
- Patients with oral lichen planus have a 50-fold increased risk for oral cancer.
- Acitretin is first-line therapy in patients with cutaneous lichen planus, and topical corticosteroids are first-line therapy in patients with mucosal erosive lichen planus.

Bacterial Infections

The most common skin infections observed in the outpatient setting include cellulitis, folliculitis, and impetigo. Increasingly more of these infections are caused by community-acquired methicillin-resistant *Staphylococcus aureus* (MRSA), especially in patients who have had close recent contact with persons having a history of a similar infection, including household members, athletic teams, prison inmates, and military personnel. Practitioners should obtain cultures whenever possible and consider MRSA as a cause for these infections, particularly in patients in whom the infection is not improving as expected (24).

Cellulitis is an infection of the dermis and subcutaneous tissues, marked by warmth, erythema, and advancing borders. Erysipelas is a specific type of cellulitis that does not involve the subcutaneous tissues, and, unlike cellulitis, is well demarcated and often associated with marked swelling of the skin. Cellulitis commonly occurs at breaks in the skin, including those caused by tinea infections, trauma, ulcerations, or wounds. Other risk factors for cellulitis include lymphedema, edema, or venous insufficiency. No part of the body is spared from cellulitis, but the legs and digits are the most commonly areas affected. The differential diagnosis for cellulitis primarily includes deep venous thrombosis, but other noninfectious causes for this condition, such as contact dermatitis, insect bites, or drug or foreign-body reactions, are also possible.

Other infectious differential diagnoses of cellulitis include septic arthritis and osteomyelitis. In otherwise-healthy patients, the most common infectious organisms responsible for cellulitis are *S. aureus* or β-hemolytic streptococci. Initial empiric treatment of cellulitis depends on whether MRSA infection is suspected. In patients in whom the suspicion for MRSA is not high, a penicillinase-resistant penicillin, first-generation cephalosporin, macrolide, or fluoroquinolone, is usually effective. In patients in whom MRSA is suspected, empiric therapy with trimethoprim-sulfamethoxazole, clindamycin, doxycycline, or minocycline is appropriate. The usual course of treatment for cellulitis is 14 days, but therapy should be continued for 3 days after acute inflammation has ceased. Patients with this skin condition who have diabetes, are immunocompromised, or have signs of systemic toxicity should be treated with parenteral cefazolin, nafcillin, clindamycin, or vancomycin. Certain measures can help to prevent recurrences of cellulitis, including use of protective clothing if cuts and abrasions occur in the area where the cellulitis occurred, treatment of tinea pedis infections, and use of prophylactic antibiotics, such as erythromycin, clindamycin, or penicillin, in patients in whom more than two episodes of cellulitis occur per year. For patients with foot lymphedema, careful hygiene and prophylactic penicillin can prevent recurrent cellulitis. This prophylactic approach might also be effective in patients with arm lymphedema, but quality studies in this area are sparse (25).

Folliculitis is a superficial or deep infection or inflammation limited to the hair follicles. Superficial folliculitis, in which a hair is often visible in the center, may be tender or painless, and heals without scarring. Factors that contribute to the onset of folliculitis include *S. aureus* nasal carriage, treatment with antibiotics or corticosteroids that are predisposing to candidal folliculitis, and exposure to a hot tub or whirlpool with inadequate levels of chlorine ("hot tub" folliculitis caused by *Pseudomonas aeruginosa*). These lesions usually resolve spontaneously, but topical antibiotics or benzoyl peroxide can also be used. In patients with frequent episodes of folliculitis, monthly nasal mupirocin (off-label use) twice daily for 5 days can reduce recurrences. A furuncle is a manifestation of deep folliculitis, sometimes without a pustule on the surface, which causes follicular swelling and erythema. *S. aureus* is the most likely causative organism of this infection, and application of warm compresses to promote drainage is usually effective in these patients. Oral antibiotics, including first-generation cephalosporins, penicillinase-resistant penicillins, macrolides, and fluoroquinolones, also can be used to treat furuncles, with adjustment in type of empiric antibiotic depending on whether the presence of MRSA infection is suspected. If treatment of folliculitis is not effective, surgical drainage and analysis of a culture of the lesions for the presence of MRSA are indicated.

Impetigo is a superficial vesiculopustular infection that usually occurs on the face and exposed extremities. It often occurs in warm, humid environments, and poor personal hygiene can promote its spread among family members. The classic appearance of impetigo consists of groups of vesicles or pustules that have an oozing or adherent yellow crust, often occurring at the site of prior breaks in the skin. This condition can rarely present as erosions, a cluster of erosions, or bullous lesions (the latter more common in infants). The most likely causative organism of impetigo is Group A Streptococcus or *S. aureus*. A recent review found that topical mupirocin or fusidic acid is equally effective as or more effective than oral antibiotics in patients with limited impetigo (26). For treatment of extensive impetigo, it is unclear whether systemic antibiotics are superior to topical agents. Penicillin is less effective than other antibiotics, and local resistance patterns and the suspicion of MRSA infection are treatment considerations.

KEY POINTS

- Cultures should be obtained whenever possible and methicillin-resistant *Staphylococcus aureus* (MRSA) infection considered as a causative organism in patients with cellulitis, folliculitis, and impetigo.

- Cellulitis occurs commonly at breaks in the skin, including those caused by tinea infections, trauma, ulcerations, or wounds.

- When MRSA infection is suspected, empiric therapy with trimethoprim–sulfamethoxazole, clindamycin, doxycycline, or minocycline is appropriate.

- Factors that contribute to the onset of folliculitis include *S. aureus* nasal carriage, antibiotic or corticosteroid treatment that might predispose a patient to candidal folliculitis, and exposure to a hot tub or whirlpool with inadequate levels of chlorine.

- Application of warm compresses to promote drainage is usually effective in patients with furuncles, a manifestation of deep folliculitis.

- Impetigo is characterized by groups of vesicles or pustules usually occurring on the face and exposed extremities, often at the site of prior breaks, with an oozing or adherent yellow crust.

- Topical mupirocin or fusidic acid are effective as or more effective than oral antibiotics in patients with limited impetigo.

Herpes Zoster

Herpes zoster infection is the reactivation of the varicella virus in a single cutaneous nerve that coincides with emotional stress, fatigue, immunosuppressive drugs, radiation, or lymphoma. This infection travels along the nerve from its dormant location in the dorsal root ganglion to the skin. There is a 10% to 20% lifetime occurrence of herpes zoster infection in those who have had chickenpox, and the incidence increases with age. Patients with herpes zoster infection may have pain and constitutional symptoms first, with continuation of pain possible for several months after the lesions resolve, especially in the elderly. Virus can be cultured from the lesions that develop over several weeks, first from swollen plaques, then from purulent vesicles, and finally from crusted lesions. Some patients with this infection also have a viremia in which 20 to 30 scattered vesicles may appear, distant to the involved dermatome. Herpes zoster lesions occurring on the eye, eyelid, and forehead indicate cranial nerve V involvement (herpes ophthalmicus) (**Figure 11**). Corneal ulceration and scarring can occur in this setting, and referral to an ophthalmologist is recommended. Vesicles occurring on either the tip or side of the nose (Hutchinson's sign) in the setting of herpes ophthalmicus are more likely indicative of infection in the deep structures of the eye, because this sign indicates nasociliary nerve-branch involvement. The Ramsay-Hunt syndrome is characterized by otologic zoster, a polycranial neuropathy involving several cranial nerves in which the virus is dormant in the geniculate ganglion. Findings of this syndrome include vesicles in the auditory canal and on the ear, ear pain, and facial paralysis. The differential diagnosis for zoster includes herpes simplex, contact dermatitis, or cellulitis, and pain is less likely with the latter two disorders. Herpes simplex infection

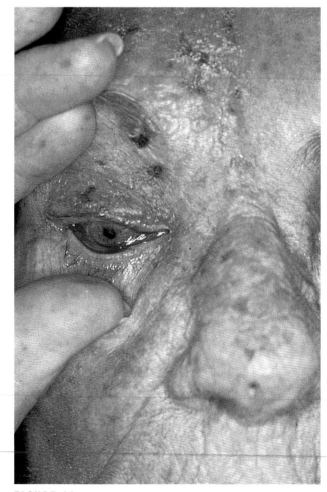

FIGURE 11.
Herpes zoster affecting the ophthalmic branch of the trigeminal nerve.

is the obvious diagnosis in patients with a recurring rash, but this rash is not usually dermatomal. Bell's palsy is a common presentation of either herpes simplex or herpes zoster without rash.

Nonmedical treatment for zoster includes the application of cold compresses to suppress bacterial growth and remove crust. Acyclovir, famciclovir, or valacyclovir can decrease pain, vesicle formation, and viral shedding in patients with herpes zoster if administered within the first 72 hours after onset, and this is essential treatment for reducing ocular involvement. Early treatment with oral corticosteroids can speed healing and resolve acute neuralgia in these patients.

Postherpetic neuralgia, in which pain is present after the rash begins healing, occurs in approximately 9% to 34% of patients with herpes zoster, and the incidence increases with age. Spontaneous resolution of postherpetic neuralgia is common, particularly in the first 6 months after presentation; however, medical treatment may be indicated for pain that interferes with functioning or sleep. Although acute treatment of zoster with antiviral agents can reduce its incidence, acute treatment with prednisone does not have this effect. Tricyclic antidepressants (off-label use) can reduce severity, duration, and prevalence of postherpetic neuralgia, especially when initiated early in the course of the illness, but side effects can limit their use. Several studies have demonstrated decreased pain and improved sleep in patients with postherpetic neuralgia who took gabapentin (27). Most studies evaluating other treatments for postherpetic neuralgia, including opioids, lidocaine patch, and capsaicin, are small; heterogeneous, better-constructed trials are needed in this area (see also Reference 27). One study reported that immunization of immunocompetent adults older than age 60 years reduces the incidence and severity of zoster and postherpetic neuralgia during an average follow-up period of 3 years (28).

KEY POINTS

- There is a 10% to 20% lifetime incidence of herpes zoster in those who have had chickenpox, and the incidence increases with age.

- Herpes zoster lesions occurring on the eye, eyelid, and forehead indicate cranial nerve V involvement (herpes ophthalmicus).

- Vesicles occurring on either the tip or side of the nose (Hutchinson's sign) in the setting of herpes ophthalmicus are more likely indicative of infection in the deep structures of the eye.

- Acyclovir, famciclovir, or valacyclovir can decrease pain, vesicle formation, and viral shedding in patients with herpes zoster if administered within the first 72 hours after onset and is essential treatment for reducing ocular involvement.

- Several studies have demonstrated decreased pain and improved sleep in patients with postherpetic neuralgia who took gabapentin.

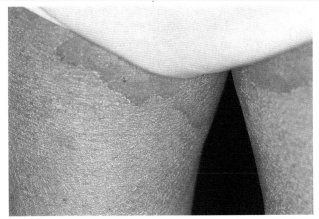

FIGURE 12.
Tinea cruris.

Superficial Fungal Infections

Superficial fungal infections, or tinea, are classified by body part. These dermatophytes, or ringworm fungi, can only survive in dead keratin of the skin, hair, and nails and not on mucosal surfaces. Superficial skin infection is the rule in patients with superficial fungal infections, except in immunocompromised patients in whom deep skin infections can occur. Genetic susceptibility may predispose a patient to these infections, and they are not usually transmitted to spouses.

Typically, the lesion in superficial fungal infections has an active border of infection and inflammation, sometimes with vesicles and scale. The presence of fungi and diagnosis can be confirmed by evaluation of potassium hydroxide (KOH) slide preparation. Tinea pedis (of the feet) is characterized by the classic ringworm pattern, maceration between the toe nails, or coverage of the entire sole (or palm) with a fine, silvery white scale ("moccasin ringworm" if on the feet). Pitted keratolysis can mimic tinea pedis, although this disorder is caused by a bacterial infection in the setting of hyperhidrosis. It differs from tinea pedis by its circular or longitudinal pits limited mostly to the weight-bearing portions of the feet. Tinea cruris (of the groin) (**Figure 12**) usually begins unilaterally and occurs more commonly in men than in women. The differential diagnosis of tinea cruris includes intertrigo, a mixture of bacterial and fungal infection in the moist folds of the skin; and erythrasma, a superficial bacterial infection that does not have an advancing border and is usually uniformly brown and scaly. Tinea corporis ("ringworm") involves the face, trunk, and extremities, and the size and degree of inflammation can vary. Pityriasis rosea is the most important differential diagnosis of tinea corporis, but the scaly skin of the pityriasis lesion is not located at the advancing border as it is in tinea corporis. Tinea barbae (of the beard) often is accompanied by folliculitis and pseudofolliculitis (ingrown hairs).

Treatment of any of the tinea infections requires topical creams twice daily for at least 2 weeks, with continuation of therapy at least 1 week after resolution of the lesions. For more refractory cases and tinea barbae, oral agents should be used. Griseofulvin, terbinafine, or itraconazole (off-label use) are treatment options in patients with tinea barbae, with careful monitoring of liver function necessary in patients with pre-existing hepatic impairment or in whom prolonged treatment is required.

The four main patterns of onychomycosis or nail infection include distal nail-bed thickening and subungual debris; superficial invasion of the nail bed without thickening; infection throughout the nail bed beginning from the cuticle and developing outward, with transverse white bands and separation of the nail from the bed; and candidal infection of all nails in a patient with mucocutaneous candidiasis. Psoriasis is the most common disease confused with onychomycosis.

Treatment of onychomycosis is recommended in patients with peripheral vascular disease or diabetes mellitus to prevent development of cellulitis (29). Patients may also seek treatment of onychomycosis for cosmetic reasons. The Food and Drug Administration has approved griseofulvin, terbinafine, and itraconazole for treatment of this condition, and the latter two can be given in a pulse-dosing regimen. Mycologic cure rates are 55% to 60% for griseofulvin; 76% to 78% for terbinafine; and 59% to 63% for continuous itraconazole and 63% to 75% for pulse-dosed itraconazole over approximately 1 year (30). Clinical cure rates (defined by the nail appearance) can be somewhat lower than mycologic cure rates, because a nail may not always return to its normal appearance after treatment. Ciclopirox is a topical lacquer approved for treatment of onychomycosis. Cure rate with the use of this agent is low (approximately 14%), and recurrence after discontinuation of treatment is common, but topical treatment is recommended as initial therapy when superficial invasion of the nail bed is noted without nail thickening.

KEY POINTS

- Treatment of any of the tinea infections requires administration of topical creams twice daily for at least 2 weeks, with continuation of therapy at least 1 week after resolution of the lesions.
- Griseofulvin, terbinafine, or itraconazole are treatment options in patients with tinea barbae, with careful monitoring of liver function necessary in patients with pre-existing hepatic impairment or with prolonged treatment.
- Treatment of onychomycosis is recommended in patients with peripheral vascular disease or diabetes to prevent development of cellulitis.

Head Lice and Scabies

Pediculosis (head lice) and scabies are closely related conditions caused by arthropods. They are transmitted by person-to-person contact, require similar treatment, and necessitate similar environmental measures. Pediculus humanus capitis (head louse) is a human parasite transmitted by person-to-person contact. Pruritis is the primary symptom of this disorder; excoriations and pyoderma may also occur. The diagnosis of head lice is established by identifying crawling lice in the scalp or hair. Lice egg cases are called *nits* and are found sticking to the hair shaft in patients with lice. Nits are generally easier to see than lice because they are often found in the occipital or retroauricular portions of the scalp (31, 32).

Patients with scabies, an infection of the parasitic mite *Sarcoptes scabiei*, have a pruritic, papular rash with excoriations. In patients with scabies, burrows are more common on the hands and wrists, and papular or nodular lesions are more common in the groin, waist, antecubital fossa, and axillae. The head and neck are usually spared in these patients. A history of pruritis (especially at night), a classic rash, and pruritis in household or sexual contacts are adequate for establishing a diagnosis (**Figure 13**). The identification of mites on microscopic examination of skin shavings is diagnostic of scabies.

Permethrin 1% insecticide in the form of a shampoo is the drug of choice for head lice, and permethrin 5% cream is the treatment of choice for scabies. Permethrin cream is applied to the entire body from the neck down after bathing and is washed off in 8 to 14 hours. Re-treatment is not necessary unless new lesions develop within 10 days. Permethrin is an over-the-counter medication. Adverse effects include pruritis and stinging on application. This drug is a pregnancy category B drug, but safety in women who are breast-feeding is unknown. Lindane 1% is an alternative treatment to permethrin for head lice and scabies, but its use is limited by the potential for neurotoxicity. Institution of environmental control measures in response to both conditions includes decontamination of linens, towels, and clothing used in the previous 4 days. Items that cannot be washed in hot water should be dry-cleaned or sealed in a plastic bag for 5 days. Household and sexual contacts should follow the same cleaning procedures as persons who have lice or scabies.

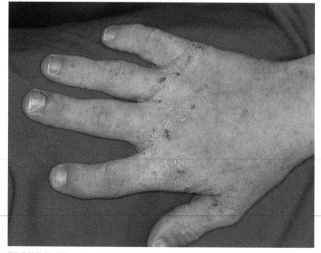

FIGURE 13.
Patient with scabies.

Skin Cancer

Skin cancer is more common than all other cancers combined, representing a major public health issue. The three most common skin cancers are basal cell carcinoma (BCC), squamous cell carcinoma (SCC), and malignant melanoma. BCC and SCC are nonmelanomatous skin cancers (NMSC). In 2003 in the United States alone, an estimated one million new cases of BCC and SCC were reported, with an additional 54,200 new diagnoses of malignant melanoma reported. The CDC estimates approximately 9800 Americans died of skin cancer in 2003. Early diagnosis of malignant melanoma can be life saving and requires a high vigilance for inspecting skin lesions and aggressive treatment when indicated.

Risk factors for all skin cancers include light-colored hair, skin, and eyes; a personal or family history of skin cancer; chronic exposure to the sun; a history of sunburns early in life; and certain types of moles or a large number of moles, including freckles. Immunosuppressed transplant recipients are highly susceptible to aggressive, fast-growing NMSC. Patients should be encouraged to watch for changes in moles and bring them to the attention of their physicians early. The United States Preventive Services Task Force has found insufficient evidence to support routine screening for or counseling about skin cancers. Sunscreen and protective wear are reasonable protective strategies and should be encouraged for anyone considered to be at high risk for skin cancer even though evidence supporting such strategies is insufficient. Although sunscreen use is associated with a decreased incidence of SCC, it has no effect on the development of BCC, and there are no direct data on sunscreen use and the development of melanoma.

For any suspicious lesion, it is important to record whether it is a primary or recurrent lesion, the location, size, general description of its borders, and an estimate of its growth rate. The approach to treatment depends greatly on whether the lesion is considered to be at low or high risk for metastasis. For low-risk lesions, superficial ablation with elec-trodissection and curettage or cryotherapy is sufficient. For high-risk lesions, a full-thickness technique is required, including Moh's micrographic surgery, excisional removal, or radiotherapy (33).

BCCs can be classified into four types of lesions: nodular, superficial, keratotic, and sclerotic. This type of lesion almost never metastasizes but can cause extensive local destruction if left untreated. They occur predominantly on exposed sites, particularly around the nose and inner canthus (**Figure 14**). Early nodular lesions are flesh-colored, dome-shaped nodules, often with adjacent telangiectasias, and occasionally with a pearly translucent surface. As BCC grows, the central area often ulcerates, with its characteristic rolled edge. Shave biopsy is the preferred method for establishing a diagnosis of BCC, because tumor depth is not an essential factor in determining treatment for BCC. The nodular and superficial types of this disease are characterized histologically by superficial growth and are generally considered low-risk lesions. The keratotic and sclerotic types are high-risk tumors, requiring a full-thickness biopsy approach.

SCC is a malignancy of the keratinocytes. This type of skin cancer is usually found on sun-damaged skin (**Figure 15**). The lesions in SCC are hyperkeratotic, ulcerated, and fast growing, with a 2% to 6% incidence of metastasis. Higher-risk SCC lesions grow noticeable within 1 to 3 months, show deeper tissue invasion, have ill-defined borders, and are less differentiated on biopsy. The size of SCC is important, with lesions >2 cm having a two- to threefold increased risk for recurrence and metastasis, respectively. Lesions on the face, ears, and vertex of the scalp are more prone to recurrence and metastasis, whereas those on the trunk and extremities are generally considered to be at low-risk for recurrence and metastasis. A punch biopsy is preferred over a shave biopsy for suspicious SCC, because the depth of tissue on biopsy directly influences treatment options.

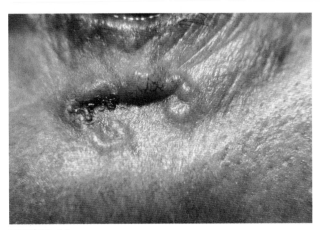

FIGURE 14.

Typical basal cell carcinoma of the lower eyelid with rolled border and telangiectasia.

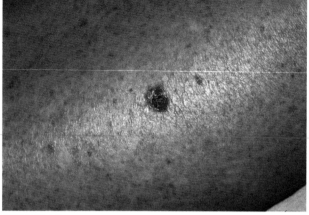

FIGURE 15.
Squamous cell carcinoma.

TABLE 49 Characteristics of Skin Lesions Suspicious for Malignant Melanoma

A — Asymmetry	Any asymmetry; inability to draw a center line
B — Border	Ill defined border, blurring of lesion from normal skin
C — Color	Very dark, black, or variegated with multiple colors contained in a single lesion
D — Diameter	Greater than diameter of pencil eraser, >6 mm

Malignant melanoma is the most deadly of the skin cancers and is increasing more rapidly than are other types of cancer. It currently accounts for 5% of all new cancer cases in men and 4% of all new cancer cases in women. A recent meta-analysis confirms that intermittent exposure to sunlight and a history of sunburns increase the risk for melanoma. Suspicion of melanoma should be high for any lesion failing two of the four "ABCD" characteristics (**Table 49**). The four main varieties of malignant melanoma are lentigo maligna melanoma, superficial spreading melanoma, acral lentiginous melanoma, and nodular melanoma, the first three types of which have an initial superficial growth phase representing the optimal time for identifying and excising lesions. Nodular melanoma is often aggressive and invades deep into the skin layers early. Shave biopsy, cryotherapy, and curettage of a suspected melanoma lesion are contraindicated in these patients; instead, excision biopsy is required. Once a diagnosis of melanoma is established, staging and frequent follow up are required. A thorough history and physical examination, including total skin examination and assessment for lymphadenopathy, are critical in patients with melanoma. Most melanomas recur within the first 3 years of diagnosis but can recur even 15 years later. Survivors of melanoma who have disease higher than stage I benefit from a comprehensive follow-up strategy (34).

Warts

Warts, caused by more than 100 types of human papillomavirus, are transmitted to the self or others by touch, to the soles of feet from moist communal areas, and to the area around the nails from nail biting. Warts may be associated with latent, subclinical, or clinical infection and may resolve spontaneously, within weeks, months, or years, because of individual variations in cell-mediated immunity; however, warts can also last a lifetime.

Warts grow in cylindrical projections, creating a mosaic pattern, with loss of normal skin lines. The differential diagnosis of warts includes corns, which can be distinguished from warts by superficial paring of the surface with a surgical blade. Although warts contain central black dots that bleed with paring, a corn contains a translucent central core. Also among the differential diagnoses of warts is *black heel*, a cluster of petechiae appearing as blue-black dots that occur when patients participate in sports requiring sudden stopping or turning. Close inspection of such lesions reveals normal skin lines, and superficial paring of these petechiae does not result in bleeding.

Warts occur in many forms. Common warts are usually fleshy colored lesions on the hands. Flat warts are slightly elevated flat-topped papules that are pink or brown and occur commonly on the forehead, mouth, backs of hands, and in shaved areas. Filiform or digitate warts, often seen on the face, develop fingerlike projections from a base. Plantar warts on the feet often occur at the point of maximum pressure, and a callous often forms around them.

There is minimal evidence indicating which treatment is best for common warts. Simple topical treatments containing salicylic acid appear to be effective and safe, and no clear evidence has found that cryotherapy is a more effective wart treatment than simple topical therapy (35). Periungual warts can be quite resistant to therapy. Cryotherapy can result in nail matrix destruction and nail distortion and must be used carefully in patients with warts. Patients should be warned that contact with the blister fluid from cryotherapy could spread the causative virus. Plantar warts require treatment only if they are painful because these warts can resolve spontaneously. Other non–Food and Drug Administration-approved treatments that may be considered for resistant and recurrent warts include imiquimod, with up to an 80% cure rate with topical administration, or mumps or candidal antigens, with a 72% to 74% cure rate with intralesional injection (36).

Treatment of filiform warts has not been well studied, and there are no evidence-based recommendations regarding treatment; brief applications of liquid nitrogen are often effective in these patients. Flat warts are often resistant to treatment with topical salicylic acid and often occur in sensitive locations, such as the face. A single randomized trial of 0.05% tretinoin cream was effective in treating flat warts, with an 85% cure rate when applied daily until exfoliation occurred (see also Reference 36).

KEY POINTS

- **Warts grow in cylindrical projections, creating a mosaic pattern, with loss of normal skin lines.**

- **Cryotherapy can result in nail matrix destruction and nail distortion and must be used carefully in patients with warts.**

- **In patients with warts, contact with the blister fluid from cryotherapy can spread the causative virus.**

- **A single randomized trial of 0.05% tretinoin cream was effective in treating flat warts, with an 85% cure rate when applied daily until exfoliation occurred.**

Alopecia

Alopecia consists of generalized or patchy hair loss, usually from the scalp, but occurring in other sites as well. Possible causes for alopecia are listed in **Table 50**. The most common cause of localized or patchy hair loss is alopecia areata, which accounts for almost 2% of all newly diagnosed cases of alopecia seen by dermatologists yearly. Alopecia areata is associated with atopy and other autoimmune processes, including thyroid disease, vitiligo, and diabetes mellitus, and it is also common in patients with Down's syndrome. Patients with alopecia areata have a well-demarcated, completely bald area with no signs of inflammation, desquamation, or scarring.

Complete loss of scalp hair is called alopecia totalis, whereas complete loss of all bodily hair is called alopecia universalis. Pitted and ridged nails are frequently associated with alopecia areata.

TABLE 50 Differential Diagnosis of Alopecia
Diffuse Hair Loss
Male pattern baldness
Telogen effluvium (postpartum, fever, "stress")
Syphilis
SLE
Hypothyroidism, hypopituitarism
Nutritional (iron deficiency)
Drug induced (cytotoxic, anticoagulants, vitamin A and analogues)
Congenital hair shaft defects
Trichotillomania
Alopecia areata
Localized Patchy Hair Loss
Alopecia areata
Fungal infections, including kerion
Chronic discoid lupus erythematosus
Follicular lichen planus
Traction (ponytail styles, use of harsh chemicals/implements)

SLE = systemic lupus erythematosus.

Alopecia areata is thought to be a T-cell–mediated autoimmune process that is usually self-limited. Evaluation of patients with this disorder should include the use of Wood's light to rule out fungal infections. Intralesional corticosteroids can help stimulate growth but are not routinely recommended in patients with alopecia areata. New topical immunomodulating drugs and biologic therapies for alopecia areata are in development, including anthralin and others (37).

Androgen-dependent hair loss or male-pattern baldness is common, and its incidence increases with age. There is usually a genetic predisposition to the age of onset and severity of the baldness in these patients. A small proportion of postmenopausal women may also have this type of baldness. Conventional medical treatments for male-pattern baldness include oral finasteride or topical preparations of 2% or 5% minoxidil. Spironolactone and flutamide have been tried in this setting but without conclusive evidence on efficacy (38, 39).

Cutaneous disorders may lead to irreversible hair loss. These include fungal or bacterial folliculitis, discoid lupus erythematosus, and lichen planopilaris. Scarring bullous disorders and skin malignancy may also be implicated in hair loss. Culture and biopsy of the affected skin are necessary to rule out infectious causes.

Telogen effluvium is a common cause of nonpermanent alopecia, a condition of increased hair shedding. On examination, 25 to 50 hairs can be removed with a gentle pull in patients with this disorder, confirming the premature conversion of growth-phase hair follicles to a resting/shedding "telogen" phase. This phenomenon is the result of an idiosyncratic drug reaction and can occur with any and all drugs. Telogen effluvium is also associated with febrile illnesses, childbirth, chronic systemic disease, administration of heparin, emotional stress, and hormonal problems.

Other causes of hair loss include drug-induced alopecia (**Table 51**), lichen planus, and trichotillomania or traction alopecia. A careful history and physical examination, including microscopic examination of the hair bulb and shaft, can help to establish the diagnosis in patients with hair loss. A white bulb on hair shaft examination suggests telogen effluvium, whereas midshaft fractured hairs are more prominent in patients with tinea capitis, in those who have experienced environmental/external factors causing hair loss, or in those with systemic disease. The hallmark of alopecia areata, alopecia totalis, and alopecia universalis are exclamation-point hairs identified by microscopy.

KEY POINTS

- Patients with alopecia areata have a well-demarcated, completely bald area, with no signs of inflammation, desquamation, or scarring in the affected area.
- Patients with complete loss of scalp hair should undergo evaluation with a Wood's light to rule out fungal infections.
- Conventional medical treatments for male-pattern baldness include oral finasteride or topical preparations of 2% or 5% minoxidil.
- Twenty-five to 50 hairs can be removed with a gentle pull in patients with increased hair shedding.
- Telogen effluvium may be associated with febrile illnesses, childbirth, chronic systemic disease, administration of heparin, emotional stress, or hormonal problems.
- The hallmark of alopecia areata, alopecia totalis, and alopecia universalis are exclamation-point hairs identified by microscopy.

Bites and Stings

Of the millions of species of insects on earth, most neither bite nor sting. In most people, insect bites or stings cause a local inflammatory reaction that subsides within a few hours. Insect and arthropod venoms can produce blisters (blister beetles, certain stinging caterpillars, or millipedes), may be neurotoxic (black and brown widow spiders, bark scorpions, certain ticks, *Hymenoptera*, and wheel bugs), or may destroy tissue (*Hymenoptera*, fire ants, ground scorpions, mites, chiggers, wheel bugs, and brown recluse spiders).

Insect bites or stings can be dangerous because they cause anaphylaxis in certain susceptible individuals, the biting or stinging insects are vectors for disease, and the venom may be locally destructive or neurotoxic. Most clinically significant allergic reactions induced by bug bites are from yellow jackets (Vespula species). Mosquitoes can transmit many diseases,

TABLE 51 Drugs That Commonly Cause Alopecia	
Cytotoxic Drugs	Cyclophosphamide
	Mercaptopurine derivatives
	Colchicines
	Adriamycin
Anticoagulants	Heparin
	Warfarin
Antithyroid drugs	Thiouracil
	Carbimazole
Others	Lithium
	Interferon
	β-Blockers
	Excessive vitamin A and synthetic retinoids
	Ethionamide

including malaria, yellow fever, eastern equine encephalitis, Japanese encephalitis, La Crosse encephalitis, St. Louis encephalitis, West Nile virus, western equine encephalitis, Dengue fever, and Rift Valley fever. Tick-borne illnesses include Lyme disease (**Figure 16**), Rocky Mountain spotted

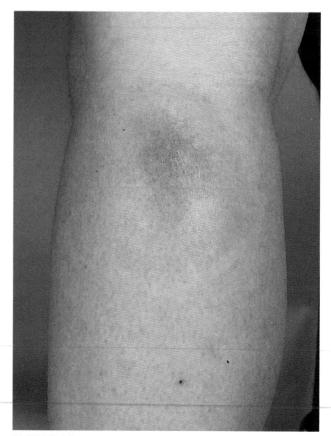

FIGURE 16.
Lyme disease, with the characteristic erythema migrans skin lesion.

fever, babesiosis, ehrlichiosis, tick typhus, tularemia, and Southern tick–associated rash illness. Brown recluse spider bites can cause extensive local tissue destruction. The syndrome occurring after a black widow spider bite is called lacrtodectism. During the first 24 hours after a bite by one of these spiders, patients may develop muscle spasms near the bite and then autonomic stimulation with headache, dizziness, diaphoresis, tachypnea, tachycardia, and hypertension. Scorpion venom causes immediate pain and swelling at the site of the bite, and the pain may last for days. Systemic symptoms in these patients include vomiting, diarrhea, and parasympathetic stimulation with sweating, hypertension, hypersalivation, and priapism. Larger amounts of venom can damage the heart, produce pulmonary edema and respiratory paralysis, or result in acute pancreatitis. Death is rare in patients who have been bitten by scorpions.

For most bug bites and stings, local administration of ice is sufficient treatment. Topical lotions, such as calamine lotion, can help decrease pruritis as can systemic antihistamines. Cleaning the wound caused by spider bites with soap and water, followed by application of ice, is appropriate. Most lesions in patients bitten by spiders heal without scarring. Necrotic ulcers from spider bites are managed as pressure ulcers are managed, with debridement and maintenance of a moist healing environment. Most lesions heal without scarring in these patients. For systemic reactions to black widow and scorpion venom, antivenom is available.

KEY POINTS

- **Most clinically significant allergic reactions induced by bug bites are from yellow jackets.**

- **During the first 24 hours after a black widow spider bite, patients may develop muscle spasms near the bite and then autonomic stimulation with headache, dizziness, diaphoresis, tachypnea, tachycardia, and hypertension.**

- **For most bug bites and stings, local administration of ice is sufficient treatment, with application of topical lotions and systemic antihistamines for decreasing pruritis.**

- **The wound resulting from a spider bite should be cleaned with soap and water, followed by ice application.**

References

1. Yosipovitch G, Greaves MW, Schmelz M. Itch. Lancet. 2003;361:690-4. [PMID: 12606187]

2. Agero AL, Verallo-Rowell VM. A randomized double-blind controlled trial comparing extra virgin coconut oil with mineral oil as a moisturizer for mild to moderate xerosis. Dermatitis. 2004;15:109-16. [PMID: 15724344]

3. Zirwas MJ, Seraly MP. Pruritus of unknown origin: a retrospective study. J Am Acad Dermatol. 2001;45:892-6. [PMID: 11712035]

4. Twycross R, Greaves MW, Handwerker H, Jones EA, Libretto SE, Szepietowski JC, et al. Itch: scratching more than the surface. QJM. 2003;96:7-26. [PMID: 12509645]

5. Smith KJ, Skelton HG, Yeager J, Lee RB, Wagner KF. Pruritus in HIV-1 disease: therapy with drugs which may modulate the pattern of immune dysregulation. Dermatology. 1997;195:353-8. [PMID: 9529556]

6. Kaplan AP. Clinical practice. Chronic urticaria and angioedema. N Engl J Med. 2002;346:175-9. [PMID: 11796852]

7. Grattan C, Powell S, Humphreys F, . Management and diagnostic guidelines for urticaria and angio-oedema. Br J Dermatol. 2001;144:708-14. [PMID: 11298527]

8. MacKie R. Clinical Dermatology: An Illustrated Textbook. 4th ed. Oxford: Oxford University Press. 2001.

9. Nelson HS, Reynolds R, Mason J. Fexofenadine HCl is safe and effective for treatment of chronic idiopathic urticaria. Ann Allergy Asthma Immunol. 2000 May;84(5):517-22. [PMID: 10831005]

10. Feldman S, Careccia RE, Barham KL, Hancox J. Diagnosis and treatment of acne. Am Fam Physician. 2004;69:2123-30. [PMID: 15152959]

11. Haider A, Shaw JC. Treatment of acne vulgaris. JAMA. 2004;292:726-35. [PMID: 15304471]

12. Loden M, Buraczewska I, Edlund F. Irritation potential of bath and shower oils before and after use: a double-blind randomized study. Br J Dermatol. 2004;150:1142-7. [PMID: 15214901]

13. Williams HC. Clinical practice. Atopic dermatitis. N Engl J Med. 2005;352:2314-24. [PMID: 15930422]

14. FDA Talk Paper. FDA issues public health advisory informing health care providers of safety concerns associated with the use of two eczema drugs, Elidel and Protopic [U.S. Food and Drug Administration Web site]. March 10, 2005. Available at: http://www.fda.gov/bbs/topics/ANSWERS/2005/ANS01343.html. Accessed on June 29, 2005.

15. Saripalli YV, Gadzia JE, Belsito DV. Tacrolimus ointment 0.1% in the treatment of nickel-induced allergic contact dermatitis. J Am Acad Dermatol. 2003;49:477-82. [PMID: 12963912]

16. Amrol D, Keitel D, Hagaman D, Murray J. Topical pimecrolimus in the treatment of human allergic contact dermatitis. Ann Allergy Asthma Immunol. 2003;91:563-6. [PMID: 14700441]

17. Schon MP, Boehncke WH. Psoriasis. N Engl J Med. 2005;352:1899-912. [PMID: 15872205]

18. Pardasani AG, Feldman SR, Clark AR. Treatment of psoriasis: an algorithm-based approach for primary care physicians. Am Fam Physician. 2000;61:725-33, 736. [PMID: 10695585]

19. Lebwohl M. Psoriasis. Lancet. 2003;361:1197-204. [PMID: 12686053]

20. Gupta AK, Ryder JE, Nicol K, Cooper EA. Superficial fungal infections: an update on pityriasis versicolor, seborrheic dermatitis, tinea capitis, and onychomycosis. Clin Dermatol. 2003;21:417-25. [PMID: 14678722]

21. Powell FC. Clinical practice. Rosacea. N Engl J Med. 2005;352:793-803. [PMID: 15728812]

22. van Zuuren EJ, Graber MA, Hollis S, Chaudhry M, Gupta AK. Interventions for rosacea. Cochrane Database Syst Rev. 2004:CD003262. [PMID: 14974010]

23. Cribier B, Frances C, Chosidow O. Treatment of lichen planus. An evidence-based medicine analysis of efficacy. Arch Dermatol. 1998;134:1521-30. [PMID: 9875189]

24. Fridkin SK, Hageman JC, Morrison M, Sanza LT, Como-Sabetti K, Jernigan JA, et al. Methicillin-resistant Staphylococcus aureus disease in three communities. N Engl J Med. 2005;352:1436-44. [PMID: 15814879]

25. Badger C, Seers K, Preston N, Mortimer P. Antibiotics / anti-inflammatories for reducing acute inflammatory episodes in lymphoedema of the limbs. Cochrane Database Syst Rev. 2004:CD003143. [PMID: 15106193]

26. Koning S, Verhagen AP, van Suijlekom-Smit LW, Morris A, Butler CC, van der Wouden JC. Interventions for impetigo. Cochrane Database Syst Rev. 2004:CD003261. [PMID: 15106198]

27. **Plaghki L, Adriaensen H, Morlion B, Lossignol D, Devulder J.** Systematic overview of the pharmacological management of postherpetic neuralgia. An evaluation of the clinical value of critically selected drug treatments based on efficacy and safety outcomes from randomized controlled studies. Dermatology. 2004;208:206-16. [PMID: 15118369]

28. **Oxman MN, Levin MJ, Johnson GR, Schmader KE, Straus SE, Gelb LD, et al.** A vaccine to prevent herpes zoster and postherpetic neuralgia in older adults. N Engl J Med. 2005;352:2271-84. [PMID: 15930418]

29. **Roberts DT, Taylor WD, Boyle J.** Guidelines for treatment of onychomycosis. Br J Dermatol. 2003;148:402-10. [PMID: 12653730]

30. **Gupta AK, Ryder JE, Johnson AM.** Cumulative meta-analysis of systemic antifungal agents for the treatment of onychomycosis. Br J Dermatol. 2004;150:537-44. [PMID: 15030339]

31. **Flinders DC, De Schweinitz P.** Pediculosis and scabies. Am Fam Physician. 2004;69:341-8. [PMID: 14765774]

32. **Ko CJ, Elston DM.** Pediculosis. J Am Acad Dermatol. 2004;50:1-12; quiz 13-4. [PMID: 14699358]

33. **Martinez JC, Otley CC.** The management of melanoma and nonmelanoma skin cancer: a review for the primary care physician. Mayo Clin Proc. 2001;76:1253-65. [PMID: 11761506]

34. **Garbe C, Paul A, Kohler-Spath H, Ellwanger U, Stroebel W, Schwarz M, et al.** Prospective evaluation of a follow-up schedule in cutaneous melanoma patients: recommendations for an effective follow-up strategy. J Clin Oncol. 2003;21:520-9. [PMID: 12560444]

35. **Gibbs S, Harvey I, Sterling JC, Stark R.** Local treatments for cutaneous warts. Cochrane Database Syst Rev. 2003:CD001781. [PMID: 12917913]

36. **Micali G, Dall'Oglio F, Nasca MR, Tedeschi A.** Management of cutaneous warts: an evidence-based approach. Am J Clin Dermatol. 2004;5:311-7. [PMID: 15554732]

37. **Price VH.** Therapy of alopecia areata: on the cusp and in the future. J Investig Dermatol Symp Proc. 2003;8:207-11. [PMID: 14582675]

38. **Carmina E, Lobo RA.** Treatment of hyperandrogenic alopecia in women. Fertil Steril. 2003;79:91-5. [PMID: 12524069]

39. **Sinclair R, Wewerinke M, Jolley D.** Treatment of female pattern hair loss with oral antiandrogens. Br J Dermatol. 2005;152:466-73. [PMID: 15787815]

EYE DISORDERS

RECENT ADVANCE

- **Clinical differentiation of bacterial from viral conjunctivitis**

Red Eye

Acute red eye is the most frequently encountered eye problem by primary care physicians. The primary causes of red eye include viral and bacterial conjunctivitis, subconjunctival hemorrhage, allergic conjunctivitis, eyelid abnormalities, episcleritis and scleritis, acute angle-closure glaucoma, uveitis, and keratitis; of these, the most common is conjunctivitis, primarily viral. Only a few causes of red eye require urgent (scleritis, anterior uveitis, and viral keratitis) or emergent (acute angle-closure glaucoma and bacterial keratitis) referral to an ophthalmologist. Red eye consists of categories of entities with or without ocular pain and/or visual loss. The combination of red eye, ocular pain, and visual loss may be an indication for an urgent or emergent referral to an ophthalmologist (**Table 52**) (1).

Conjunctivitis is a common cause of red eye and can occur secondary to bacterial or viral infections, allergies, chemical exposure, or a tear deficiency. Viral conjunctivitis is characterized by presentation in one eye, but this condition commonly spreads to the other eye within 2 days and remains contagious for 2 weeks (**Figure 17**). Blurred vision is secondary to tearing in these patients (2). The infectious process in viral conjunctivitis is usually self-limited, although treatment with topical antibiotics is common.

Bacterial conjunctivitis is caused by a range of gram-positive and gram-negative organisms and is characterized by presentation in one eye, but this condition often spreads to involve the other eye and is associated with purulent discharge. Empirical treatment with broad-spectrum topical antibiotics is indicated (gentamicin 0.3% or tobramycine 0.3%) in patients with bacterial conjunctivitis, with referral to an ophthalmologist appropriate for those in whom no improvement occurs within 1 week. Hyperacute bacterial conjunctivitis with abrupt onset is usually associated with a gonococcal infection in sexually active adolescents or adults. Immediate referral to an ophthalmologist is indicated in these patients. Treatment of a gonococcal infection requires topical and systemic antibiotics. *Chlamydia trachomatis* infection, a sexually transmitted disease, can lead to inclusion conjunctivitis, requiring treatment with oral antibiotics. Inclusion conjunctivitis is usually caused by exposure to the genital tract of an asymptomatic patient who is infected with *C. trachomatis*. Patients with this infection have a preauricular node on the infected side of the eye, and a prominent follicular response in the conjunctival fornix. Oral treatment with tetracycline, erythromycin, or doxycycline for 14 days is indicated in patients with this infection. Sexual partners of patients with *C. trachomatis* should

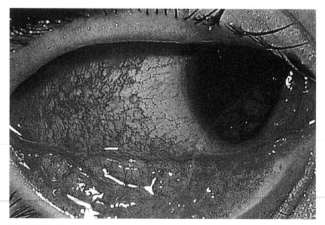

FIGURE 17.
Conjunctivitis.

TABLE 52 Clinical Presentation of Red Eye

Clinical Entity	Ocular pain	Visual loss	Urgent or emergent referral to ophthalmologist indicated
Viral and bacterial conjunctivitis	No	No	No
Subconjunctival hemorrhage	No	No	No
Allergic conjunctivitis	No	No	No
Episcleritis	Yes	No	No
Scleritis	Yes	Yes	Urgent
Acute angle-closure glaucoma	Yes	Yes	Emergent
Anterior uveitis	Yes	Yes	Urgent
Viral and bacterial keratitis	Yes	Yes	Viral—urgent; bacterial—emergent

also receive treatment. This treatment is contraindicated in pregnant women and children.

A recent prospective cohort study provided empirical evidence on how to distinguish viral from bacterial conjunctivitis clinically. In this study of adults who had uncomplicated infectious conjunctivitis with no acute vision loss, contact lens use, or ocular pain, early morning "glued" eyes was independently associated with bacterial conjunctivitis, whereas viral conjunctivitis as defined by culture results was associated with itching and previous history of conjunctivitis (3, 4).

Subconjunctival hemorrhage is a common cause of red eye characterized by unilateral, localized, and sharply circumscribed redness without discharge or pain. Exacerbating factors of this condition include trauma, bleeding disorders, anticoagulation therapy, hypertension, and episodes of prolonged coughing or vomiting. The disorder resolves spontaneously in 2 to 3 weeks. In patients in whom symptoms do not resolve, referral to an ophthalmologist is indicated.

Allergic conjunctivitis is characterized by red, itching, and tearing eyes and nasal congestion. Topical and systemic antihistamines and over-the-counter antihistamine and vasoconstrictor eyedrops can provide symptomatic relief for short-term use in these patients.

Red eye may also be caused by eyelid abnormalities. A *stye*, an acute external hordeolum, is an infection of Moll's gland along the lashline. Blepharitis is an acute or chronic eyelid inflammation often associated with conjunctival inflammation. Blepharitis may occur secondary to a seborrheic process, allergic disorders, or bacteria. Treatment of styes and blepharitis consists of warm compresses and topical antibiotics. Referral to an ophthalmologist is indicated in patients in whom a response to treatment is not shown.

A pterygium is a benign, degenerative, conjunctival lesion, occurring in persons who spend time outdoors in hot and dusty climates. It is characterized by acute eye redness, inflammation, and irritation. The lesion in pterygium is soft and yellowish. Treatment of this disorder consists of artificial tears used for lubrication. Emergent referral to an ophthalmologist is indicated in patients in whom the lesion invades the cornea.

Episcleritis is a chronic, recurrent, and self-limited condition causing inflammation of the episcleral vessels. The episclera is located beneath the conjunctiva and over the sclera. Episcleritis may occur secondary to collagen vascular disorders, granulomatous disease, metabolic disorders, and infectious agents. Patients with episcleritis have eye redness and pain, but vision is not affected. Oral NSAIDs are appropriate for symptomatic relief in these patients, but the process is typically self-limited. Persistent episcleritis requires referral to an ophthalmologist. Patients with scleritis have focal or diffuse eye redness with pink sclera, ocular pain, and impaired vision. Urgent referral to an ophthalmologist is indicated in patients with this condition.

Acute angle-closure glaucoma results from closure of a preexisting narrow anterior chamber angle and occurs most commonly in the elderly. This condition is an ocular emergency; optic nerve atrophy and vision loss can occur within hours of onset (see Glaucoma section).

Uveitis is characterized by inflammation of the iris (iritis), ciliary body (cyclitis), and choroids (choroiditis). Anterior uveitis (iritis and cyclitis) may be characterized by acute red eye, pain, photophobia, and blurred vision in the involved eye. The pupil is constricted and may be irregular or sluggish to light in these patients. Anterior uveitis may be granulomatous or nongranulomatous and can lead to glaucoma, papillary abnormalities, cataract formation, and macular dysfunction. Urgent referral to an ophthalmologist is required in patients with suspected uveitis. Treatment involves the use of corticosteroids and immunosuppressive therapy.

Keratitis is characterized by red eye, pain, photophobia, tearing, and reduced vision. It can be caused by various factors, including dry eyes, topical medications, and viral and bacterial infections. In patients with keratitis, a ciliary flush is typically found on physical examination, and the use of a slit lamp is required to confirm the diagnosis. Urgent referral to an ophthalmologist is indicated in patients with viral keratitis. Bacterial keratitis is an ophthalmologic emergency.

Age-related Macular Degeneration and Vision Impairment

Various physiologic processes can lead to vision impairment. The most common causes of visual impairment are age-related macular degeneration (AMD), glaucoma, cataracts, and diabetic retinopathy. This section focuses on AMD and diabetic retinopathy (see also Glaucoma and Cataracts sections). AMD is the leading cause of blindness in persons older than 65 years. It is a degenerative disorder of the retinal pigment epithelium and neurosensory retina characterized by the presence of drusen, accumulations of acellular debris that appear as yellow spots on the macula as identified on ophthalmoscopic examination. Dry (non-neovascular) AMD is characterized by the presence of soft drusen, pigmentary abnormalities, and geographic atrophy on the macula. Wet (neovascular) AMD is an exudative process characterized by choroidal neovascularization, pigment epithelial detachment, or disciform scarring. The wet form of AMD accounts for only 15% of cases of AMD but is more severe than the dry form and responsible for most AMD-related visual loss.

Diabetic retinopathy occurs in the nonproliferative form (characterized by microaneurysms, intraretinal hemorrhages, and retinal edema) and the proliferative form (characterized by newly formed blood vessels from the optic disc, retina, or iris) of AMD.

Population-based studies estimate the prevalence of AMD in developed countries to be 1.7% to 1.9%. The prevalence increases with age to 7.8% in individuals aged 75 years or older, according to the Beaver Dam Eye study (5). The risk factors for AMD are older age, female sex, white race, cigarette smoking, and low dietary intake of carotenoids. Genetic and familial factors may also be involved in the development of this disease. The prevalence of diabetic retinopathy is 2.5% in adults 18 years or older in the United States. In comparison, the prevalence of cataracts is 17% in adults older than aged 40 years.

At least 40% of blindness or visual impairment is preventable or treatable. Although not supported by evidence-based clinical trials, broad consensus supports periodic vision evaluation of asymptomatic adults, especially in older adults. Persons with diabetic retinopathy should be examined by an eye care professional. Smoking cessation is beneficial for prevention of cataracts, AMD, and diabetic retinopathy. Control of hyperglycemia and hypertension decreases the risk for diabetic retinopathy in patients with diabetes.

AMD is characterized by unilateral presentation with gradual or sudden central vision loss, fading colors, visual distortions, difficulty seeing faces, and the need for increased light. Macular retinal changes include drusen, localized deposits of extracellular material that appear as yellow spots on ophthalmoscopic examination. Small drusen are commonly present on the macula with aging, but large and numerous drusen are associated with AMD. Diabetic retinopathy is characterized by symptoms of distorted near-vision and blurry or obstructed visual fields. Ophthalmologic examination in patients with diabetic retinopathy indicates retinal edema, hemorrhages, and exudates. Patients who have these symptoms require a thorough examination performed by an eye care professional.

A Cochrane review found a benefit with antioxidants (β-carotene and vitamins C and E) and zinc supplementation in progression to advanced AMD (6). Photodynamic therapy is effective in preventing visual loss for patients with choroidal neovascularization due to AMD. Although only 10% of patients with AMD have the exudative form of this disease, exudative AMD accounts for 80% to 90% of cases of severe vision loss from AMD. Treatment of diabetic retinopathy includes effective glycemic and hypertensive control to prevent progression. Effective surgical interventions for diabetic retinopathy include laser photocoagulation and vitrectomy.

Vision impairment is associated with decreased functional status and quality of life. The prognosis of exudative AMD is guarded, but complete blindness is rare in patients with this disease, and peripheral vision is spared. Vision loss from AMD and diabetic retinopathy can be reduced through screening and effective early interventions. Patients who are visually impaired require routine ophthalmologic follow-up examinations.

Effective surgical interventions for diabetic retinopathy include laser photocoagulation and vitrectomy.

Glaucoma

Glaucoma is an optic neuropathy that can cause progressive visual field loss, leading to irreversible blindness. Primary open-angle glaucoma is the most common type of glaucoma. Among Americans 40 years of age and older, primary open-angle glaucoma accounts for 6.4% of blindness in whites, 36.8% in blacks, and 28.6% in Hispanics (7). The prevalence of this disease in this age group is estimated to be 1.9% (95% CI, 1.75 to 1.96) (8), and the prevalent number of cases is expected to increase from 2.22 million in 2002 to 3.6 million by 2020 owing to the aging of the population. Less frequently, glaucoma results from acute angle closure, congenital causes, or secondary to uveal changes, trauma, corticosteroids, proliferative retinopathy, and other ocular syndromes. The strongest risk factors for open-angle glaucoma include increased (>21 mm Hg) intraocular pressure (IOP), increased age, family history, and race. Blacks have an age-adjusted prevalence nearly three times higher than that of whites. Additional risk factors for this disease include a decreased central corneal thickness, increased cup-to-disc ratio (>0.4), and severe myopia. Early-stage primary open-angle glaucoma is asymptomatic, with patients initially noting decreased peripheral vision or blind spots, seeing halos around lights, or having difficulty adapting to darkness. Decreased central visual acuity is a late finding of primary open-angle glaucoma. A diagnosis of glaucoma is established by identification of characteristic optic neuropathy and visual field loss. Funduscopic examination in these patients reveals thinning of the optic disc rim, with an increased cup-to-disc ratio and abnormalities in the retinal nerve-fiber layer. Because many patients with primary open-angle glaucoma (25% to 50%) have normal IOP (normal-tension glaucoma), this disorder is no longer defined by an elevated IOP, although IOP is a risk factor for primary open-angle glaucoma. However most patients with ocular hypertension will not develop glaucoma.

Evidence-based guidelines have found insufficient evidence to determine whether routine screening for primary open-angle glaucoma prevents visual impairment (9), although patients at high risk for visual impairment could receive a referral to an eye specialist for a comprehensive evaluation (10). Screening for IOP has limited effectiveness; visual field testing and assessment of the optic disc and retinal fiber layer are necessary to increase the likelihood of detecting glaucoma.

Increased IOP is the only modifiable risk factor for primary open-angle glaucoma; treatments lowering IOP can limit or prevent vision loss. Topical and oral medications (**Table 53**) increase aqueous outflow (prostaglandin analogues and cholinergic agonists,) or decrease aqueous production (α-adrenergic agonists, carbonic anhydrase inhibitors, and β-blockers), whereas laser trabeculoplasty and surgical trabeculectomy increase aqueous outflow. Prostaglandin analogues have become the first-line medical treatment in patients with primary open-angle glaucoma because they effectively reduce IOP, can be taken once daily, and have minimal systemic side effects. Applying punctal compression or gently closing the eyelid for several minutes after administering topical medications can reduce systemic side effects.

A randomized trial has shown that topical medications can prevent the onset of primary open-angle glaucoma in patients with just ocular hypertension (11). At 60-month follow-up, 4.4% of the treatment group progressed to primary open-angle glaucoma versus 9.5% of the untreated controls (hazard ratio = 0.40, 95% CI, 0.27 to 0.59). A recent trial of patients with newly diagnosed primary open-angle glaucoma reported those who received immediate laser trabeculoplasty and topical betaxolol experienced a 17% reduction (hazard ratio = 0.50, 95% CI, 0.35 to 0.71) in disease progression after 6 years of follow-up compared with those who received delayed treatment (12). Factors associated with disease progression included a higher baseline IOP, bilateral disease, and older age. Clinical trials have shown similar visual field outcomes in patients with primary open-angle glaucoma who received initial surgical or laser treatment versus aggressive medical management, although cataracts occurred more frequently in patients who underwent surgery (13). Ocular hypotensive medications are appropriate first-line treatments for reducing IOP, although surgery or laser treatments are options for patients in whom medications are ineffective or poorly tolerated. Patients with primary open-angle glaucoma require lifelong monitoring and treatment.

Acute angle-closure glaucoma results from closure of a preexisting narrow anterior chamber angle and occurs most commonly in the elderly. Presenting symptoms include eye pain, headache, blurry vision, and, occasionally, nausea and vomiting. In patients with acute angle-closure glaucoma, the eye is red, the pupil may be dilated and poorly reactive to light, the cornea is hazy, and IOP is elevated. Precipitating factors of this disorder include darkness (leading to mydriasis), stress, and use of sympathomimetic or anticholinergic medications. Acute angle-closure glaucoma is an ocular emergency; optic nerve atrophy and vision loss can occur within hours without treatment. Immediate ocular hypotensive medications are effective in preserving vision in patients with acute angle-closure glaucoma, but definitive therapy requires surgery or laser treatment, and these patients should receive a referral to an ophthalmologist for urgent care.

TABLE 53 Medications That Reduce Intraocular Pressure		
Drug Action	**Selected Examples**	**Most Common Systemic Side Effects**
Agents That Suppress Aqueous Outflow		
β-Adrenergic blockers	Betaxolol (β-1 selective) Carteolol (intrinsic sympathomimetic activity) Levobunolol (nonselective) Metipranolol (nonselective) Timolol (nonselective)	Bradycardia, hypotension, heart failure, bronchospasm
α-2 Adrenergic agonists	Apraclonidine Brimonidine	Headache, fatigue, drowsiness, dry mouth
Carbonic anhydrase inhibitors	Dorzolamide (topical) Brinzolamide (topical) Acetazolamide (oral) Methazolamide (oral)	Nausea, loss of appetite and taste, diarrhea, fatigue, paresthesias, renal calculi, blood dyscrasias
Agents That Increase Aqueous Outflow		
Prostaglandin analogues	Latanoprost Travoprost Unoprostone	Myalgia, arthralgia, back pain, chest pain; rash, upper respiratory infections
Cholinergic agonists	Pilocarpine Carbachol	Flushing, headache, dizziness, chills, gastrointestinal disturbances, diaphoresis, urinary frequency, weakness, rhinitis

Adapted from Weinreb RN, Khaw PT. Primary open-angle glaucoma. Lancet 2004: 363:1711-20; and Goldzweig CL, Rowe S, Wenger N, MacLean CH, Shekelle PG. Preventing and managing visual disability in primary care. JAMA 2004; 291:1497-1502.

KEY POINTS

- The strongest risk factors for open-angle glaucoma include increased intraocular pressure, increased age, family history, and race.

- Blacks have an age-adjusted prevalence for open-angle glaucoma nearly threefold higher than that of whites.

- Signs of early-stage primary open-angle glaucoma are decreased peripheral vision or blind spots, seeing halos around lights, or having difficulty adapting to darkness.

- Funduscopic examination in patients with primary open-angle glaucoma shows thinning of the optic disc rim, with an increased cup-to-disc ratio, and abnormalities in the retinal nerve-fiber layer.

- Treatments lowering intraocular pressure can limit or prevent vision loss in patients with primary open-angle glaucoma.

- Topical medications can prevent the onset of primary open-angle glaucoma in patients with just ocular hypertension.

- Patients with newly diagnosed primary open-angle glaucoma who received immediate laser trabeculoplasty and topical betaxolol experienced a 17% reduction in disease progression after 6 years of follow-up compared with those who received delayed treatment.

- Presenting symptoms of acute angle-closure glaucoma include eye pain, headache, blurry vision, and, occasionally, nausea and vomiting.

Cataracts

A cataract is an acquired or congenital opacification of the lens of the eye that can impair vision. Cataracts are the second leading cause of blindness (9%) and the most common cause of low vision (50%) in Americans older than 40 years. An estimated 20.5 million (17.2%) Americans in this age range have cataracts, whereas another 6.1 million (5.1%) have undergone cataract surgery. By 2020, the prevalence of Americans with cataracts is expected to reach 30.1 million, and 9.5 million are expected to have undergone cataract surgery. Women have a significantly higher age-adjusted prevalence of cataracts than do men (OR = 1.37, 95% CI, 1.26 to 1.50). There are no significant racial differences among women with cataracts, but the age-adjusted prevalence is significantly higher in white men (OR = 1.09, 95% CI 1.02 to 1.16) than black men.

Risk factors for cataracts include aging, sun exposure, diabetes, smoking, alcohol consumption, and corticosteroid use (14). A meta-analysis concluded that cataract risk might be elevated in older patients with asthma who use inhaled corticosteroids, although evidence was insufficient to determine whether type of preparation or dose was associated with this risk (15). The use of systemic corticosteroids is associated with an increased incidence of posterior subcapsular cataracts. Neither vitamin E nor β-carotene supplements were effective in reducing the incidence or progression of age-related cataracts in randomized controlled trials (16, 17).

Cataracts cause blurred vision; glare with fluorescent lighting, bright sunlight, and night driving; fading colors; and difficulty reading in dim light. This visual disorder usually progresses slowly, with vision deteriorating over months to years. Cataracts are classified by their clinical appearance (nuclear, cortical, and posterior subcapsular) and can be identified by ophthalmoscopy or slit-lamp examination.

The definitive treatment for cataracts is outpatient surgical removal with synthetic intraocular lens implantation. Cataract surgery is indicated in patients in whom vision loss interferes with performance of activities of daily living. Nearly 90% of patients who undergo cataract surgery are expected to have postoperative visual acuity of 20/40 or better. Serious postoperative complications occur infrequently, including endophthalmitis (0.13%), bullous keratopathy (0.3%), intraocular lens malposition/dislocation (1.1%), macular degeneration (1.5%), and retinal detachment (0.7%). Initial cataract surgery and subsequent surgery on the second eye are both cost-effective, with costs per quality-adjusted life-year below $4000 (18).

KEY POINTS

- Cataract risk may be elevated in older patients with asthma who use inhaled corticosteroids.
- Systemic corticosteroids are associated with an increased incidence of posterior subcapsular cataracts.
- Cataracts cause blurred vision; glare with fluorescent lighting, bright sunlight, and night driving; fading colors; and difficulty reading in dim light.
- The definitive treatment for cataracts is outpatient surgical removal with synthetic intraocular lens implantation.

Corneal Abrasions and Foreign Bodies

Corneal abrasions are defined as defects in the epithelial surface of the cornea caused by mechanical trauma (including contact lenses), infection, or spontaneous breakdown of the corneal surface. When a foreign body causes the corneal abrasion, there can be remnant foreign bodies in the eye, the presence of which significantly increases the risk for infection and the integrity of the cornea and, potentially, other structures of the eye. Corneal epithelial disruption can also occur spontaneously and is generally considered within the category of corneal abrasions. Corneal abrasions constitute 10% to 50% of cases of acute eye disorders in patients evaluated in emergency rooms, primary care offices, and occupational healthcare facilities. Contact lens wearers have a higher risk for developing pseudomonal keratitis, a fulminant infection that can rapidly destroy the cornea within 24 hours, and warrant management that is different from that provided to noncontact lens wearers.

Corneal abrasions typically are characterized by pain and a sensation of a foreign body in the eye. Patients with corneal abrasions also complain of an inability to open the eye. In the evaluation of patients with corneal abrasions, the history helps to determine whether the eye injury was caused by a traumatic abrasion; however, foreign body–related trauma may not be evident to patients in whom small particles (for example, sand, grinding particles, and rust) are responsible for the trauma. Prior corneal abrasion is a risk factor for recurrent spontaneous erosions, and such patients also typically present with nighttime pain or pain on awakening in the morning (that is, during rapid eye movement sleep).

The physical examination in patients with corneal abrasions includes an evaluation for visual acuity and identification of infiltrate, opacity, foreign body, extraocular muscle dysfunction, or evidence of penetrating trauma. Fluorescein staining is useful in evaluating the extent of corneal disruption in patients with corneal abrasions. In this type of testing, fluorescein stains the basement membrane exposed by epithelial defects, which is evaluated with a Wood's lamp or the blue filter on an ophthalmoscope. A branching pattern may indicate a progressive herpetic infection and warrants referral to an ophthalmologist, whereas a punctuate pattern is consistent with contact lens trauma. In patients in whom infection is suspected (for example, from a nonsterile foreign substance or in contact lens wearers), daily observation is necessary to evaluate for ulceration or infiltrate. Corneal infiltrates or ulcers, visual acuity impairment, purulent discharge, or progression of symptoms after 24 hours warrants immediate referral to an ophthalmologist.

Drug treatment of corneal abrasions focuses on pain control and includes short-acting narcotics with acetaminophen; topical NSAIDs (for example, ketorolac) (19); and topical antibiotics, such as erythromycin or sulfacetamide and ofloxacin or ciprofloxacin (four times daily for 3 to 5 days) for contact lens wearers to protect against *Pseudomonas aeruginosa* infection. Antibiotic ointment is preferred in patients with corneal abrasions because it functions as a soothing lubricant. Although no rigorous evidence exists assessing the efficacy for this practice, antibiotic therapy is used in this setting to protect against possible infectious processes that could result in rapid and permanent visual compromise. Topical anesthetics or corticosteroids may delay healing and are contraindicated in patients with corneal abrasions. Lubricant drops (methylcellulose) should be used prophylactically in patients with recurrent erosions.

Nonpharmacologic treatment of corneal abrasion includes remaining in a dark room and avoiding eye rubbing. Eye patches are not necessary in the treatment of this condition (and are contraindicated in contact lens wearers) given the preponderance of evidence suggesting that they prolong healing despite sometimes easing pain (20). If a foreign body is identified in the eye, an attempt at removal with simple irrigation is reasonable, but if the attempt is unsuccessful, referral to an ophthalmologist for removal of the foreign body is appropriate.

Simple corneal abrasions usually require no follow-up because they generally heal rapidly within 24 hours.

Dry Eyes and Excessive Tearing

Tears function to maintain the functional and structural integrity of the ocular superficial tissues, specifically the corneal and conjunctival epithelium. Tear film is constituted by a lipid outer layer excreted by the meibomian glands, an aqueous middle layer (the dominant portion of the tear film) secreted by the lacrimal glands located at the upper outer portion of the orbit, and the inner mucinous layer secreted by the conjunctival goblet cells. Tears drain from the orbit through the punctum, located in the medial portion of the eyelid, which drain into the canalicular system, and ultimately drain into the nose through an opening under the inferior nasal turbinate. Tears flow by way of gravity and pressure induced by eyelid closure.

Dry Eyes

Keratoconjunctivitis sicca is the condition of lacrimal gland dysfunction in which insufficient production of the aqueous portion of tears occurs, resulting in dry eyes. This condition can be due to aging, connective tissue disease involving autoimmune destruction of the lacrimal gland (for example, Sjogrens syndrome), or anticholinergic medication use. Mucin deficiency within tears can be caused by vitamin A deficiency or goblet cell destruction from chemical burns or primary skin disorders. Because continuous bathing of the eyeball with tears depends on eyelid movement, any disorder of the eyelid or extrusion of the eyeball, such as exophthalmos, may also cause dry eyes due to excessive air exposure of the eye without sufficient tear replenishment.

The typical symptoms of patients with dry eyes include burning, grittiness, or foreign-body sensations. Patients with dry eyes also occasionally have corneal abrasions or even ulcers with a concomitant red eye. Ocular sicca is exacerbated by smoking, decreased humidity, and prolonged activities requiring focused visual attention (driving or computer work) and tends to worsen as the day progresses. Associated history including dry mouth, joint pains, medications (specifically antihypertensive agents, tricyclic antidepressants, or antihistamines), and history of connective tissue disease are important considerations in these patients. The physical examination of patients with dry eyes should focus on the effectiveness of eyelid closure and other signs of connective tissue disease. Confirmation of insufficient aqueous tear production is performed with the Schirmer test, which is considered positive if <5 mm of filter paper is wet after the paper is placed on the lower eyelid with the eyes closed for 5 minutes. In patients in whom Sjogrens syndrome is suspected, an antinuclear antibody assay should be performed (95% sensitivity) and, in those who test positive for this syndrome, assays for the presence of anti-Ro (SS-A) and anti-La (SS-B) antibodies (>90% sensitivity) should be performed. Lip biopsy is considered the gold standard in the diagnosis of Sjogrens syndrome but is rarely necessary (21).

Patients with dry eyes should first receive treatment of any epithelial defects caused by this condition followed by symptomatic management consisting of artificial tear substitutes (for example methylcellulose, 0.5% or 1%), which can be used as often as necessary, and behavioral measures, including humidifying air and wearing protective eye cover (for example, goggles or glasses with side chambers to protect against wind). Patients with dry eyes have an increased risk for bacterial conjunctivitis and blepharitis (for example, *Staphylococcus aureus*); therefore, antibiotics should be used liberally in these patients in the presence of red eyes or eyelid inflammation. In extreme cases of dry eyes that are not responsive to moisture preservation, secretagogue receptors can be used. These agents stimulate muscarinic receptors of the lacrimal glands. Cevimeline (30 mg, three times daily) is preferable to pilocarpine (5 mg, 4 times daily) because it has a longer half-life and fewer side effects than pilocarpine. Referral to an ophthalmologist is indicated in patients who do not respond to symptomatic therapy, have visual disturbance, or have persistent red eye. The long-term clinical course of these patients is one of chronic-recurrent symptoms, with symptom reduction with regular use of artificial tears.

Excessive Tearing

Excessive tearing is caused by excessive tear production or impaired tear drainage. Excessive tear production is typically caused by inflammation of the ocular or periocular tissues (for example, conjunctivitis or blepharitis), although dry eyes can occasionally trigger a reflex tearing that can alternate with dry eyes. Dysfunctional tear drainage is most commonly caused by sagging of the lower eyelid, which blocks access of tears to the punctum and is largely a function of aging or of any soft-tissue obstruction of the nasolacrimal drainage system (for example,

TABLE 54 Eye Emergencies Requiring Referral to an Ophthalmologist

Diagnosis	Red Eye	Pain	Vision Loss
Hyperacute bacterial conjunctivitis	+	–	–
Abrupt onset, copious purulent discharge, rapid progression, bright red conjunctiva, marked lid swelling with aching and tenderness; usually gonococcal; requires immediate empiric topical and systemic antibiotics for gonococcal infection			
Acute angle-closure glaucoma	+	+	+
Farsighted and older persons susceptible; symptoms often occur in evening due to decreased ambient light → mydriasis → iris folds block angle and inhibit drainage of aqueous humor → rapidly increased IOP, moderate-severe pain, halos around lights due to corneal edema; involved eye firmer palpation than uninvolved eye; pupil moderately dilated 4 to 6 mm, nonreactive diffuse erythema most pronounced in circumcorneal area (limbus); deepness of pain, nausea, vomiting may distract from evaluation of eyes and lead to missed diagnosis			
Acute anterior uveitis (iritis, iridocyclitis) with hypopyon or hyphema (urgent referral for uncomplicated iritis)	+	+	+
Inflammation of iris, ciliary body, anterior uvea; usually no foreign body sensation; aching pain, photophobia, blurred vision; young or middle-aged persons; usually requires slit-lamp examination but hypopyon or hyphema may be visible at base of anterior chamber; diffuse erythema prominent at limbus; mucopurulent drainage with hypopyon; sluggish to a reactive constricted pupil			
Complicated corneal abrasion: associated with contact lenses, corneal trauma, infiltrate or ulcer, purulent discharge, vision worsened by >1 line on Snellen chart, worsened defect at 24 h	+	+	+/–
Corneal abrasion associated with contact lenses is especially susceptible to infectious keratitis. Corneal trauma: flat chamber by pen-light examination, hyphema, irregular pupil			
Bacterial keratitis	+	+	+/–
Mucopurulent discharge; punctuate corneal lesions; positive fluorescein staining			
Temporal arteritis	–	+	+
May rarely present bilaterally; +/- symptoms of polymyalgia rheumatica; scalp and temple pain and tenderness; afferent papillary defect (see nonarteritic ischemic optic neuropathy below). Additional management: empiric corticosteroids awaiting biopsy			
Optic Neuritis	–	+	+
Usually found in younger patients; may be associated with multiple sclerosis; vision loss over hours to days; +/– ocular pain on eye movement; afferent papillary defect			
Periorbital cellulitis with abscess (fluctuant eyelid)	–	+	+
If no abscess, treat empirically with anti-staphylococcal antibiotic. Refer emergently for abscess drainage. Spread to orbital structures (orbital cellulitis) is unlikely due to preseptal fascia			
Orbital cellulitis	–	+	+
Usually from maxillary and ethmoid sinuses or penetrating trauma; fever, lid edema, rhinorrhea, sinusitis followed by headache, orbital pain, tenderness to palpation, then dark erythema, proptosis, conjunctival hyperemia, chemosis, pain and limitation of eye movement; vertical or horizontal globe displacement with abscess. Complications include subperiosteal, orbital, or brain abscess, cavernous sinus thrombosis, meningitis, blindness due to proptosis, increased IOP, venous congestion, or direct extension to optic nerve			
Cavernous sinus thrombosis	–	+	+
Acute, subacute, or chronic thrombophlebitis with infection spread from nasal area, paranasal sinuses, ears, tonsils, teeth; eyelid edema and chemosis initially → proptosis and edema of bridge of nose; +/- ophthalmoplegia due to venous congestion; progression can involve cranial nerves III IV ,VI (ophthalmoplegia), V, and VII (pain, paralysis); pupil usually fixed and dilated but may be small			
Vitreous hemorrhage	–	–	+
Commonly associated with diabetes or trauma; red reflex and retinal detail obscured with direct ophthalmoscope			
Serous or hemorrhagic macular disease	–	–	+
Choroidal neovascular membranes and age-related macular degeneration			
Retinal detachment	–	–	+
Diagnosis usually requires indirect ophthalmoscopy but white billowing retina can sometimes be seen by direct ophthalmoscopy			
Retinal vein occlusion	–	–	+
Intraretinal hemorrhages may be diffuse throughout fundus or localized to distribution quadrant of a vein branch			
Central retinal artery occlusion	–	–	+
May be preceded by amaurosis fugax, profound vision loss, afferent pupillary defect, pale fundus with "cherry-red spot" in the macula, possible "boxcar" appearance to arteries. Additional management: interim relief of vasospasm by 1) ocular/globe massage with direct pressure for 5 s, and release for 5 s; or 2) increased Pco$_2$ by having patient breathe into a paper bag for 10 min/h			
Nonarteritic ischemic optic neuropathy	–	–	+
Idiopathic disease more common than temporal arteritis, may be due to diabetes, hypertension, or systemic vascular disease. Additional management includes empiric systemic corticosteroids while awaiting biopsy and results			

IOP = intraocular pressure. *Symptom or sign present (+) or absent (–).

atresia, infection, tumor, or turbinate disease). Obstruction of the nasolacrimal system causes stasis, which can predispose patients to bacterial infections, such as dacryocystitis.

The treatment of excessive tearing consists of mechanical manipulation of the nasolacrimal system by placement of frequent, moderate pressure on the medial nasolacrimal portion of the eye with clean hands and antibiotic therapy for evidence of infection. Patients who are recalcitrant to treatment can consider surgical options to improve the patency or function of the punctum or the canaliculi.

KEY POINTS

- The typical symptoms of patients with dry eyes include burning, grittiness, or foreign-body sensations.
- Symptomatic management of patients with dry eyes consists of artificial tear substitutes and behavioral measures.
- Confirmation of insufficient aqueous tear production is performed with the Schirmer test.
- An antinuclear antibody assay should be performed in patients with suspected Sjogrens syndrome.
- Patients with dry eyes have an increased risk for bacterial conjunctivitis and blepharitis.
- The treatment of excessive tearing consists of mechanical manipulation of the nasolacrimal system and antibiotic therapy for evidence of infection.

Eye Emergencies

The main challenge in managing patients with acute eye problems is accurately distinguishing emergencies needing immediate (same day as presentation) or urgent (1 to 2 days after presentation) referral to an ophthalmologist from problems that can be managed in a general medicine setting or electively referred. In general, an initial diagnosis and treatment without referral is appropriate in patients in whom vision is not affected, pupil reactivity is normal, opening and holding open the eye is possible despite a foreign-body sensation, and there is no corneal opacity. Patients with marked distress accompanied by nausea/vomiting and headache (from possible acute angle-closure glaucoma); red eye with severe eye pain or impaired vision or visual defect; and those with hypopyon or hyphema require emergent referral. Hypopyon is a white or yellowish-white accumulation of leukocytes, inflammatory cells, and purulent material in the anterior chamber of the eye. Hyphema is blood in the anterior chamber of the eye. Both disorders form inferiorly, with pooling caused by gravity. Topical corticosteroids should never be administered empirically in these patients without the guidance of an ophthalmologist because of the risk for misdiagnosis of infection and delay in diagnosis of other critical eye problems.

Specific diagnoses that require emergent referral include thermal and chemical burns and those described in **Table 54** (see page 91) (22-26). For thermal or chemical burns, the immediate first step is copious irrigation with normal saline at body temperature, with water as a second resort. Acid rapidly penetrates the cornea and anterior chamber, but damage is relatively self-limiting because of visible secondary protein precipitation, which blocks further penetration. Duration of initial irrigation should be 15 to 20 minutes in these patients. Alkaline burns are more destructive than thermal or chemical burns because hydroxyl ions combine with cellular-membrane lipids to produce ongoing cellular destruction; duration of initial irrigation should be 30 minutes in these patients. Patients who have pterygium with corneal invasion, vision impairment, and scleritis should receive urgent referral to an ophthalmologist (see Red Eye section).

KEY POINT

- Patients with marked distress accompanied by nausea/vomiting and headache, red eye with severe eye pain or impaired vision or visual defect, and those with hypopyon or hyphema require emergent referral.

References

1. **Leibowitz HM.** The red eye. N Engl J Med. 2000;343:345-51. [PMID: 10922425]
2. **Shingleton BJ, O'Donoghue MW.** Blurred vision. N Engl J Med. 2000;343:556-62. [PMID: 10954765]
3. **Rietveld RP, van Weert HC, ter Riet G, Bindels PJ.** Diagnostic impact of signs and symptoms in acute infectious conjunctivitis: systematic literature search. BMJ. 2003;327:789. [PMID: 14525879]
4. **Rietveld RP, ter Riet G, Bindels PJ, Sloos JH, van Weert HC.** Predicting bacterial cause in infectious conjunctivitis: cohort study on informativeness of combinations of signs and symptoms. BMJ. 2004;329:206-10. [PMID: 15201195]
5. **Rowe S, MacLean CH, Shekelle PG.** Preventing visual loss from chronic eye disease in primary care: scientific review. JAMA. 2004;291:1487-95. [PMID: 15039416]
6. **Evans JR.** Antioxidant vitamin and mineral supplements for slowing the progression of age-related macular degeneration. Cochrane Database Syst Rev. 2006 Apr 19;(2):CD000254. Review. [PMID: 16625532]
7. **Congdon N, O'Colmain B, Klaver CC, Klein R, Munoz B, Friedman DS, et al.** Causes and prevalence of visual impairment among adults in the United States. Arch Ophthalmol. 2004;122:477-85. [PMID: 15078664]
8. **Friedman DS, Wolfs RC, O'Colmain BJ, Klein BE, Taylor HR, West S, et al.** Prevalence of open-angle glaucoma among adults in the United States. Arch Ophthalmol. 2004;122:532-8. [PMID: 15078671]
9. **Fleming C, Whitlock EP, Beil T, Smit B, Harris RP.** Screening for primary open-angle glaucoma in the primary care setting: an update for the U.S. preventive services task force. Ann Fam Med. 2005;3:167-70. [PMID: 15798044]
10. **Tuulonen A, Airaksinen PJ, Erola E, Forsman E, Friberg K, Kaila M, et al.** The Finnish evidence-based guideline for open-angle glaucoma. Acta Ophthalmol Scand. 2003;81:3-18. [PMID: 12631014]

11. Kass MA, Heuer DK, Higginbotham EJ, Johnson CA, Keltner JL, Miller JP, et al. The Ocular Hypertension Treatment Study: a randomized trial determines that topical ocular hypotensive medication delays or prevents the onset of primary open-angle glaucoma. Arch Ophthalmol. 2002;120:701-13; discussion 829-30. [PMID: 12049574]

12. Heijl A, Leske MC, Bengtsson B, Hyman L, Bengtsson B, Hussein M, et al. Reduction of intraocular pressure and glaucoma progression: results from the Early Manifest Glaucoma Trial. Arch Ophthalmol. 2002;120:1268-79. [PMID: 12365904]

13. Weinreb RN, Khaw PT. Primary open-angle glaucoma. Lancet. 2004;363:1711-20. [PMID: 15158634]

14. Asbell PA, Dualan I, Mindel J, Brocks D, Ahmad M, Epstein S. Age-related cataract. Lancet. 2005;365:599-609. [PMID: 15708105]

15. Leone FT, Fish JE, Szefler SJ, West SL. Systematic review of the evidence regarding potential complications of inhaled corticosteroid use in asthma: collaboration of American College of Chest Physicians, American Academy of Allergy, Asthma, and Immunology, and American College of Allergy, Asthma, and Immunology. Chest. 2003;124:2329-40. [PMID: 14665517]

16. McNeil JJ, Robman L, Tikellis G, Sinclair MI, McCarty CA, Taylor HR. Vitamin E supplementation and cataract: randomized controlled trial. Ophthalmology. 2004;111:75-84. [PMID: 14711717]

17. Christen WG, Manson JE, Glynn RJ, Gaziano JM, Sperduto RD, Buring JE, et al. A randomized trial of beta carotene and age-related cataract in US physicians. Arch Ophthalmol. 2003;121:372-8. [PMID: 12617708]

18. Busbee BG, Brown MM, Brown GC, Sharma S. Cost-utility analysis of cataract surgery in the second eye. Ophthalmology. 2003;110:2310-7. [PMID: 14644712]

19. Weaver CS, Terrell KM. Evidence-based emergency medicine. Update: do ophthalmic nonsteroidal anti-inflammatory drugs reduce the pain associated with simple corneal abrasion without delaying healing? Ann Emerg Med. 2003;41:134-40. [PMID: 12514694]

20. Flynn CA, D'Amico F, Smith G. Should we patch corneal abrasions? A meta-analysis. J Fam Pract. 1998;47:264-70. [PMID: 9789511]

21. Kassan SS, Moutsopoulos HM. Clinical manifestations and early diagnosis of Sjogren syndrome. Arch Intern Med. 2004;164:1275-84. [PMID: 15226160]

22. Yanofsky NN. The acute painful eye. Emerg Med Clin North Am. 1988;6:21-42. [PMID: 3278885]

23. Howes DS. The red eye. Emerg Med Clin North Am. 1988;6:43-56. [PMID: 3278886]

24. Zun LS. Acute visual loss. Emerg Med Clin North Am. 1988;6:57-72. [PMID: 3278887]

25. Cavalier JP. When moments count... the two eye emergencies that demand instant intervention. RN. 1981;44:41-3. [PMID: 6913103]

26. Brunette DD, Bennett SR. Neuro-ophthalmologic emergencies. Emerg Med Clin North Am. 1988;6:1-20. [PMID: 3278882]

EAR, NOSE, MOUTH, AND THROAT DISORDERS

Hearing Loss

Hearing loss can be sensorineural, conductive, or mixed. Sensorineural hearing loss involves the inner ear, cochlea, or auditory nerve. Conductive hearing loss is caused by a mechanical obstruction, blocking sound waves from reaching the inner ear (for example, cerumen impaction, middle ear fluid, or fixation of the ossicular chain).

In the evaluation of patients with hearing loss, the history should focus on whether the hearing loss is acute or chronic, bilateral or unilateral, progressive or stable, or associated with pain, drainage, trauma (including barotrauma and chronic or acute noise exposure), prior ear surgery, family history of hearing problems, exposure to ototoxic agents, tinnitus, or vertigo.

Acute hearing loss usually requires emergent referral. Causes of acute hearing loss include acoustic neuroma, meningioma, trauma (temporal bone fracture), meningitis, viral or suppurative labyrinthitis, systemic or local inflammatory disease, and drugs (aminoglycosides and cisplatin), but most cases are idiopathic. Several trials have demonstrated improved outcome in patients with acute hearing loss who received oral corticosteroids compared with those who received placebo or no treatment; treatment consists of immediate oral corticosteroid therapy (30 to 60 mg orally, rapidly tapered dose over 1 to 2 weeks) and emergent referral (1, 2).

In unilateral hearing loss, the Rinne and Weber tests with a 512-Hz tuning fork help to distinguish between conductive and sensorineural disease (3). In the Weber examination, the vibrating fork is held midline on the vertex, forehead, or nose; patients perceive louder sound in the good ear with sensorineural loss and louder sound in the worse ear with conductive hearing loss. The Rinne test is more accurate than the Weber test for detecting conductive hearing loss and is performed by touching the vibrating fork to the mastoid tip (bone conduction) of each ear and then holding it over the external auditory canal (air conduction). Bone and air conduction can be compared by having patients maintain each position for 2 seconds and asking them which position produces the louder sound or timing how long the sound is heard. With normal hearing or sensorineural hearing loss, hearing is better with air conduction; with conductive hearing loss, hearing is better with bone conduction.

The most common cause of chronic sensorineural hearing loss (>90%) is the aging ear (presbycusis). This condition is usually gradual, bilateral, worse in the presence of high-frequency sound, and may be accompanied by tinnitus. In older adults, presbycusis is related to a significant burden of illness relating to depression, social isolation, and functional decline (see also Reference 1 and 2). Although the evidence is clear that treatment of this condition improves function and quality of life, presbycusis is typically under-diagnosed, possibly because patients are unwilling to admit to having hearing difficulty, and because screening tests for hearing loss are imperfect.

Screening tests for presbycusis include the subjective whispered-voice test and the Hearing Handicap Inventory for the Elderly-Screening self-administered questionnaire (HHIE, **Table 55**) and objective audioscopy (4) (see also Reference 2). The HHIE-S captures functional hearing loss (patient-perceived disability), whereas the whispered-voice

TABLE 55 Self-Administered Screening Version of the Hearing Handicap Inventory for the Elderly*

Does a hearing problem cause you to feel embarrassed when meeting new people?

Does a hearing problem cause you to feel frustrated when talking to members of your family?

Do you have difficulty hearing when someone speaks in a whisper?

Do you feel handicapped by a hearing problem?

Does a hearing problem cause you difficulty when visiting friends, relatives, or neighbors?

Does a hearing problem cause you to attend religious services less often than you would like?

Does a hearing problem cause you to have arguments with family members?

Does a hearing problem cause you difficulty when listening to TV or radio?

Do you feel that any difficulty with your hearing limits or hampers your personal or social life?

Does a hearing problem cause you difficulty when in a restaurant with relatives or friends?

*Scoring: yes = 4 points, sometimes = 2 points, no = 0 points. Probability of impaired hearing: total score of ≤8 = 13%; score of 10 to 24 = 50%; score of 26 to 40 = 84% probability.

test and audioscopy identify physiologic hearing loss. Whispered-voice tests can accurately detect hearing loss but cannot be standardized among examiners. Handheld audioscopes cost $500 to $800, allow examination of the external auditory canal, require little training, and can be used by ancillary, or midlevel, health care providers. Currently, presbycusis screening by HHIE-S and audioscopy in patients older than 55 to 60 years every 1 to 3 years is recommended (see also Reference 2).

Treatment of chronic conductive hearing loss consists of removal of the obstruction. Some patients can be managed in a general medicine setting, such as those with cerumen impaction or those who have taken ototoxic drugs, whereas others require referral, such as those with chronic otitis media, perforated tympanic membrane, or cholesteatoma.

Referral for formal audiologic testing can help to establish a diagnosis of conductive versus sensorineural hearing loss and identify various hearing-assistive devices available to patients, such as telephone or pocket amplifiers, hearing aids, visual or tactile alerts for doorbells, telephones, and smoke alarms, and referral for working dog companions. Patients with hearing loss can also be educated about making social accommodations, including avoiding situations with high ambient noise levels and asking others to speak slowly and in a lower-pitched versus higher-pitched voice. In addition, cochlear nerve transplantation, developed for children, is increasingly applicable for profound bilateral sensorineural hearing loss in adults. This procedure involves sound received through a miniaturized microphone that is transmitted to a processor for conversion to electrical energy that directly stimulates the auditory nerve through an electrode array implanted in the cochlea (5).

General medicine practitioners should be aware of when patients are noncompliant in using hearing aids prescribed by certified audiologists and understand the difficulties patients may have in using them effectively (see also Reference 2).

KEY POINTS

- Screening tests for presbycusis include the whispered-voice test, the Hearing Handicap Inventory for the Elderly-Screening self-administered questionnaire, and audioscopy.
- Cochlear nerve transplantation, developed for children, is increasingly applicable for use in adults with profound bilateral sensorineural hearing loss.

Tinnitus

Subjective tinnitus is the perception of sound in the absence of an external acoustic stimulus. The sound in tinnitus is variably described as ringing, whistling, hissing, or buzzing and may be continuous or intermittent. Tinnitus is most often reported as high-pitched, loud, and asymmetric. With the less-common objective tinnitus, patients and examiners can hear real sounds, such as abnormal vascular flow, which may cause pulsatile sounds, whereas palatal spasm or contractions of the tensor tympani or stapedius muscles may create clicking sounds. An estimated 50 million Americans have tinnitus, with 25% of them reporting this symptom interferes in the performance of their activities of daily living. Prevalence of tinnitus increases with age and is more common in men than women and in whites than blacks. Only 1% to 2% of the population, however, has severely debilitating tinnitus. Tinnitus is most bothersome to patients with physical immobility, sleeplessness, pain, depression, or social isolation.

Tinnitus is rarely caused by a serious medical condition. Associated hearing loss and pulsatile, persistent (>3 months), or debilitating tinnitus are indications for further evaluation. Diagnostic assessment and treatment of tinnitus should focus on the causes described in **Table 56**. Treating cerumen impaction, otitis media, or Meniere's disease, and discontinuing potentially responsible drugs may relieve subjective tinnitus. Audiologic testing is routinely recommended in patients with subjective tinnitus. Clinically bothersome tinnitus is often associated with hearing impairment and may improve with the use of hearing aids or cochlear implants or otologic surgery for conductive hearing loss; some patients also benefit from sound-masking devices, which are generators worn behind the ear that produce low-level noise that can reduce the perception of tinnitus (evaluated during audiologic testing) (6). Preventing further hearing loss by limiting exposure to noise and ototoxic drugs is routinely recommended in these patients. Depression frequently coexists in

TABLE 56 Causes of Subjective and Objective Tinnitus

Type	Causes
Subjective Tinnitus	
Otologic	Noise-induced hearing loss, presbycusis, otosclerosis, otitis, impacted cerumen, sudden deafness, Menière's syndrome, barotrauma
Neurologic	Head injury, whiplash, multiple sclerosis, acoustic neuroma, pseudotumor cerebri
Infectious	Chronic otitis media
Drug-related	Salicylates, non-steroidal anti-inflammatory drugs, aminoglycoside antibiotics, loop diuretics, and chemotherapeutic agents
Other	Temporomandibular joint dysfunction
Objective Tinnitus	
Pulsatile	Carotid stenosis, arteriovenous malformations, vascular tumors, valvular heart disease, high cardiac output states
Muscular or anatomic	Palatal myoclonus, spasm of stapedius or tensor tympani muscle, patulous eustachian tube

patients with tinnitus, and antidepressant drugs (only tricyclic agents have been evaluated) may be helpful in reducing symptom-related disability; however, no treatment for tinnitus is considered to be uniformly effective. Recent randomized controlled trials have shown that misoprostol and botulinum toxin A injections significantly improve the loudness in tinnitus, but the sample sizes in these studies were small and follow-up durations limited. A systematic review (7) found no evidence that gingko biloba was beneficial in treating tinnitus, and another meta-analysis found no consistent evidence for the effectiveness of tocainide, iontophoresis of lidocaine, carbamazepine, benzodiazepines, tricyclic antidepressants, sound maskers, electrical stimulation, magnetic stimulation, ultrasound, biofeedback, acupuncture, hypnosis, psychotherapy, or antihistamines (8) in treating tinnitus. Tinnitus retraining therapy to habituate patients to the sounds associated with this disorder has also not been proven effective. Patients with tinnitus may be referred to the American Tinnitus Association for information and support (http://www.ata.org).

KEY POINTS

- Associated hearing loss and pulsatile, persistent (>3 months), or debilitating tinnitus are indications for further evaluation.
- Hearing aids, cochlear implants, otologic surgery for conductive hearing loss, and sound-masking devices may be helpful in patients with clinically bothersome tinnitus resulting in hearing impairment.

Otitis Media and Externa

Otitis Media

Otitis media is generally categorized as acute (either serous or suppurative) or chronic. It occurs uncommonly in adults, but its management approach is similar to that used in children. Risk factors for otitis media include age (younger for acute otitis media, and older for chronic otitis media), smoking, altered immune defenses, allergic rhinitis, and chronic eustachian tube dysfunction.

In patients with otitis media and infection, the most common organisms include *Streptococcus pneumoniae*, *Haemophilus influenza*, and *Moraxella catarrhalis*. Mycoplasma and gram-negative rods are uncommon in this disorder but cause specific notable syndromes. For example, malignant otitis is caused by *Pseudomonas aeruginosa*, typically occurring in patients with diabetes mellitus or in those who are otherwise immunocompromised, and bullous myringitis (a vesicular eruption on the tympanic membrane) is often caused by mycoplasma. Viruses responsible for otitis media include respiratory syncitial virus, influenza viruses, rhinoviruses, and adenoviruses.

The symptoms of otitis media are ear pain, decreased conductive hearing, and evidence of middle-ear effusion on otoscopy. With serous otitis, bulging alone may occur without clouding, and with suppurative otitis, bulging-associated clouding of the tympanic membrane occurs. Mastoiditis can occur with extension of the infectious process and is characterized by tenderness to palpation of the mastoid. Chronic otitis media can be suppurative or associated with the formation of excess squamous epithelium concatenated into a mass (that is, a cholesteatoma), which can then erode into surrounding structures. This compressive process causes otorrhea, pain, hearing loss, or neurologic symptoms. Up to 30% of hearing loss in older patients is related to reversible cerumen impaction or chronic otitis media; therefore, evaluation for chronic otitis by otoscopic examination to identify opacification of the tympanic membrane, erythema, or purulence in the canal, is indicated when an older adult patient is evaluated for signs of hearing loss.

The general principles of management of acute otitis media are watchful waiting, decongestant therapy (topical or systemic), and pain control; antibiotic therapy should be reserved for patients in whom evidence of purulent otitis exists (that is, opacification of the tympanic membrane with intense erythema, or purulent drainage in the canal), or in those in whom symptoms of congestion and eustachian tube dysfunction do not respond to treatment.

Antibiotic treatment of otitis media includes amoxicillin as first-line therapy, macrolides (erythromycin, clarithromycin, and azithromycin) in patients who are allergic to penicillin, and broad-spectrum antibiotics (amoxicillin-clavulanate and cefuroxime) in patients who do not respond to amoxicillin or who have a high resistance to penicillin for the treatment of streptococcal pneumonia. Myringotomy is rarely needed for adults but may be indicated for recalcitrant effusions in patients with otitis media.

Follow-up of these patients is not necessary unless symptoms persist or progress. Rare complications of otitis media include meningitis, epidural abscess, brain abscesses, lateral sinus thrombosis, cavernous vein thrombosis, and carotid artery thrombosis.

Otitis Externa

Otitis externa is a common disorder affecting at least 1 in 10 people in their lifetime. Bacterial infections are the most common cause of this disorder, with the typical causative pathogens being *Staphylococcus aureus* and *P. aeruginosa* (one third of these pathogens are polymicrobial), although contact or atopic allergic dermatitis and fungal infection with *Candida* or *Aspergillus* can also cause otitis externa. Risk factors for otitis externa include excessive ear cleaning, ear itching, or water exposure, and auricular devices, such as headphones, hearing aids, or ear covers.

The typical symptoms of this disorder are pain, pruritus, discharge, occlusive hearing loss, and pain with auricular movement or pressure. More severe cases of otitis externa can cause canal obstruction from edema of the auricular canal tissue. The severity of the pain and occlusion, and the presence of systemic progression of the infection (for example, fever) are factors determining necessity of otolaryngologic consultation. Fungal infections in otitis externa typically exude a black or white moldy substance.

Topical drops are the mainstay of treatment in most patients with this disorder. The focus of treatment should be acidification of the canal with agents such as acetic acid drops (white vinegar); decreasing occlusion and inflammation with agents such as corticosteroid drops; and halting bacterial growth with bacteriostatic agents such as alcohol, or with bactericidal agents. The most commonly prescribed bactericidal agent is a combination preparation of neomycin plus polymyxin, which is also appropriate for treating staphylococcal and pseudomonal infections. The principal side effect of these bactericidal agents is neomycin-induced contact dermatitis. The typical dosing regimen is three to six drops, three to four times daily, with treatment duration of 7 to 21 days depending on persistence of symptoms. In patients with otitis externa, a corticosteroid (triamcinolone 0.1%) plus acetic acid (75% cure rate at 2 weeks) was found to be equally effective as a corticosteroid (dexamethasone) plus an antibiotic (polymyxin plus neomycin; 82% cure rate), both combinations of which were found to be substantially more effective than acetic acid alone (57% cure rate) (9). Recurrence rates were twofold higher in patients with otitis externa who received acetic acid alone (45% vs. 23%).

Fungal infections can be treated with sulfanilamide powder or clotrimazole 1% solution, both of which are over-the-counter drugs, administered twice daily for 14 days. Eczema treatment consists of topical corticosteroid drops administered twice daily for 14 days, followed by a tapered dose.

Nonpharmacologic treatment of otitis media involves canal evacuation of cerumen and detritus, and purulent drainage, either mechanically or with a cleansing agent such as hydrogen peroxide. If severe occlusion prevents the passage of drops into the inner canal, a cotton wick can be passed through the occlusion to allow for better seepage of the drops past the occlusion.

Lack of prompt resolution, systemic involvement, or evidence of extension of infection to bony or intracranial structures as demonstrated by radiographs or neurologic findings are signs warranting prompt referral to an ear, nose, and throat specialist.

KEY POINTS

- In patients with otitis externa, a corticosteroid plus acetic acid was found to be as effective as a corticosteroid plus an antibiotic, both combinations of which were found to be substantially more effective than acetic acid alone in treating this disorder.

- Nonpharmacologic treatment of otitis media involves canal evacuation of cerumen and detritus and purulent drainage, either mechanically or with a cleansing agent.

Upper Respiratory Infections and Bronchitis

Upper Respiratory Infections

Upper respiratory infections (URIs) of the nasopharyngeal tree are extremely common, occurring up to two to three times in each adult annually and accounting for 40% of all days lost from work and $3.5 billion in lost productivity and treatment costs. These infections are otherwise mostly benign, self-limited conditions, lasting typically 3 to 7 days. However, while patients are ill, they experience considerable decrements in health-related quality of life (10), rendering

URIs cumulatively responsible for many person-days of disability annually. The cause of URIs is overwhelmingly viral in origin, with rhinovirus, coronavirus, and respiratory syncytial virus accounting for most infections; these infections are typically transmitted through direct contact or aerosolized particles, with an incubation period of 24 to 72 hours. The major risk factors for infection and excessive morbidity from URIs are overcrowding, age (young and old), malnutrition, and immunocompromised health states. Although not proven, rational preventive measures against URIs include hand washing, airway cover, and fastidious disposal of nasal secretions. Medicinal preventive measures, such as vitamins C or E or echinacea, are not supported by strong evidence. The typical symptoms and course of URIs are initial nasal congestion, rhinorrhea, and scratchy throat, all of which subside in 3 to 5 days, whereas the onset of cough occurs later in the course of illness, around days 2 to 4. The duration of illness in patients with URIs is up to 2 weeks in 25% of cases. Bacterial rhinosinusitis superinfection occurs in 1% to 3% of cases.

The principal diagnostic dilemma in patients with URI symptoms is determining the presence of a bacterial superinfection requiring antibiotics. Although clinical features of URI do not have good test characteristics, recent consensus statements recommend using the duration (>7 days) or the presence of signs or symptoms that increase the likelihood for sinusitis, such as fever, upper-tooth or facial pain, or purulent secretions (see Sinusitis section) to determine the need for antibiotics. Imaging studies are reserved for patients with recalcitrant, prolonged sinusitis, who are unresponsive to at least two courses of antibiotics or for those in whom there is suspicion of influenza based on time of year, recent contacts, or myalgias.

Management of patients with URIs consists largely of symptomatic therapy. Evidence supports the use of pseudoephedrine, cromolyn sodium, and ipratropium for congestion, rhinorrhea, and sneezing, although the relative efficacy of each agent is unknown because no head-to-head trials comparing these treatments have been conducted. The evidence for antitussives, antihistamines, zinc, and echinacea indicate no benefit, marginal benefit, or a poor side-effect–to–benefit ratio, and most of these trials have significant methodologic flaws; therefore, the routine use of these agents is not recommended. Antiviral agents such as nasal interferon are currently being studied. Heated humidified air has been found efficacious in improving URI symptoms.

Acute Bronchitis

Acute bronchitis is a syndrome of inflammation of the bronchi characterized clinically by a cough that is usually productive and associated with a URI; fever is uncommon, and, if present, suggests a pneumonitis. Other diagnoses that can mimic this syndrome are reactive airways dysfunction syndrome, gastroesophageal reflux disease, and postnasal drip in the setting of a URI or allergic rhinitis. Most cases of acute

bronchitis are viral in origin, with influenza, parainfluenza, coronavirus, and rhinovirus accounting for most infections, yet most patients who have this syndrome are treated with antibiotics in practice (11). There has been a robust effort to reduce inappropriate antibiotic use in patients with acute bronchitis. With the exception of acute bronchitis in the setting of underlying pulmonary disease, the only bacterial infection that requires antibiotic therapy (erythromycin 400 mg, four times daily for 7 to 14 days) is *Bordetella pertussis*, which is typically characterized by a barking or paroxysmal cough in the setting of URI symptoms lasting longer than 2 weeks. Pertussis is increasing in incidence in adults and often is misdiagnosed as bronchitis. The diagnosis of pertussis is best confirmed with a throat swab with polymerase chain reaction testing or culture.

Symptomatic treatment of acute bronchitis is the same as for URI management. There is insufficient evidence to prescribe bronchodilators routinely in patients with this syndrome.

KEY POINTS

- Indications of sinusitis warranting antibiotics are duration of signs or symptoms for >7 days or the presence of fever, upper-tooth or facial pain, or purulent secretions.
- Heated humidified air has been found efficacious in improving URI symptoms.
- Besides acute bronchitis in the setting of underlying pulmonary disease, the only bacterial infection requiring antibiotic therapy is *Bordetella pertussis*.
- The diagnosis of pertussis is best established with a throat swab and polymerase chain reaction testing or culture.

Cerumen Impaction

Cerumen is the natural cleansing mechanism of the ear, but with age-related changes in thickness and clearance time, prevalence of impaction may be as high as 35% in elderly patients, thus contributing to chronic or acute hearing deficits by conduction loss. Monthly use of a softening agent or ceruminolytic for 10 minutes followed by gentle lavage with an ear syringe can prevent impaction. Impaction should be treated only in patients with symptoms, such as worsened hearing, ear pain, fullness or itching, dizziness or vertigo, or unexplained fever, or when examination of the tympanic membrane is necessary.

In the primary care setting, the approach to cerumen impaction includes softening agents or ceruminolytics, either for 10 to 15 minutes or three times daily for 3 to 7 days, followed by lavage and curettage if needed (12). Softening agents include distilled water, hydrogen peroxide, or household oils (mineral, olive, vegetable, baby oil). Ceruminolytics including 0.5% acetic acid, combined mineral oil and hydrogen peroxide, and docusate sodium (8 to 10 drops of 1% solution in 30-mL dropper bottle for 10 minutes [off-label use]) were superior to triethanolamine polypeptide oleate or more expensive agents such as carbamide peroxide in patients with cerumen impaction. Triethanolamine polypeptide oleate is associated with allergic reactions. Current evidence does not indicate superiority of one agent to another; large, well-designed randomized trials in this area are needed. (13, 14)

Lavage for cerumen impaction should be performed gently, with water or saline at body temperature, using an ear syringe or 10- to 20-mL syringe with a short length of intravenous tubing directed at any visible break in the cerumen of the posterior-superior canal wall when the auricle is pulled up and back (left ear at 1:00, right ear at 11:00). The primary risk of irrigation is retained water behind remaining cerumen, with possible secondary infection and skin maceration. Overaggressive lavage can cause worsened pain, hearing loss, and tympanic perforation. Lavage should be stopped if pain, nausea, or vertigo occurs. Once cerumen is softened, suction can be used in conjunction with lavage or curettage.

Blunt curettes or cerumen spoons should be used under direct visualization by otoscopy with an operating head and only for impaction in the distal third, or fibrocartilaginous portion, of the canal. The curette should be advanced past softened cerumen and then gently pulled back. Curettage should not be used in the proximal two thirds of the canal or in uncooperative patients.

Contraindications to cerumen removal in the primary care setting include otitis externa, which should be first treated with a topical otic antibiotic and corticosteroids; history of severe otic infection associated with purulent otorrhea and severe otalgia; history of ear or mastoid surgery; presence of myringotomy tubes; presence of perforated tympanic membrane (from a prior head trauma or associated with a history of sudden, pronounced hearing loss); or possible compromised integrity of the tympanic membrane. Additional indications for referral to an otolaryngologist include severely swollen canal, purulent or necrotic material, resistant impaction, severe pain or vertigo during disimpaction, persistent acute hearing loss, and history of chronic impaction.

KEY POINTS

- **Ceruminolytics including 0.5% acetic acid, combined mineral oil and hydrogen peroxide, and docusate sodium, appear superior to triethanolamine polypeptide oleate or more expensive agents in patients with cerumen impaction.**

- **Contraindications to cerumen removal include otitis externa, history of severe otic infection, history of ear or mastoid surgery, presence of myringotomy tubes, presence of perforated tympanic membrane, or compromised integrity of the tympanic membrane.**

Epistaxis

Epistaxis occurs commonly, with a lifetime prevalence of approximately 60%, and is usually benign and self-limited. The source of epistaxis is usually anterior; 80% of cases occur in the Kiesselbach's plexus, where the circulation areas of branches of three arteries converge in the nasal septum. Most epistaxis (80%) is idiopathic or involves trauma, hyperemia with allergic or viral rhinitis, intranasal drug use, foreign body, and oral antiplatelet drugs or anticoagulation. Unusual causes of epistaxis include hereditary hemorrhagic telangiectasia (Osler-Weber-Rendu disease), familial platelet and coagulation disorders, aneurysms of head and neck vessels, and nasal tumors.

In patients in whom fluid resuscitation and airway management are not necessary, management includes pressure, cold pack, examination, chemical cautery with a silver nitrate stick, and packing (15). Pressure should be applied, possibly by the patient, to the distal third of the nose for 5 to 20 minutes. Additional maneuvers include administration of phenylephrine or oxymetazoline spray for vasoconstriction; expectorating, rather than swallowing, blood to prevent nausea and vomiting; insertion of a plug of cotton swab, gauze pad, or tissue paper; and application of a cold pack across the bridge of the nose. Because elevated blood pressure is possibly the result of distress rather than cause of the bleeding in patients with epistaxis, control of high blood pressure in these patients is controversial, and rapid lowering of blood pressure may not be tolerated.

The nasal passages of patients with epistaxis should be anesthetized before examination, with cotton swabs soaked in local anesthetic. The nasal examination requires good lighting, a nasal speculum, and patients sitting with the chin slightly raised. Tilting the head back obscures proper visualization of nasal anatomy. Clots can be removed with gentle nose blowing, suction, or a cotton swab.

In patients in whom no bleeding site is obvious, pressure alone is usually sufficient to stop the bleeding. Anterior nosebleeds should be chemically or electrically cauterized. The nose should be packed in patients in whom an anterior nose bleed continues—with consideration to the horizontal orientation of nasal floor—with a commercially available nasal tampon or ribbon gauze impregnated with petroleum jelly, with or without 3% bismuth tribromophenate, or polymyxin B-bacitracin zinc-neomycin ointment. Tampons, which expand on contact with blood, should be applied with lubricant jelly or antibiotic ointment before insertion; after insertion, dripping saline onto the tampon helps promote full expansion, and a small amount of topical vasoconstrictor may further help stop bleeding. For ribbon gauze, bayonet forceps are used to pack the folded layers as far into the posterior nasal cavity as possible. Although there is no evidence that nasal tampons or ribbon gauze is superior to the other in treating patients with nosebleeds, tampons are simpler and more efficient for use in these patients. Complications of packing include septal hematomas or abscesses, sinusitis, pressure necrosis, and neurogenic syncope during the procedure. Leaving packing in place for 3 days may facilitate clot formation, but leaving packing in place for longer durations confers a risk for pressure necrosis, toxic shock syndrome, and infection. Prophylactic antistaphylococcal topical or oral antibiotics are recommended in patients with epistaxis and nasal packing, although it is unclear whether these agents prevent rare toxic shock syndrome in the setting of packing. If bleeding persists or recurs, packing the contralateral nasal cavity may be helpful.

Indications for referral to an otorhinolaryngologist include posterior nosebleeds, which require a more complicated packing technique and the need for electrocautery. Urgent referral is indicated in patients in whom bleeding is not controlled or recurs within 24 to 48 hours for possible endoscopic arterial ligation or angiographic embolization. Patients who may not be compliant with prompt follow-up, those who are elderly or frail, and most with posterior packing may require hospitalization.

Besides warfarin, aspirin, and NSAIDs, other medications implicated in epistaxis include selective serotonin reuptake inhibitors, cytotoxic chemotherapy, antifungals, fluoroquinolone antibiotics, sildenafil, valproic acid, high-dose vitamin E, and oral contraceptives (16). Routine coagulation studies are usually normal and of little help in these patients except in those taking warfarin or with a history suggestive of an underlying bleeding disorder. Discontinuing oral antiplatelet drugs for several days is of unclear benefit in patients with epistaxis. Patients with epistaxis who are receiving anticoagulation and have a therapeutic INR can probably continue warfarin therapy. Temporary interruption of warfarin can be considered in patients with an INR ≥4. Available topical clotting agents for epistaxis include tranexamic acid, fibrin glue, hemostatic gel tamponades, or a combination of alginic acid and oxidized cellulose.

KEY POINTS

- Elevated blood pressure may be the result of distress from epistaxis rather than its cause, and these patients may not tolerate rapid lowering of blood pressure.

- The nose should be packed in patients with a continuing anterior nosebleed with a nasal tampon or ribbon gauze impregnated with petroleum jelly, with or without 3% bismuth tribromophenate, or polymyxin B-bacitracin zinc-neomycin ointment.

- Leaving packing in place for 3 days may facilitate clot formation, but leaving packing in place for longer durations confers a risk for pressure necrosis, toxic shock syndrome, and infection.

- Prophylactic antistaphylococcal topical or oral antibiotics are recommended in patients with epistaxis and nasal packing.

Sinusitis

Acute sinusitis, more appropriately called rhinosinusitis, consists of inflammation of one or more paranasal sinuses accompanied by nasal mucosal inflammation. Rhinosinusitis usually is caused by viral infections, and much less often by allergies, local irritants, or anatomic abnormalities. Overall, approximately 2% of cases of viral rhinosinusitis are complicated by bacterial infection, including 15% of patients evaluated in the ambulatory care setting. Rhinosinusitis is 1 of the 10 most frequently diagnosed conditions in ambulatory care, accounting for 25 million office visits in 1995, and the fifth leading diagnostic indication for prescribing antibiotics.

Most community-acquired bacterial infections are caused by *Streptococcus pneumoniae* or *Haemophilus influenzae*. Dental disease or instrumentation can cause anaerobic infections. Immunocompromised patients are at risk for fungal infections, and gram-negative organisms are associated with nosocomial infections (nasal intubation or a decreased level of consciousness).

Patients with acute rhinosinusitis have symptom duration of less than 4 weeks, with symptoms consisting of nasal congestion, purulent nasal secretions, sinus tenderness, and facial pain. Acute viral rhinosinusitis generally resolves within 7 to 10 days, and about two thirds of cases of bacterial rhinosinusitis resolve without treatment within 1 month. Serious complications of rhinosinusitis, including meningitis, brain abscess, and periorbital cellulitis, are rare, although the precise risk for progression to these conditions is unknown. Distinguishing acute bacterial infection from prolonged viral rhinosinusitis can be quite difficult. Purulent nasal secretions, maxillary toothache, poor response to decongestants, pain on bending forward, abnormal transillumination, and air-fluid levels or opacification on plain radiography of the sinuses are the strongest predictors for bacterial infection. Symptoms that persist for more than 10 to 14 days or worsen after 5 to 7 days suggest a bacterial cause as do fever and severe unilateral maxillary pain with swelling or erythema (17).

Numerous clinical decision rules have been developed to identify patients with bacterial rhinosinusitis to reduce inappropriate antibiotic use. Consensus guidelines suggest that antibiotics are appropriate for patients with moderately severe symptoms who meet the clinical diagnostic criteria for acute bacterial rhinosinusitis. These criteria consist of symptom duration of 7 days or more, maxillary tooth or facial pain or tenderness (especially unilateral), and purulent nasal secretions (18). However, likelihood ratios associated with positive clinical signs and symptoms range from only 1.1 to 5.5, and clinical studies, which have been limited by lack of an acceptable gold standard (sinus aspirate culture) and variable symptom durations, have not rigorously evaluated these criteria. Although the presence of air-fluid levels or complete sinus opacification is 80% sensitive and 85% specific for bacterial rhinosinusitis, routine sinus radiography is not recommended.

Meta-analysis has shown that antibiotics improve cure rates of acute maxillary sinusitis and provide symptomatic relief. After 10 to 14 days of treatment with antibiotics, symptoms in 81% of patients with maxillary sinusitis were cured or improved compared with 66% in those who received placebo (absolute benefit, 15%; number needed to treat = 7). Amoxicillin, doxycycline, and trimethoprim-sulfamethoxazole are considered appropriate first-line treatments in patients with rhinosinusitis, but the increasing antibiotic resistance of *S. pneumoniae* and *H. influenzae* may alter therapeutic decisions (19). Although adjuvant therapies, including oral and nasal decongestants, antihistamines, mucolytics, and nasal corticosteroids, are frequently used for treating acute rhinosinusitis, randomized trials have not shown convincing evidence for their efficacy (20).

Extended-spectrum antibiotics, CT sinus imaging, and/or referral to an otolaryngologist may be appropriate in patients in whom symptoms do not respond to first-line antibiotics or in those with severe symptoms. Fluoroquinolones, macrolides, and second- and higher-generation cephalosporins are no more effective than the less-expensive amoxicillin-clavulanate in patients with rhinosinusitis. Patients with recurrent or refractory symptoms may need to undergo evaluation for opportunistic infections, immunodeficiency, and structural abnormalities.

KEY POINTS

- The criteria for bacterial sinusitis are symptom duration ≥7 days, maxillary tooth or facial pain or tenderness (especially unilateral), and purulent nasal secretions.

- After 10 to 14 days of treatment with antibiotics, symptoms in 81% of patients with maxillary sinusitis were cured or improved compared with 66% in those who received placebo.

- Extended-spectrum antibiotics, CT sinus imaging, and/or referral to an otolaryngologist may be appropriate in patients with sinusitis in whom symptoms do not respond to first-line antibiotics or in those with severe symptoms.

Rhinitis

Rhinitis is an inflammation of the nasal mucosal membranes that causes rhinorrhea, nasal itching, sneezing, nasal congestion, and postnasal drainage. Allergic rhinitis, which can be seasonal or perennial, occurs when inhaled allergens bind IgE receptors in sensitized patients, leading to release of inflammatory mediators. Nonallergic causes of rhinitis include acute viral infections, idiopathic rhinitis (a nonallergic reaction to nonspecific irritants), atrophic rhinitis (occurring in elderly patients), and rhinitis medicamentosa. Allergic rhinitis is asso-

ciated with impaired quality of life and may be a risk factor for asthma.

Symptoms triggered by pollen or animals, summertime symptoms, personal history of hay fever, or family history of allergy strongly suggest allergic rhinitis, with positive likelihood ratios ranging from 3 to 6 for each factor (**Table 57**) (21). The presence of pain, bleeding, fever, cough, purulent discharge, and unilateral symptoms suggest an alternative diagnosis or complication.

Patients with allergic rhinitis may receive empirical treatment with medications, including antihistamines, decongestants, nasal corticosteroids, anticholinergics, antileukotrienes, and cromolyn sodium, a mast-cell stabilizer. Numerous controlled trials have shown that oral antihistamines effectively relieve allergic symptoms; however, only the nonsedating antihistamines also improved quality of life and reduced work and activity impairment. Somnolence, dry mouth, dizziness, and headache were the most commonly reported adverse events, although almost exclusively with sedating antihistamines. Nonsedating antihistamines cause less somnolence but are more expensive. Controlled trials have shown that combining oral decongestants, such as pseudoephedrine, with oral antihistamines improved rhinitis symptoms more than either agent alone or placebo. The most common side effects from oral decongestants were headache and insomnia, but oral sympathomimetic agents may also elevate blood pressure and worsen lower urinary tract symptoms in men with benign prostatic hyperplasia (22).

Nasal corticosteroids produce significantly greater relief of nasal symptoms than oral (sedating and nonsedating) or topical H_1-receptor antagonists for perennial and seasonal allergic rhinitis (23). Minimal inhaler side effects include nasal irritation and epistaxis; septal perforation is an exceedingly rare complication, and nasal corticosteroids do not cause adrenal suppression. Nasal corticosteroids are also more effective than oral antihistamines for as-needed symptomatic relief of seasonal rhinitis (24); however, approximately half of patients require an antihistamine combined with a nasal corticosteroid for optimal symptomatic control. Leukotriene receptor antagonists are slightly more effective than placebo, are as effective as oral antihistamines, but are less effective than nasal corticosteroids in improving nasal symptoms and quality of life in patients with seasonal allergic rhinitis (25). Cromolyn sodium is more effective in treating seasonal than perennial allergic rhinitis.

When empiric treatment fails, diagnostic allergy testing may be appropriate to guide allergen avoidance or immunotherapy. Removing dust mites with an acaricide, high-efficiency particulate air filters, or environmental control programs, and removing pets from the bedroom may reduce rhinitis symptoms (26). Immunotherapy reduces symptoms during treatment, and benefits may persist for 6 years. Allergy tests may also be helpful in patients in whom the pretest

TABLE 57 Accuracy of Medical History for the Diagnosis of Allergic Rhinitis

Medical History	Question	Positive Likelihood Ratio	Negative Likelihood Ratio
Triggers	Do you have nasal symptoms from pollen or animals?	6.69	0.15
	Do weeds increase symptoms?	6.53	0.65
	Are symptoms from animals?	4.22	0.34
	Do cats or dogs affect nasal symptoms?	4.21	0.81
	Do trees increase symptoms?	4.86	0.52
	Does grass increase symptoms?	3.95	0.40
	Do house dust, house dust mites, or pollen affect symptoms?	3.34	0.39
History	Have you had hay fever?	4.80	0.58
	Have you had positive tests for allergies?	3.47	0.56
Family history	Family member with asthma, eczema, or allergic rhinitis?	3.41	0.70
Months of	Are your symptoms worse in summer?	3.33	0.52
the year	Do you have seasonal exacerbations?	1.59	0.59
General	Do you think you are allergic?	3.12	0.33

Reprinted with permission from Gendo K, Larson EB. Ann Intern Med. 2004;140(4):278-89. Copyright © 2004 American College of Physicians.

probability for allergic rhinitis is low, because the positive likelihood ratios are consistently high, and a positive test could lead to treatment.

Patients with nonallergic rhinitis may respond to topical antihistamines such as azelastine; nasal corticosteroids; topical anticholinergics such as ipratropium; and cromolyn sodium. Rhinitis-causing URIs most commonly are viral, although 2% are complicated by bacterial infections. A meta-analysis found that antibiotic treatment in patients with a rhinitis-causing URI did not reduce symptoms compared with placebo while significantly increasing the risk for adverse events (27).

KEY POINTS

- Oral antihistamines effectively relieve allergic symptoms, but only the nonsedating antihistamines also improve quality of life and reduce work and activity impairment in patients with rhinitis.
- Combining oral decongestants with oral antihistamines improved rhinitis symptoms more than either agent alone or placebo.
- Nasal corticosteroids produce significantly greater relief of nasal symptoms than oral (sedating and nonsedating) or topical H_1-receptor antagonists for perennial and seasonal allergic rhinitis.
- Leukotriene receptor antagonists are slightly more effective than placebo, are as effective as oral antihistamines, but are less effective than nasal corticosteroids in improving nasal symptoms and quality of life in patients with seasonal allergic rhinitis.

Dental Disease

Although dental care is not usually in the domain of general medicine practitioners, patients sometimes have oral complaints that are dental in nature, and some dental diseases can progress to require medical treatment (28). In the absence of trauma, dental pain is usually a result of infection, of either the tooth or gingiva. The local anatomic barriers of bone, muscle, and fascia determine the routes of spread of infection. The crown of each tooth is covered in enamel and projects above the gum line. The tooth's enervation and blood supply enter from the apex, forming the pulp in the center of the tooth. Below the gum line, the tooth has roots that extend into the alveolar bone of the mandible or maxilla. The tooth is held in place by a periodontal membrane that allows for slight movement of the tooth. Infections of the pulp can produce abscesses of the mandibular or maxillary bone or osteomyelitis, extend into the maxillary sinuses, or spread along the oral fascia. Disease spread can extend into the orofacial area or deeper into the peripharyngeal spaces of the head and neck. The superficial orofacial spaces include buccal, submental, masticator, canine, and infratemporal areas. The location of the swelling can often pinpoint the tooth involved. Infection of the superficial oral spaces results in local swelling, tenderness, and erythema. Infection from maxillary molars spreads to the temporal space, whereas that in the mandibular molars spreads to the sublingual space. The bicuspid teeth often cause infection in the buccal space, and the mandibular incisors cause infection in the submental parotid space. Infection can spread from the tooth throughout the mouth, or hematogenously, particularly in susceptible individuals.

The deeper areas for infection include the submandibular, lateral, and retropharyngeal spaces. Infection from these areas can spread intracranially, resulting in meningitis or subdural empyema or caudally resulting in aspiration, obstruction, or necrotizing mediastinitis; any of these conditions can cause very serious medical complications.

Dental infections usually begin with a tooth carie. A carie is an erosion of the enamel and dentin caused by acid secreted by oral bacteria, commonly *Streptococcus mutans.* Caries are asymptomatic unless they extend into the pulp or result in inflammation or abscesses in surrounding gingival tissue. Cavities extending into the pulp may be associated with jaw pain or headache, but these patients usually report symptoms that are intermittent and worsen with hot, cold, or sweet foods. A referral to a dentist is appropriate for patients with caries and no other cause of pain. Pulpitis, an infection of the tooth's pulp, can be treated by filling the caries on early identification but may require a root canal (removal and filling of the pulp) or tooth extraction. The dental pulp can also be infected hematogenously (almost exclusively after mechanical irritation of the pulp) or by spread from an adjacent infected tooth. Because this area of the tooth is a closed space, inflammation can quickly result in necrosis of the pulp.

Infections localized to the gums (gingivitis), periodontal membrane, or teeth require management by a dentist. In patients with infections that have spread to the superficial oral spaces, the most important treatment is surgical drainage and removal of necrotic tissue. Needle aspiration can help identify the causative infectious organism in these patients and allow for drainage. In addition, antibiotics often are used in this setting to halt local spread and prevent hematogenous dissemination. In immunocompetent patients, the use of penicillin remains appropriate because most organisms are sensitive to this agent. Clindamycin or metronidazole is appropriate in patients who are allergic to penicillin. Other possible choices include doxycycline, cefoxitin, or cefotetan, depending on results from cultures. For immunosuppressed patients, double coverage with an aminoglycoside and a broad-spectrum antibiotic, such as ceftizoxime, cefotaxime, piperacillin, or imipenem, is indicated.

Trauma to the tooth can result in loosening of the tooth. Treatment of minimally loose teeth consists of a soft diet for a few days, but markedly mobile teeth require routine dental referral. Adult teeth that are completely avulsed can be successfully reimplanted, with best results occurring when reimplantation is performed within 30 minutes of the trauma. The best way to transport a completely avulsed tooth for treatment is to place it back in its socket. Dedicated tooth transport media are available and can maintain cell viability for 12 to 24 hours. The best alternative to these transport media is milk.

Management of patients with fractures that do not expose the pulp (class 1 or 2) consists of placement of a gauze covering on the tooth and nonurgent dental referral. Patients with fractures that expose the pulp should receive a prompt dental referral.

Oral Lesions

Ulcers

Aphthous ulcers are painful lesions that are localized, shallow, and round, often with a whitish appearance (**Figure 18**). They are among the most common ulcers in North America. The etiology of aphthous ulcers is unknown; they are not caused by the herpes simplex virus.

The differential diagnosis of ulcers is mainly between aphthous ulcers of uncertain etiology and those accompanying Behcet's disease, which is a connective-tissue disease characterized by recurrent oral and genital ulcers. Although patients with recurrent aphthous ulcers are healthy, patients with Behcet's disease have other systemic manifestations, including genital aphthae, ocular disease, skin lesions, neurologic disease, vascular disease, or arthritis. HIV infection can also cause recurrent, often severe, aphthous ulcers. In immunocompetent hosts, these ulcers heal in 10 to 14 days without scarring but often recur. Most individuals experience fewer attacks of these ulcers as they age.

Treatment of aphthous ulcers is largely symptomatic with topical analgesics. Some evidence suggests that amlexanox, an over-the-counter, 5% oral paste, results in quicker healing than with placebo. Thalidomide has been found to be useful in treating severe aphthous ulcer disease in patients with HIV

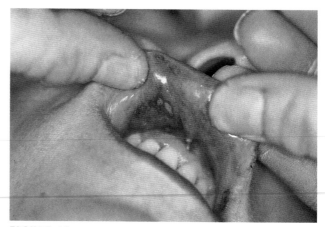

FIGURE 18.
Aphthous ulcer.

infection. Recalcitrant lesions, particularly those associated with Bechet's disease, can be treated with intralesional or oral corticosteroids, in addition to colchicine, dapsone, pentoxifylline, interferon alfa, and levamisole.

Oral Infections

Many infections involve the mouth, including candidiasis (thrush), herpes simplex virus, varicella, coxsackievirus (foot and mouth disease), syphilis, and HIV. Candidiasis is common, particularly in infants, denture wearers, after broad-spectrum antibiotic use, in association with inhaled corticosteroids, and in individuals with immunodeficiency caused by chemotherapy, radiation, or disease. The most common form of this infection appears as white plaques on the oral surface, although it may appear as erythema under dentures. Candidiasis can also cause painful fissuring at the corners of the mouth, known as cheilitis or perleche. This infection is usually treated with topical antifungal agents consisting of nystatin swish and swallow or clotrimazole troche for 1 to 2 weeks. Immunosuppressed patients and those with severe oral candidiasis may require systemic therapy, usually fluconazole.

Oral Tumors

Most oral cancers are squamous cell carcinomas and are associated with tobacco and alcohol use. The incidence of squamous cell carcinoma is more than 200 times higher in heavy smokers and drinkers than in patients who do neither. The United States Preventive Services Task Force does not recommend for or against routine screening of adults for oral cancer because there is insufficient evidence to indicate screening of high-risk individuals would result in better outcomes. A biopsy should be performed on any nonhealing ulcer and any persistent papule, plaque, erosion, or mass in the mouth, particularly in patients with risk factors for oral cancer. Oral leukoplakia is a precancerous lesion, consisting of a white patch or plaque of the oral mucosa. Like most precancerous lesions, it is associated with a spectrum of transformation from hyperplasia, to dysplasia, and then to carcinoma in situ. It is estimated that up to 20% of such lesions will progress to carcinoma within 10 years.

Melanoma is another type of oral malignancy. A biopsy should be performed on any pigmented oral lesion, particularly those with irregular borders, variegation in color, or changing size, to rule out this disease.

Mucocutaneous Manifestations of Autoimmune Diseases

Systemic lupus erythematosus (SLE) is commonly characterized by mucocutaneous manifestations. Characteristic lesions with erythema, atrophy, and depigmentation commonly occur on the lips, and irregularly shaped plaques, erosions, ulcers, and erythema may involve the oral mucosa in patients with SLE.

More than 90% of patients with Stevens-Johnson syndrome have mucosal involvement that may include painful oral lesions. Other autoimmune diseases that can produce oral lesions include SLE, Reiter's syndrome (also known as reactive arthritis), bullous pemphigoid, pemphigus vulgaris, and cicatricial pemphigoid. Although commonly involving the mouth, these lesions usually are associated with bullae in other locations of the body. Biopsy is indicated when oral bullae are present in patients with autoimmune disorders.

KEY POINTS

- Thalidomide has been found to be useful in treating severe aphthous ulcer disease in patients with HIV infection.
- Recalcitrant oral ulcers, particularly those associated with Bechet's disease, can be treated with intralesional or oral corticosteroids, in addition to colchicine, dapsone, pentoxifylline, interferon alfa, and levamisole.
- A biopsy should be performed on any nonhealing ulcer and any persistent papule, plaque, erosion, or mass in the mouth, particularly in patients with risk factors for oral cancer.
- Oral leukoplakia is a precancerous lesion, characterized by a white patch or plaque of the oral mucosa, with eventual transformation to carcinoma in situ.
- A biopsy to rule out melanoma should be performed on any pigmented oral lesion, particularly those with irregular borders, variegation in color, or changing size.
- More than 90% of patients with Stevens-Johnson syndrome have mucosal involvement that may include painful oral lesions.

Pharyngitis

Pharyngitis, defined as direct infection of pharyngeal tissue, is the sixth most common reason patients visit physicians. Viral infections, particularly rhinovirus, are the most common cause of pharyngitis. Epstein–Barr virus–associated mononucleosis and acute retroviral syndrome are relatively uncommon viral causes of pharyngitis. The most common bacterial organisms implicated in pharyngitis are group A β-hemolytic streptococcus (GABHS), *Chlamydia pneumoniae*, and *Mycoplasma pneumoniae*; less than 1% of pharyngitis is caused by *Neisseria gonorrhoeae* or *Corynebacterium diphtheriae*.

It is important to detect the presence of GABHS because this bacterial pathogen causes 5% to 15% of acute pharyngitis in adults, and antibiotic therapy may be beneficial in these patients (29). Although untreated GABHS usually lasts for fewer than 10 days, it is associated with a risk for developing rheumatic fever, acute glomerulonephritis, and suppurative complications, including peritonsillar and retropharyngeal abscesses. The gold standard diagnostic test for suspected

GABHS is throat culture, although lower sensitivity may result from improper collection and laboratory technique, and lower specificity may result in patients who are chronic carriers of GABHS. In addition, throat culture results are not available for 24 to 48 hours after testing is performed. Rapid antigen detection tests provide immediate results in patients with suspected GABHS, and the newer optical immunoassays have a sensitivity of 88% and a specificity of 94%.

Penicillin is the preferred antibiotic treatment for patients with GABHS, and erythromycin is recommended for those with penicillin allergy. Antibiotics initiated within the first 2 to 3 days of symptom onset reduce symptom duration by approximately 1 day; antipyretic, analgesic, and gargle agents are also recommended as supportive therapies in these patients. Although treatment also reduces contagion in patients with GABHS within 24 hours, this is less relevant in adults who do not have intensive exposure to children. Antibiotics significantly reduce the risk for acute rheumatic fever in patients with GABHS, but this complication occurs rarely in North America, and the number needed to treat (NNT) for benefit exceeds 3000, with the NNT for prevention of clinically significant carditis even higher. Although antibiotics reduce the risk for suppurative complications in patients with GABHS, these are also rare outcomes that have often developed by the time of initial presentation. There is insufficient evidence to determine whether antibiotic treatment prevents acute glomerulonephritis in patients with GABHS.

More than 70% of adults seeking care for acute pharyngitis receive antibiotics, most often, broad-spectrum agents; however, indications for antibiotics in adults, even with confirmed GABHS, are less than compelling (30). Practice guidelines to limit inappropriate antibiotic use in healthy adults have focused on the presence of clinical findings and laboratory test results. The Centers for Disease Control guidelines emphasize using the validated Centor score as criteria for antibiotic use in patients with pharyngitis (**Table 58**), which assigns one point each for the presence of tonsillar exudates, tender anterior cervical adenopathy or lymphadenitis, absence of cough, and history of fever (31) (**Table 59**). The sensitivity and specificity of three or four clinical criteria are both 75% compared with performing a throat culture (32). No further testing or treatment is recommended in adults who meet none or only one of the Centor criteria. Patients who meet more of these criteria can be empirically treated or treated only if results from a rapid antigen detection test are positive. Previous guidelines recommended empiric antibiotic treatment for patients meeting 3 or 4 of these criteria or antibiotics for those meeting 2 or 3 criteria who also have positive rapid antigen detection test results.

However, a prospective observational study found that empirically treating adults with Centor scores of 3 or 4 could lead to 44% of patients receiving unnecessary antibiotics (33). Applying the Infectious Disease Society of America guidelines that recommend use of antibiotics only in adults with clinical findings suggestive of GABHS and positive rapid antigen test results could reduce the rate of unnecessary antibiotic use to

2%; however, at least 20% of patients with positive cultures would not receive antibiotics under these guidelines, although the clinical consequences of such a scenario are considered negligible (34). A cost-effectiveness analysis also found that empirical treatment for suspected GABHS was less effective than rapid-testing strategies, although performing a throat culture was found to be the most effective and least expensive strategy in these patients when the GABHS prevalence was 10% (35). A subsequent trial found that the optimal management strategy for GABHS was to routinely perform rapid antigen detection tests for patients with Centor scores greater than 1 and treat only those with positive results (36). A recent decision analysis further concluded that patients with Centor scores of 3 or 4 who have negative rapid antigen testing should then undergo throat cultures to guide treatment decisions (37).

TABLE 58 Centor Clinical Prediction Rule for Diagnosing GABHS in Adults (Posttest probabilities)

Points*	Likelihood Ratio	Pretest probability of GABHS (%)			
		5	15	25	50
0	0.16	1	2	5	14
1	0.3	2	5	9	23
2	0.75	4	12	20	43
3	2.1	10	27	41	68
4	6.3	25	53	68	86

Reprinted with permission from Ebell MH, et al. JAMA 2000; 284:2912-8.

*One point assigned for each of the following characteristics: history of fever, anterior cervical adenopathy, tonsillar exudates, and absence of cough.

GABHS = group A β-hemolytic streptococcus.

TABLE 59 Principles of Appropriate Antibiotic Use for Acute Pharyngitis in Adults

All patients with pharyngitis should be offered appropriate doses of analgesics, antipyretics, and other supportive care
Physicians should limit antimicrobial prescriptions to patients who are most likely to have GABHS as indicated by:
Presence of more than one clinical criterion of tonsillar exudates, anterior cervical lymphadenopathy, absence of cough, history of fever and positive rapid antigen detection test or GABHS throat culture
No treatment indicated for patients with 0 or 1 clinical criterion for GABHS
The preferred antimicrobial agent for treatment of acute GABHS pharyngitis is penicillin, or erythromycin in penicillin-allergic patients
Rationale for treatment is to prevent rare sequelae of rheumatic fever, acute glomerulonephritis, and suppurative complications; decrease contagion; and reduce symptom duration

Data are from References 31 and 37.

GABHS = group A β-hemolytic streptococcus.

Hoarseness

Hoarseness directly implicates the larynx and is a sign of a multitude of disorders. When recent in onset, hoarseness is most commonly caused by bacterial or viral infection but can also be attributed to overuse; drugs, particularly those that cause dryness; foreign body; laryngeal spasm; and burns (inhalation or aspiration). Allergies and smoking are the most frequent causes of intermittent or recurrent hoarseness. Stridor suggests edema and inflammation of the vocal folds and warrants urgent airway evaluation when found in patients with hoarseness. Treatment for acute hoarseness consists of rest and avoidance of exposure to irritants. Moisture and cough suppression can help limit further irritation, but there is no definitive benefit to these therapies.

Chronic hoarseness, defined as hoarseness lasting for more than 2 weeks, requires direct visualization of the laryngeal structures. Benign causes of hoarseness include gastroesophageal reflux disease, hypothyroidism, goiter, rheumatoid arthritis, laryngeal polyps, and infections, such as tuberculosis, syphilis, and histoplasmosis. Malignancies of the larynx, pharynx, esophagus, and, even chest when there is entrapment of the left recurrent laryngeal nerve, may also be implicated in hoarseness. Patients with a history of neck surgery, particularly of the thyroid and parathyroid, can experience hoarseness from recurrent laryngeal nerve paralysis even years postoperatively. Hoarseness following endotracheal intubation occurs commonly in critically ill patients but usually resolves 3 to 5 days after removal of the endotracheal tube.

Evaluation of hoarseness should begin with a careful history of trauma and exposures, including to oral and inhaled tobacco products. A complete oropharyngeal and neck examination as well as a mirror laryngoscopy, a simple bedside maneuver that directly visualizes the vocal cords, are appropriate in patients with hoarseness. Once the vocal cords are visible, patients should be asked to make high-pitched tones and hold them for a few seconds, which facilitates visualization of the cords as they open and close and identification of any structural abnormalities.

Treatment of chronic hoarseness depends on the underlying cause. For laryngeal paralysis or injury, nerve-grafting and transplant procedures have been used to restore function.

Hiccups

A hiccup, defined as spasmodic contraction of the diaphragm followed by abrupt closure of the glottis, is thought to be a reflex arc involving the phrenic and vagus nerves and the central nervous system. Hiccups are most commonly a benign and transient condition. Hiccups are most likely to occur secondary to peripheral irritation of the vagus and phrenic nerves, such as that resulting from gastric distention, sudden changes in gastrointestinal temperatures, alcohol use, tobacco use, an intrathoracic mass compressing on these nerves, or an intraabdominal or intrathoracic mass irritating the diaphragm. Less common are central nervous system (mass lesion, demyelinating condition, infarcts, or infections), metabolic (uremia, alcohol intoxication, or anesthesia), and psychogenic causes (largely attributable to anxiety) of hiccups.

A workup is required in patients with persistent hiccups, roughly defined as those lasting more than 48 hours, to rule out more serious underlying causes. Imaging and laboratory studies relevant to the history and physical examination findings are appropriate in patients with hiccups (38).

Institution of nonpharmacologic therapies should be the first step in management of patients with hiccups. Reflex-arc provocation maneuvers can break the persistent reflex-arc cycle; these include breath-holding, pharyngeal irritation (pulling on the tongue or direct application of sugar to the pharynx), and startle maneuvers. Pharmacologic measures for which there is sufficient evidence of efficacy include antidopaminergic agents, such as intravenous or oral chlorpromazine 25 to 50 mg, 3 to 4 times daily; metoclopramide 10 mg, 3 times daily; and baclofen 10 mg, 3 times daily. Otherwise, only observational data support the use of anticonvulsant therapy (carbamazepine, valproate, or phenytoin), methylphenidate, tricyclic antidepressants, cannabinoids, and nefopam in the treatment of hiccups. Extreme measures for intractable hiccups, defined as those lasting more than 2 weeks, include phrenic nerve block and even-breath pacing using an electrical stimulator of the phrenic nerve.

References

1. **Bogardus ST Jr, Yueh B, Shekelle PG.** Screening and management of adult hearing loss in primary care: clinical applications. JAMA. 2003;289:1986-90. [PMID: 12697802]

2. **Yueh B, Shapiro N, MacLean CH, Shekelle PG.** Screening and management of adult hearing loss in primary care: scientific review. JAMA. 2003;289:1976-85. [PMID: 12697801]

3. **McGee S.** Evidence-based physical diagnosis. New York: WB Saunders; 2001.

4. **Pirozzo S, Papinczak T, Glasziou P.** Whispered voice test for screening for hearing impairment in adults and children: systematic review. BMJ. 2003;327:967. [PMID: 14576249]

5. **Copeland BJ, Pillsbury HC 3rd.** Cochlear implantation for the treatment of deafness. Annu Rev Med. 2004;55:157-67. [PMID: 14746514]

6. **Vernon JA.** Masking devices and alprazolam treatment for tinnitus. Otolaryngol Clin North Am. 2003;36:307-20 [PMID: 12856299]

7. **Hilton M, Stuart E.** Ginkgo biloba for tinnitus. Cochrane Database Syst Rev. 2004:CD003852. [PMID: 15106224]

8. **Dobie RA.** A review of randomized clinical trials in tinnitus. Laryngoscope. 1999;109:1202-11. [PMID: 10443820]

9. **van Balen FA, Smit WM, Zuithoff NP, Verheij TJ.** Clinical efficacy of three common treatments in acute otitis externa in primary care: randomised controlled trial. BMJ. 2003;327:1201-5. [PMID: 14630756]

10. **Linder JA, Singer DE.** Health-related quality of life of adults with upper respiratory tract infections. J Gen Intern Med. 2003;18:802-7. [PMID: 14521642]

11. **Steinman MA, Landefeld CS, Gonzales R.** Predictors of broad-spectrum antibiotic prescribing for acute respiratory tract infections in adult primary care. JAMA. 2003;289:719-25. [PMID: 12585950]

12. **Grossan M.** Safe, effective techniques for cerumen removal. Geriatrics. 2000;55:80, 83-6. [PMID: 10659076]

13. **Hand C, Harvey I.** The effectiveness of topical preparations for the treatment of earwax: a systematic review. Br J Gen Pract. 2004;54:862-7. [PMID: 15527615]

14. **Guest JF, Greener MJ, Robinson AC, Smith AF.** Impacted cerumen: composition, production, epidemiology and management. QJM. 2004;97:477-88. [PMID: 15256605]

15. **Kucik CJ, Clenney T.** Management of epistaxis. Am Fam Physician. 2005;71:305-11. [PMID: 15686301]

16. **Choudhury N, Sharp HR, Mir N, Salama NY.** Epistaxis and oral anticoagulant therapy. Rhinology. 2004;42:92-7. [PMID: 15224636]

17. **Scheid DC, Hamm RM.** Acute bacterial rhinosinusitis in adults: part I. Evaluation. Am Fam Physician. 2004;70:1685-92. [PMID: 15554486]

18. **Hickner JM, Bartlett JG, Besser RE, Gonzales R, Hoffman JR, Sande MA, et al.** Principles of appropriate antibiotic use for acute rhinosinusitis in adults: background. Ann Intern Med. 2001;134:498-505. [PMID: 11255528]

19. **Scheid DC, Hamm RM.** Acute bacterial rhinosinusitis in adults: part II. Treatment. Am Fam Physician. 2004;70:1697-704. [PMID: 15554487]

20. **Williams JW Jr, Aguilar C, Cornell J, Chiquette ED, Makela M, Holleman DR, et al.** Antibiotics for acute maxillary sinusitis. Cochrane Database Syst Rev. 2003:CD000243. [PMID: 12804392]

21. **Gendo K, Larson EB.** Evidence-based diagnostic strategies for evaluating suspected allergic rhinitis. Ann Intern Med. 2004;140:278-89. [PMID: 14970151]

22. Management of allergic and nonallergic rhinitis. Summary, Evidence Report/Technology Assessment: Number 54, May 2002. Available at: http://www.ahrq.gov/clinic/epcsums/rhinsum.htm. Accessed on December 30, 2004.

23. **Yanez A, Rodrigo GJ.** Intranasal corticosteroids versus topical H1 receptor antagonists for the treatment of allergic rhinitis: a systematic review with meta-analysis. Ann Allergy Asthma Immunol. 2002;89:479-84. [PMID: 12452206]

24. **Kaszuba SM, Baroody FM, deTineo M, Haney L, Blair C, Naclerio RM.** Superiority of an intranasal corticosteroid compared with an oral antihistamine in the as-needed treatment of seasonal allergic rhinitis. Arch Intern Med. 2001;161:2581-7. [PMID: 11718589]

25. **Wilson AM, O'Byrne PM, Parameswaran K.** Leukotriene receptor antagonists for allergic rhinitis: a systematic review and meta-analysis. Am J Med. 2004;116:338-44. [PMID: 14984820]

26. **Sheikh A, Hurwitz B.** House dust mite avoidance measures for perennial allergic rhinitis. Cochrane Database Syst Rev. 2001:CD001563. [PMID: 11687117]

27. **Arroll B, Kenealy T.** Antibiotics for the common cold. Cochrane Database Syst Rev. 2002:CD000247. [PMID: 12137610]

28. **Douglass AB, Douglass JM.** Common dental emergencies. Am Fam Physician. 2003;67:511-6. [PMID: 12588073]

29. **Del Mar CB, Glasziou PP, Spinks AB.** Antibiotics for sore throat. Cochrane Database Syst Rev. 2004:CD000023. [PMID: 15106140]

30. **Bisno AL.** Acute pharyngitis. N Engl J Med. 2001;344:205-11. [PMID: 11172144]

31. **Snow V, Mottur-Pilson C, Cooper RJ, Hoffman JR; American Academy of Family Physicians; American College of Physicians-American Society of Internal Medicine; Centers for Disease Control.** Principles of appropriate antibiotic use for acute pharyngitis in adults. Ann Intern Med. 2001;134:506-8. [PMID: 11255529]

32. **Ebell MH, Smith MA, Barry HC, Ives K, Carey M.** The rational clinical examination. Does this patient have strep throat? JAMA. 2000;284:2912-8. [PMID: 11147989]

33. **McIsaac WJ, Kellner JD, Aufricht P, Vanjaka A, Low DE.** Empirical validation of guidelines for the management of pharyngitis in children and adults. JAMA. 2004;291:1587-95. [PMID: 15069046]

34. **Bisno AL, Gerber MA, Gwaltney JM Jr, Kaplan EL, Schwartz RH.** Practice guidelines for the diagnosis and management of group A streptococcal pharyngitis. Infectious Diseases Society of America. Clin Infect Dis. 2002;35:113-25. [PMID: 12087516]

35. **Neuner JM, Hamel MB, Phillips RS, Bona K, Aronson MD.** Diagnosis and management of adults with pharyngitis. A cost-effectiveness analysis. Ann Intern Med. 2003;139:113-22. [PMID: 12859161]

36. **Humair JP, Revaz SA, Bovier P, Stalder H.** Management of acute pharyngitis in adults: reliability of rapid streptococcal tests and clinical findings. Arch Intern Med. 2006; 166: 640-4. [PMID: 16567603]

37. **Singh S, Dolan JG, Centor RM.** Optimal management of adults with pharyngitis—a multi-criteria decision analysis. BMC Med Inform Decis Mak. 2006; March 13;6:14 [PMID: 16533386]

38. **Kolodzik PW, Eilers MA.** Hiccups (singultus): review and approach to management. Ann Emerg Med. 1991;20:565-73. [PMID: 2024799]

MENTAL HEALTH

Depression

Depression occurs commonly in patients who are evaluated by general medicine practitioners. Most patients with depression undergo evaluation for physical, rather than emotional, complaints, reporting an average of seven physical symptoms as currently bothersome compared with two reported by patients who are not depressed. In addition, depressed patients report greater stress, more functional impairment, and describe the symptoms as more severe compared with those who are not depressed. This somatization results in an exhaustive search for a non–mental health diagnosis. Consequently, only approximately 30% of these patients are recognized as depressed at presentation, with rates of recognition of depression, even after 5 years, as low as 50%.

The direct and indirect costs of depression to individuals, their families, and society are enormous. Depressed patients experience markedly worse functioning in all aspects of life. In addition to having more physical symptoms than those who are not depressed, they have higher rates of health care utilization, hospitalization, and work impairment, and excessive mortality. Depression occurs at higher rates in patients with cardiovascular disease, neurologic disorders, cancer, diabetes, and several other chronic medical disorders compared with the nondepressed population. The presence of depression worsens the outcomes of comorbid medical diseases.

The biologic basis for depression involves imbalances in norepinephrine, serotonin, and/or dopamine in the brain. There is also evidence of a genetic component to this disorder, with elevated rates of depression in those with first-degree relatives who were depressed and high rates of concordance among twins. Depression produces changes in many physiologic processes, including autonomic dysfunction, increased insulin resistance and platelet aggregation, and decreased cellular immunity.

There are four categories of depression relevant to medical populations: major depression, minor depression (also known as sub-threshold depression), bipolar disorder, and dysthymia. Major depression requires the presence of at least five of nine depressive symptoms nearly every day for at least 2 weeks, with at least one of these symptoms being depressed mood or anhedonia. A diagnosis of minor (sub-threshold) depression is established when two to four symptoms are present. Dysthymia is a more chronic, lower-intensity disorder, requiring the presence of symptoms for at least 2 years. The Nine-Item Patient Health Questionnaire (PHQ-9) (1) is a popular measure for diagnosing depression and monitoring treatment response (**Figure 19**). Bipolar disorder is marked by cyclical changes in mood, from mania or euphoria to depression. Minor depression is more common than major depression, occurring in up to 15% of primary care patients, but studies to date have been inconclusive as to whether treatment is more effective than placebo (2) in these patients. Although more than half of patients with minor depression experience remission within a few months (3), 15% progress to major depression within 1 year (4).

Medical conditions that can mimic depression include hypothyroidism, hypercalcemia, hepatitis, and renal failure. Substance abuse also commonly results in depression. Certain medications may produce depression, such as corticosteroids, interferon, and centrally acting agents. Grief is an entity that is distinct from depression. Patients experiencing a significant loss can be expected to manifest symptoms of depression as a natural, normal part of the recovery process. However, if symptoms are severe or last beyond several months, treatment of depression is warranted.

Patients with some classes of depression should probably not receive treatment in a primary care setting. Suicidal patients, particularly those with a plan for suicide, should receive referral for psychiatric evaluation, with consideration of hospitalization. Patients with psychotic features and those with a history of mania or bipolar disorder should also receive referral for psychiatric evaluation.

Depressed patients often have other psychiatric disorders. Anxiety symptoms commonly occur in depressed patients, with up to 72% having anxiety symptoms of at least moderate severity; 11% meet criteria for generalized anxiety disorder and 5% for panic disorder.

Most studies have found comparable efficacy of pharmacologic and psychotherapeutic interventions (5) and among different classes of drugs in depression treatment (6). Combining antidepressants and psychotherapy may yield better long-term outcomes in patients with more severe disease (7). Electroconvulsive therapy is reserved for situations warranting immediate change, for example, in patients profoundly suicidal or extremely malnourished. Effective psychologic treatment options include cognitive behavioral therapy, interpersonal therapy, and problem-solving therapy. Patients with a high degree of insight respond well to psychotherapy as do individuals with specific issues, such as marital difficulties or a history of childhood trauma or abuse.

The major classes of available drugs for depression (**Table 60**) include the selective serotonin reuptake inhibitors (SSRIs), tricyclic antidepressants, heterocyclics, monoamine oxidase inhibitors, and a few agents that inhibit reuptake of serotonin and norepinephrine. Because all of these agents are equally effective, initial selection is based on side-effect profile, medical and psychiatric comorbidities, patient preferences, and clinician experience. Tricyclic antidepressants have the disadvantage of having many anticholinergic side effects, necessitating a slow titration to effective dose, and can be lethal when taken in overdose. Conversely, they are quite effective at restoring rapid eye movement sleep and are useful in treating various pain and symptom syndromes, including headache, fibromyalgia, and chronic fatigue syndrome. Because they have fewer side effects than tricyclic antidepressants, SSRIs are

PATIENT QUESTIONNAIRE: PHQ-9
Nine-Symptom Checklist

Patient Name: _____   Date: _____

1. Over the *last 2 weeks,* how often have you been bothered by any of the following problems?

	Not at all	Several days	More than half the days	Nearly every day
	0	**1**	**2**	**3**
a. Little interest or pleasure in doing things	❑	❑	❑	❑
b Feeling down, depressed, or hopeless	❑	❑	❑	❑
c. Trouble falling/staying asleep, sleeping too much	❑	❑	❑	❑
d. Feeling tired or having little energy	❑	❑	❑	❑
e. Poor appetite or overeating	❑	❑	❑	❑
f. Feeling bad about yourself, or that you are a failure or have let yourself or your family down	❑	❑	❑	❑
g. Trouble concentrating on things, such as reading the newspaper or watching television	❑	❑	❑	❑
h. Moving or speaking so slowly that other people could have noticed. Or the opposite – being so fidgety or restless that you have been moving around a lot more than usual	❑	❑	❑	❑
i. Thoughts that you would be better off dead or of hurting yourself in some way	❑	❑	❑	❑

2. If you checked off <u>any</u> problem on this questionnaire so far, how <u>difficult</u> have these problems made it for you to do your work, take care of things at home, or get along with other people?

Not difficult at all	Somewhat Difficult	Very Difficult	Extremely Difficult
❑	❑	❑	❑

Total Score: _____

FIGURE 19.

Patient Questionnaire: PHQ-9 (Nine-Symptom Checklist). Depresion severity scores: 0-4 = none; 5-9 = mild; 10-14 = moderate; 15-19 = moderately severe; 20-27 = severe.

TABLE 60 Commonly Used Antidepressants

Agent	Antidepressant Therapeutic Dose Range (mg/d)	Comments
SSRIs		
Citalopram	10 to 40	Probably helpful for anxiety disorders. Possibly fewer cytochrome P-450 interactions. Generic available soon
Escitalopram	10 to 20	10-mg dose usually effective for most
Fluoxetine	10 to 40	Helpful for anxiety disorders. Long half-life good for poor adherence, missed doses. Generic available
Paroxetine	10 to 40	FDA approved for most anxiety disorders. Generic available soon. May have slightly greater fetal risk in pregnant women
Sertraline	25 to 200	FDA approved for most anxiety disorders. Safety shown after myocardial infarction
Serotonin and Norepinephrine Antagonist		
Mirtazapine	15 to 45	Few drug interactions. Less or no sexual dysfunction
		Less sedation as dose increased. May stimulate appetite (and weight gain)
Norepinephrine and Dopamine-Reuptake Inhibitor		
Bupropion	300 to 400	Stimulating. Less or no sexual dysfunction
		At higher dose, may induce seizures in persons with seizure disorder. Twice-daily dosing unless using extended release
Serotonin and Norepinephrine Reuptake Inhibitors		
Venlafaxine	75 to 300	Extended-release version can be taken every day. Helpful for anxiety disorders. Possibly fewer cytochrome P-450 interactions. May increase blood pressure at higher doses
Duloxetine	60	Similar to venlafaxine in efficacy. May be helpful in patients with painful physical symptoms associated with depression (as may be venlafaxine and tricyclic antidepressants)
Primarily Norepinephrine Reuptake Inhibitor		
Desipramine	100 to 300	Like all tricyclics, anticholinergic. Caution with benign prostatic hyperplasia or in patients with cardiovascular disease
Nortriptyline	25 to 150	Availability of reliable, valid blood levels. Results in lower orthostatic hypotension than with other tricyclics. Generic available. Cautions same as with desipramine

Adapted from MacArthur Foundation Depression Management Tool Kit (available at www.depression-primarycare.org).

SSRIs = selective serotonin reuptake inhibitors. FDA = Food and Drug Administration.

currently a more popular option in depression treatment, and, as a class, differ from each other little. Sertraline has the greatest safety data in patients with cardiovascular disease (8). Bupropion has fewer effects on sexual function and weight gain than some of the other antidepressants. Common side effects of mirtazapine are sedation and weight gain. Dual-acting antidepressants, such as venlafaxine and duloxetine, are another therapeutic option in patients with depression. Monoamine oxidase inhibitors are less commonly used in patients with depression because of concerns about enhancing sympathetic activity, drug–drug interactions, and the possibility for severe hypertension with ingestion of tyramine-containing foods.

The response to depression treatment should be monitored with instruments such as the PHQ-9 (see Figure 19) or other validated measures (9). The goal of depression therapy should not be simply improvement of symptoms but rather remission of depressive symptoms whenever possible, because patients who achieve remission have significantly lower recurrence rates than those who experience improvement of symptoms. For an initial episode of depression, 6 to 9 months of medical treatment after achievement of remission is appropriate. Patients with no response to full-dose therapy within 6 weeks should receive another medication or referral for psychotherapy. Inquiring about substance abuse, antidepressant adherence, and adverse effects is also appropriate. A lack of response to one drug in a class does not preclude a trial with another drug in the same or a different class. Because only approximately 50% of patients achieve remission with monotherapy, combination treatment, known as augmentation, may be necessary.

Adding trazodone at night to help with sleep is a common approach. Adding bupropion to SSRI therapy or instituting a combination of SSRIs and tricyclic antidepressants may be helpful, with careful monitoring, because SSRIs can increase tricyclic antidepressant levels.

KEY POINTS

- Depression worsens the outcomes of comorbid medical diseases.
- Although more than half of patients with minor depression experience remission within a few months, 15% progress to major depression within 1 year.
- Medical conditions that can mimic depression include hypothyroidism, hypercalcemia, hepatitis, and renal failure.
- Patients experiencing a significant loss manifest symptoms of depression as a normal part of the recovery process but should receive treatment for depression for severe or long-lasting symptoms.
- Sertraline has the greatest safety data in depressed patients with cardiovascular disease.
- Bupropion has fewer effects on sexual function and weight gain in patients with depression than some other antidepressants.
- Patients who achieve remission from depression have significantly lower recurrence rates than those who experience improvement of symptoms.
- Because only approximately 50% of patients achieve remission with monotherapy, combination treatment, known as augmentation, may be necessary.

Anxiety

Anxiety disorders are common and, according to the Diagnostic and Statistical Manual of Mental Disorders, Fourth Edition (DSM-IV), include acute stress disorder, agoraphobia (with or without a history of panic disorder), generalized anxiety disorder, obsessive-compulsive disorder, panic disorder (with or without agoraphobia), phobias (including social anxiety disorder), and posttraumatic stress disorder (PTSD). Generalized anxiety disorder, panic disorder, and PTSD are the most common anxiety disorders occurring in primary care patients. A phobia is a pathologic stress to external stimuli, with avoidance. It can be specific; for example, social phobia involves anxiety and avoidance of social situations due to fear of embarrassment. A more generalized phobia is agoraphobia, which is anxiety associated with being in places or situations from which escape might be difficult or embarrassing or in which help may not be available should unexpected panic-like symptoms occur. Agoraphobic fears often involve being outside the house alone; being in a crowd or standing in a line; being on a bridge; and traveling in a bus, train, or automobile. Untreated, generalized anxiety disorders

and panic disorders can develop into secondary agoraphobia. Obsessive compulsive disorder is characterized by repetitive behaviors, such as hand washing, ordering, or checking, or mental acts such as praying, counting, or repeating words silently, which a person feels compelled to perform, or performs according to rules that must be applied rigidly to prevent or reduce anxiety.

An acute stress disorder is the result of a traumatic event in persons who experienced threatened or actual serious injury or death and to which the response was intense fear and a sense of helplessness. This disorder is a common reaction to a traumatic event. Symptoms of acute stress disorder include dissociative symptoms, such as numbing, detachment, reduced awareness of one's surroundings, de-realization, or depersonalization; re-experiencing of the trauma; avoidance of associated stimuli; and significant anxiety, including irritability, poor concentration, difficulty sleeping, and restlessness. The symptoms of acute stress disorder must be present for a minimum of 2 days and a maximum of 4 weeks, occurring within 4 weeks of the traumatic event. Prognosis in these patients is very good. Reassurance that their reaction is normal and that this disorder will resolve with time may be the only necessary treatment in patients with acute stress disorder. Only few of these patients subsequently develop PSTD. Although debriefing is commonly used, there is little evidence to support its help in preventing development of PTSD.

PTSD is unique among the DSM-IV disorders in its emphasis on exposure to trauma. PTSD has a lifetime prevalence of approximately 8%. Risk factors for developing this disorder in response to an acute stress disorder include persistence of symptoms beyond 3 months, a history of prior traumatic events, lack of social support, and the presence of three or more symptoms of re-experiencing the trauma or hyperarousal after trauma; however, the ability to predict PTSD is poor. Four indicators suggestive of PTSD are 1) history of exposure to trauma, 2) persistent re-experiencing of the traumatic event, 3) avoidance of stimuli associated with the trauma, 4) and increased arousal. Treatment of patients with this disorder is best handled by mental health professionals with experience in PTSD. Cognitive behavioral therapy (CBT) combinations of exposure therapy and cognitive restructuring have produced excellent results, especially in female victims of childhood or adult sexual trauma. Psychotherapy is the treatment of choice in patients with PTSD, even with the addition of drugs to the therapeutic regimen. Sertraline and paroxetine have received Food and Drug Administration approval in the treatment of PTSD, and most clinicians supplement psychotherapy with pharmacotherapy. Up to 30% of patients with PTSD have comorbid psychiatric disorders. The screening for and treatment of depression, anxiety, and other psychiatric disorders are indicated in patients with PTSD.

Generalized anxiety disorder (GAD) is present in approximately 5% of primary care patients. A sensitive screening question for GAD is "Have you felt nervous, anxious, or on edge during more than half the days in the past month?" (10). If the answer to this question is yes, a more detailed assessment for GAD is appropriate (**Table 61**). Many medical conditions can make patients feel anxious. Some are common conditions, including hyperthyroidism, electrolyte abnormalities, renal cell carcinoma, and arrhythmias, whereas others are quite rare, such as pheochromocytoma, insulinoma, and carcinoid syndrome. Routine laboratory evaluation in patients with suspected GAD should include a complete blood count, chemistry panel, thyroid-stimulating hormone measurement, and urinalysis. Electrocardiography might be appropriate in older patients or in those with chest pain or palpitations. Anxiety can result from several drugs, both legal and illicit. Performing urine or serum toxicology studies or drug level measurements in patients in whom drugs or medications are the suspected cause of anxiety is also appropriate. The majority of patients with GAD (72%) have comorbid psychiatric diagnoses, with most of these meeting the criteria for major depression. Psychotherapy and pharmacotherapy are effective in treating patients with GAD (11). CBT is the psychotherapy of choice in these patients, although psychosocial support therapy has been shown to be effective in the primary care setting. Randomized trials have shown benefits of tricyclic, SSRI, and dual-acting (serotonin norepinephrine reuptake inhibitor) antidepressants in the treatment of various anxiety disorders (12). In addition, trials have demonstrated the efficacy of benzodiazepines, which, in the absence of a history of polydrug or alcohol abuse, may be a useful adjunct to treatment in selected patients.

Social Anxiety Disorder

Social anxiety disorder, previously known as social phobia, is common. This disorder has a lifetime prevalence rate of 13.3% and a 1-year prevalence rate of 7.9% in community samples, constituting the third most prevalent psychiatric disorder, following substance abuse and depression (13). Social phobia is an intense, irrational, and persistent fear of being scrutinized or negatively evaluated by others. Three screening questions for social anxiety disorder are (Yes/No):

1. Does fear of embarrassment cause me to avoid doing things or speaking to people?

2. Do I avoid activities in which I am the center of attention?

3. Is being embarrassed or looking stupid among my worst fears?

Social anxiety disorder often begins at a young age. The average age at onset is 15 years, and it rarely occurs initially past the age of 25 years. A high rate of psychiatric comorbidity is present in patients with social anxiety disorder, particularly depression, with rates ranging from 43% to 69%. Usually, social anxiety disorder precedes development of comorbid conditions. SSRIs are considered first-line therapy for treating

TABLE 61 Generalized Anxiety Disorder

Excessive, difficult-to-control anxiety, occurring more days than not for at least 6 months
Associated with three or more of the following:
Restlessness or feeling keyed up or on edge
Being easily fatigued
Difficulty concentrating or mind going blank
Irritability
Muscle tension
Sleep disturbance (difficulty falling or staying asleep, or restless unsatisfying sleep)
Results in significant distress or impairment in social, occupational, or other important areas of functioning
The focus of the anxiety and worry is not due to another anxiety disorder, such as PTSD, panic disorder, phobias, or other nondepressive disorders, such as somatization disorder or eating disorder
Not due to substance abuse or other medical condition (e.g., hyperthyroidism)

PTSD = posttraumatic stress disorder.

patients with this disorder, although CBT has also been shown to result in improvement (see also Reference 11) (14).

Panic Disorder

Because the symptoms of panic disorder are primarily physical, most patients with this disorder present to their primary care physicians or to emergency departments for evaluation. Patients with panic disorder are evaluated, on average, by 10 clinicians before the diagnosis is established. The alarming nature of their symptoms prompts patients with panic disorder to seek medical attention; consequently, they have very high health care utilization rates. Overall, 2% to 5% of primary care patients have panic disorder.

Panic disorder, like GAD, has very high rates of psychiatric comorbidity. Up to half of patients with panic disorder also have major depression and often also have PTSD or GAD. Untreated, many of these patients develop agoraphobia and other behavior-avoidance patterns.

Because of the somatic and alarming nature of complaints in these patients, clinicians should be attentive to the signs indicative of panic disorder. However, many medical conditions, some life-threatening, can mimic panic disorder, including angina, arrhythmias, chronic obstructive pulmonary disease, temporal lobe epilepsy, pulmonary embolus, asthma, hyperthyroidism, and pheochromocytoma. Acutely, cocaine, caffeine, and other drugs can also produce symptoms of panic. Limited diagnostic tests, such as thyroid function tests, complete blood count, and serum chemistry panels, are indicated in patients with suspected panic disorder, with a more extensive evaluation performed as determined by the history and physical examination findings.

Panic attacks are not uncommon, occurring in up to 30% of individuals during their lifetimes. In patients with a first attack who do not have comorbid psychiatric conditions, providing the diagnosis and reassurance may be sufficient. In patients with panic disorder, (**Table 62**) CBT and pharmacotherapy have been shown to be effective (15). In the primary care setting, SSRIs tend to be first-line therapy because of their low incidence of sideeffects, but tricyclic antidepressants and monoamine oxidase inhibitors are also effective. As with depression therapy, patients who do not respond to an adequate dose of therapy by 6 weeks after initiation of therapy may require a change in medications. Judicious use of benzodiazepines may also be warranted in patients with panic disorder.

TABLE 62 Panic Disorder
A panic attack is the acute onset of anxiety when one would not expect to be anxious, with four or more of:
Shortness of breath
Palpitations or racing heart
Chest pain or pressure
Sweating
Choking
Hot flashes or chills
Abdominal distress
Dizziness, unsteadiness or fainting
Paresthesias
Trembling or shaking
Feelings of unreality or depersonalization
Fear of losing control or going crazy
Fear of dying
Panic disorder is characterized by:
Four or more panic attacks in 1 month, or
Fear about having another attack or significant changes in behavior because of the attacks

KEY POINTS

- Randomized trials have shown benefits of tricyclic, SSRI, and dual-acting antidepressants in the treatment of anxiety disorders.
- Many medical conditions can mimic panic disorders, including angina, arrhythmias, chronic obstructive pulmonary disease, temporal lobe epilepsy, pulmonary embolus, asthma, hyperthyroidism, and pheochromocytoma.
- In patients with panic disorder, cognitive behavioral therapy and pharmacotherapy have been shown to be effective therapy.
- SSRIs tend to be first-line therapy in patients with panic disorder, but tricyclic antidepressants and monoamine oxidase inhibitors are also effective.

Somatization Disorder

Somatization is defined as the presentation of physical symptoms as a manifestation of psychologic distress. The difficulty for clinicians in managing patients with somatization disorder is determining when the symptoms are psychologic and not manifestations of an undiagnosed medical disease. Even after extensive evaluation, 30% to 50% of physical symptoms in primary care patients remain unexplained. Fortunately, the natural history of physical symptoms is favorable in many cases, with more than 75% reporting resolution or marked improvement in symptoms at 3 months follow-up (16). Depressive and anxiety disorders should be high among the differential diagnoses in patients who have multiple physical symptoms, particularly when findings of the history, physical examination, and selective laboratory studies do not suggest a unifying diagnosis.

According to the DSM-IV, somatoform disorders consist of conversion disorder, hypochondriasis, body dysmorphic disorder, factitious disorders and malingering, somatization disorder, and pain disorder. Except for factitious disorders and malingering, none of these involves conscious intent by the patient.

Conversion disorder is characterized by the acute onset of a symptom, usually neurologic, in response to overwhelming stress. Hypochondriasis is a state of constant, deep fear of developing a serious medical condition, with misattribution of physical symptoms. Body dysmorphic disorder is a preoccupation with an imagined or exaggerated defect in physical appearance. Patients with factitious disorders usually have a medical background and use their knowledge to feign illness. The most dramatic of this type of disorder is Munchausen syndrome, in which patients often present to multiple emergency departments with self-induced illnesses, such as surreptitious injection of insulin. Malingering patients purposefully feign symptoms and are often engaged in ongoing legal battles or have substance abuse problems.

Patients with somatization disorders are evaluated commonly in primary care (17). Although a full somatization disorder is present in less than 1% of primary care patients, 10% or more have three or more medically unexplained symptoms (18). Such patients are at higher risk for polypharmacy, unnecessary surgical procedures, extensive diagnostic testing, high health care utilization, and frequent referrals than those without this disorder.

Treatment of full or abridged forms of somatization disorder is problematic. Psychotherapy, particularly CBT, has been shown to produce some benefit in these patients (19). Although evidence for the role of pharmacotherapy in patients with somatization disorder is weaker than that for psychotherapy, antidepressants are often used because depression develops or to treat painful symptoms or functional somatic syndromes in these patients.

Eating Disorders

Numerous American teenagers see themselves as too fat. Many diet, and up to 10% report vomiting or taking laxatives to control weight. The DSM-IV cites four eating disorders: 1) anorexia nervosa, 2) bulimia nervosa, 3) binge eating disorder, and 4) eating disorder not otherwise specified (NOS). Eating disorder NOS is a diagnosis reserved for patients with deranged eating practices that do not meet the criteria for anorexia or bulimia. These disorders occur in men and women but occur less commonly in men.

Anorexia Nervosa

Overall, the rate of anorexia is approximately 3 in 1000 in the general population and 5 in 1000 among women between the ages of 15 to 21 years. There are two types of anorexia nervosa: restricting, in which patients restrict intake, and binge eating/purging, in which they binge or purge to control weight. Diagnostic criteria for this disorder consist of refusal to maintain weight within 15% of normal, fear of weight gain, distorted body image, and amenorrhea or lack of onset of menstruation. The medical complications of anorexia nervosa arise from the consequences of starvation and include anemia, osteopenia, hypotension, and arrhythmias. During the first few weeks of eating, patients with severe anorexia are at risk for the refeeding syndrome, which can include cardiac arrest and delirium. This syndrome is caused by exacerbation of hypophosphatemia, which results in depletion of intracellular adenosine triphosphate and hypoxia caused by reduced levels of erythrocyte 2,3-diphosphoglycerate. Because osteopenia is so common in these patients, daily supplementation with calcium and vitamin D is indicated. Anorexia is typically managed by multidisciplinary teams, including a medical provider, mental health provider, and nutritionist. Pharmacologic therapy has not been shown helpful in patients with anorexia per se but may be indicated for those with depression, which frequently coexists in patients with this disorder. CBT is considered first-line treatment in patients with anorexia nervosa; however, a recent review of psychotherapeutic options for this disorder suggested an urgent need for large, well-designed trials (20).

Bulimia Nervosa

Bulimia incidence peaks in college-aged students. Diagnostic criteria for this disorder are episodes of bingeing with loss of control occurring a minimum of two times per week for 3 months, followed by purging or other compensatory behavior, such as fasting, strict dieting, or excessive exercise.

Purging includes vomiting or abuse of laxatives or diuretics. Patients with bulimia usually have normal weight, but many have depression or anxiety (21). The medical complications of bulimia nervosa result from the method and frequency of purging and can involve acid-induced dental disease, esophageal tears, and electrolyte derangements. Clues for the presence of bulimia include abnormal serum potassium or bicarbonate levels in otherwise-healthy patients. Patients with this disorder respond well to psychotherapy and pharmacotherapy, the combination of which may be better than either therapy alone, although some data suggest patients prefer psychotherapy (22).

Binge Eating Disorder

Binge eating disorder is present in patients who binge at least 2 days per week for 6 months, bingeing with rapid eating, eating until uncomfortable, and feeling disgusted or guilty after the binge. Binge eating disorder does not involve purging, and the diagnosis is only made in the absence of anorexia. There are few studies on the treatment of binge eating disorder, but short-term trials suggest benefit from CBT, interpersonal psychotherapy, SSRIs, or the anticonvulsant agent topiramate (23, 24) in these patients.

References

1. **Kroenke K, Spitzer RL.** The PHQ-9: A new depression and diagnostic severity measure. Psychiatric Annals. 2002;32:509-521.

2. **Ackermann RT, Williams JW Jr.** Rational treatment choices for non-major depressions in primary care: an evidence-based review. J Gen Intern Med. 2002;17:293-301. [PMID: 11972726]

3. **Frank E, Rucci P, Katon W, Barrett J, Williams JW Jr, Oxman T, et al.** Correlates of remission in primary care patients treated for minor depression. Gen Hosp Psychiatry. 2002;24(1):12-9. [PMID: 11814529]

4. **Hermens ML, van Hout HP, Terluin B, van der Windt DA, Beekman AT, van Dyck R, et al.** The prognosis of minor depression in the general population: a systematic review. Gen Hosp Psychiatry. 2004;26:453-62. [PMID: 15567211]

5. Fava GA, Ruini C, Rafanelli C, Finos L, Conti S, Grandi S. Six-year outcome of cognitive behavior therapy for prevention of recurrent depression. Am J Psychiatry. 2004;161:1872-6. [PMID: 15465985]

6. Kroenke K, West SL, Swindle R, Gilsenan A, Eckert GJ, Dolor R, et al. Similar effectiveness of paroxetine, fluoxetine, and sertraline in primary care: a randomized trial. JAMA. 2001;286:2947-55. [PMID: 11743835]

7. Pampallona S, Bollini P, Tibaldi G, Kupelnick B, Munizza C. Combined pharmacotherapy and psychological treatment for depression: a systematic review. Arch Gen Psychiatry. 2004;61:714-9. [PMID: 15237083]

8. Glassman AH, O'Connor CM, Califf RM, Swedberg K, Schwartz P, Bigger JT Jr, et al. Sertraline treatment of major depression in patients with acute MI or unstable angina. JAMA. 2002;288:701-9. [PMID: 12169073]

9. Löwe B, Unützer J, Callahan CM, Perkins AJ, Kroenke K. Monitoring depression treatment outcomes with the patient health questionnaire-9. Med Care. 2004;42:1194-201. [PMID: 15550799]

10. Spitzer RL, Kroenke K, Williams JB. Validation and utility of a self-report version of PRIME-MD: the PHQ primary care study. Primary Care Evaluation of Mental Disorders. Patient Health Questionnaire. JAMA. 1999;282:1737-44. [PMID: 10568646]

11. Davidson JR, Foa EB, Huppert JD, Keefe FJ, Franklin ME, Compton JS, et al. Fluoxetine, comprehensive cognitive behavioral therapy, and placebo in generalized social phobia. Arch Gen Psychiatry. 2004;61:1005-13. [PMID: 15466674]

12. Kapczinski F, Lima MS, Souza JS, Schmitt R. Antidepressants for generalized anxiety disorder. Cochrane Database Syst Rev. 2003:CD003592. [PMID: 12804478]

13. Kessler RC, Chiu WT, Demler O, Merikangas KR, Walters EE. Prevalence, severity, and comorbidity of 12-month DSM-IV disorders in the National Comorbidity Survey Replication. Arch Gen Psychiatry. 2005;62:617-27. [PMID: 15939839]

14. Liebowitz MR, Gelenberg AJ, Munjack D. Venlafaxine extended release vs placebo and paroxetine in social anxiety disorder. Arch Gen Psychiatry. 2005;62:190-8. [PMID: 15699296]

15. Otto MW, Tuby KS, Gould RA, McLean RY, Pollack MH. An effect-size analysis of the relative efficacy and tolerability of serotonin selective reuptake inhibitors for panic disorder. Am J Psychiatry. 2001;158:1989-92. [PMID: 11729014]

16. Jackson JL, Passamonti M. The outcomes among patients presenting in primary care with a physical symptom at 5 years. J Gen Intern Med. 2005;20:1032-7. [PMID: 16307629]

17. Kroenke K. The interface between physical and psychological symptoms. J Clin Psychiatry Primary Care Companion. 2003;5[suppl 7]:11-18.

18. Khan AA, Khan A, Harezlak J, Tu W, Kroenke K. Somatic symptoms in primary care: etiology and outcome. Psychosomatics. 2003;44:471-8. [PMID: 14597681]

19. Kroenke K, Swindle R. Cognitive-behavioral therapy for somatization and symptom syndromes: a critical review of controlled clinical trials. Psychother Psychosom. 2000;69:205-15. [PMID: 10867588]

20. Hay P, Bacaltchuk J, Claudino A, Ben-Tovim D, Yong PY. Individual psychotherapy in the outpatient treatment of adults with anorexia nervosa. Cochrane Database Syst Rev. 2003:CD003909. [PMID: 14583998]

21. Mehler PS. Clinical practice. Bulimia nervosa. N Engl J Med. 2003;349:875-81. [PMID: 12944574]

22. Bacaltchuk J, Hay P, Trefiglio R. Antidepressants versus psychological treatments and their combination for bulimia nervosa. Cochrane Database Syst Rev. 2001:CD003385. [PMID: 11687197]

23. McElroy SL, Shapira NA, Arnold LM, Keck PE, Rosenthal NR, Wu SC, et al. Topiramate in the long-term treatment of binge-eating disorder associated with obesity. J Clin Psychiatry. 2004;65:1463-9. [PMID: 15554757]

24. Arnone D. Review of the use of topiramate for treatment of psychiatric disorders. Ann Gen Psychiatry. 2005;4:5. [PMID: 15845141]

GERIATRICS

Functional Assessment of the Elderly

There is no specific chronologic age that defines a person as elderly. However, people older than 50 years are at increased risk for conditions that may limit their functional status, and the risk for those conditions continues to increase with age. The concept of functional status assessment, in addition to the traditional classification of disease, has helped to clarify common geriatric problems. Functional status refers to a person's ability to function independently in the physical, mental, and social realms of life. Conditions of frailty that can affect functional status include impaired vision and hearing, mobility and falls, and the common geriatric syndromes of cognitive impairment, depression, malnutrition, and urinary incontinence.

Epidemiology

Among the community-based elderly, less than 10% need assistance with basic activities of daily living (ADL). Functional visual impairment among community-dwelling elderly occurs in approximately 7% of those 71 to 74 years old, increasing to 39% in those 90 years or older. Hearing loss is present in approximately 24% of persons 65 to 74 years old, increasing to 40% in those 75 years or older. Approximately 30% of community-residing elderly patients fall each year, with this rate increasing to 50% in those 80 years and older. Dementia is present in approximately 10% of those 65 years and older, increasing to 50% in community-based patients older than 85 years. The definition of dementia is based on the criterion of a clinical decline in cognitive function that interferes with work or usual social activities. Urinary incontinence is present in approximately 10% to 15% of women aged 65 years and older, increasing to 25% in men and women 85 years and older (1).

Risk Factors

The risk for functional impairment increases with age, in those with comorbid medical and psychiatric disease, and in elderly patients who are socially isolated, reside in nursing homes, or are hospitalized. The cause and effect of these associations is bidirectional.

Screening and Primary Prevention

Geriatric functional assessment can help to identify and address previously unrecognized problems to improve quality of life in older persons significantly. Some of the various geriatric assessment tools that have been developed have been adapted for use in a general internal medicine office setting. The Katz Index of Activities of Daily Living and the Barthel Index are functional assessment tools that assess basic ADL, such as eating and dressing. The Lawton & Brody Instrumental ADL Scale assesses instrumental activities, such as using the telephone or shopping (**Table 63**).

TABLE 63 Basic and Instrumental Activities of Daily Living

Index	Functional Activities Assessed
Katz Index of Basic Activities of Daily Living*	Feeding Continence Transferring Toileting Dressing Bathing
The Barthel Index†	Feeding Bathing Grooming Dressing Bowels Bladder Toilet use Transfers Mobility Stairs
Lawton & Brody Instrumental Activities of Daily Living Scale‡	Ability to use a telephone Shopping Food preparation Housekeeping Laundry Mode of transport Responsibility for own medication Ability to handle finances

*The Katz Index can be scored by assigning a score of 1 to each activity if it can be completed independently, which is defined as having no supervision, direction, or personal assistance; scores are then added for a range of 0 to 6. †The Barthel Index results in a score of 0 to 100, with higher scores reflecting independence. ‡The Lawton & Brody Instrument results in a score of 0 to 8, with a score of 8 representing independence and 0 representing total dependence for activities of daily living.

Basic and instrumental ADL tools have been validated against the gold standard of a geriatric clinical assessment and take approximately 10 minutes for office staff to administer. Patients who need help with basic ADL are unlikely to be able to live alone safely. Patients who have loss of independence for performing instrumental ADL may have significant cognitive or physical illnesses that require further evaluation. A comprehensive functional assessment can be guided by the mnemonic DEEP-IN (delirium, dementia, depression, polypharmacy side effects, vision and hearing impairments, decline in general physical performance, incontinence, and malnutrition) (2). Delirium in older persons is manifested by lethargy and decreased response to stimuli. Criteria for the diagnosis of delirium include a disturbance of consciousness or change in cognition that develops over a short period (hours or days) and often fluctuates during the course of a day. The causes of delirium are broad and include drugs, electrolyte imbalance, common infections, and pain. A return to baseline mental status after an illness may be slow among the elderly, taking months or years. Patients with suspected dementia commonly undergo screening with the Folstein Mini–Mental State Examination (MMSE); however, shorter screening tools are also available, including three-item recall, the animal-naming test, and the clock-completion test.

In the three-item recall test, the patient is asked to recall three items 1 minute after the examiner names the items.

Recall of only one or two items is considered a positive screening result for dementia and requires further evaluation. In the animal-naming test, the patient is asked to name as many animals as possible in 1 minute. Recalling fewer than 12 animals is associated with a low MMSE score (<23). In the clock-completion test, the examiner draws a circle and asks the patient to complete the clock by writing the numbers 1 to 12 within the circle. When completed correctly, each quadrant of the clock should contain three numbers. Patients with dementia tend to bunch the numbers in the right half of the circle.

Depression can be assessed by asking a single screening question: "Do you often feel sad or depressed?" The sensitivity and specificity of this screening method is 85% and 65%, respectively. The Five-Item Geriatric Depression Scale can be administered to patients who respond positively to this question (3). The questions in this screening tool ask patients whether they 1) are generally satisfied with their lives; 2) feel bored; 3) feel helpless; 4) prefer to stay home rather than go out and do new things; and 5) are currently experiencing feelings of worthlessness. Patients who respond "yes" to questions 2, 3, 4, and 5 and "no" to question 1 screen positively for depression (sensitivity: 97%; specificity: 85%; positive predictive value: 85%; negative predictive value: 97%) and require a thorough evaluation for this disorder.

Review of prescription drugs as part of the functional assessment is appropriate. Older patients taking more than four prescribed drugs are at risk for falls. Antipsychotics, antidepressants, antihypertensives, and long-acting benzodiazepines have a high association with falls.

Screening tests for hearing loss include the subjective whispered-voice test, the Hearing Handicap Inventory for The Elderly-Screening self-administered questionnaire, or an audioscope (see Ear, Nose, Mouth, and Throat Disorders section). A standard technique for the whispered-voice test consists of the examiner standing at arm's length behind a seated patient. The examiner then whispers a combination of numbers and letters, and the patient is asked to repeat the sequence. The patient passes this test by identifying at least half of the numbers or letters whispered (4). The whispered-voice test can accurately detect hearing loss but cannot be standardized among examiners.

Screening for vision impairment can be accomplished by asking patients if they have any difficulty driving, watching television, reading, or performing any other ADL because of poor eyesight. Those who answer yes can be tested using a Snellen eye chart to confirm vision impairment, with a score of <20/40 mandating further testing.

The rapid gain test assesses physical performance and requires patients to walk 3.5 m (10 ft), turn, and walk back as quickly as possible. Patients who can complete this task in less than 10 seconds have a good chance of remaining stable in ability to perform ADL for at least 1 year. In the chair risk test, patients are seated, with their hands folded on the lap, and are asked to stand up. Rising without the use of the arms is considered a passing grade. Patients who fail this test have a 40% chance of developing impairment in ability to perform ADL within 1 year.

Evaluation of patients who are at risk for falls includes asking them whether they have a history of falls. In the "Get Up and Go" test, a screening test determining falls risk, patients are asked to rise from a chair, walk 3.5 m (10 ft), turn around, walk back to the chair, and sit down. Patients who take longer than 20 seconds to complete this test are at risk for falls.

Incontinence screening involves asking two questions: "In the past year, have you ever lost your urine and gotten wet?" and "If so, have you lost your urine on at least 6 separate days?" Patients who answer yes to both questions are at high risk for incontinence.

"Have you lost 4.5 kg (10 lb) over the past 6 months without trying to do so?" is a screening question for malnutrition. Patients who respond positively to this question are at risk for malnutrition and increased risk for mortality. Other indicators of malnutrition are body weight <45 kg (<100 lb) and a BMI of <22.

Treatment

Elderly persons with functional impairments should undergo evaluation for and treatment of the underlying diagnoses (5). Primary care providers should collaborate with community resources and programs to provide patients with functional-needs assistance.

Prognosis and Follow-Up

Identifying functional status deficits in elderly patients has resulted in improved health outcomes and the ability to maintain independence in these patients. General internal medicine practices should establish systems to maintain relationships with support services in the community for the elderly. Functional status assessments can be repeated regularly in elderly patients to monitor their improvement, decline, or stability in functional status and to allow for adjustment in management approach as appropriate.

KEY POINTS

- Approximately 30% of community-residing elderly patients fall each year, with an increase to 50% in those 80 years and older.
- Dementia is present in approximately 10% of those 65 years and older, increasing to 50% in community-based patients older than 85 years.
- Criteria for the diagnosis of delirium include a disturbance of consciousness or change in cognition that develops over hours or days and often fluctuates during the course of a day.
- Patients with suspected dementia commonly undergo screening with the Folstein Mini–Mental State Examination; however, shorter screening tools include three-item recall, the animal-naming test, and the clock-completion test.

Pressure Ulcers

Pressure ulcers are common, ranging in incidence from 5% in hospitalized patients to 30% in community-dwelling patients with spinal cord injuries. Pressure ulcers consist of areas of localized damage to the skin and underlying tissue caused by pressure, shear, or friction. They occur more commonly over bony prominences and most frequently in the elderly, the immobile, and those with neurologic deficits. Other risk factors for pressure ulcers include incontinence and poor nutritional status. The extent to which pressure ulcers are preventable is not clear (6). Pressure ulcers have four stages:

Stage 1. The skin is intact, but there is evidence of pressure changes, including changes in temperature, consistency, or sensation.

Stage 2. The wound is superficial, with partial-thickness skin loss involving the epidermis or dermis.

Stage 3. There is full-thickness skin loss extending to the subcutaneous tissue.

Stage 4. There is extensive destruction, including to the muscle, bone, or supporting structures.

Although this staging system is useful for characterizing the extent of damage, it is not helpful for tracking healing because healing does not follow this pattern. The Pressure Ulcer Scale for Healing (PUSH) has been found useful in tracking healing. PUSH forms are available for clinical use and are accessible at http://www.npuap.org/push3-0.html.

Prevention of pressure ulcers focuses on identifying patients at risk and reducing pressure by changing patient positioning or using pressure-reduction devices. The following are recommendations for patients who are at risk for pressure ulcers or their families (7):

- Position should be changed at least every 2 hours to relieve pressure.
- Items should be used that can help reduce pressure (for example, pillows, sheepskin, or foam padding).
- A healthy diet, with well-balanced meals, should be maintained.
- A daily exercise regimen, including range-of-motion exercises for immobile patients, should be implemented.
- Skin should be kept clean and dry. Those with incontinence must be vigilant in limiting exposure to moisture.

Standard mattresses have been consistently outperformed by a range of foam-based, low-pressure mattresses and overlays, and by "higher-tech" pressure-relieving beds in preventing pressure ulcers (8).

Treatment of pressure ulcers includes relieving the pressure, wound debridement, treating infection, and maintaining a moist wound environment (9). Using normal saline for cleansing most pressure ulcers is recommended rather than using antiseptics. Adequate irrigation pressure is necessary for enhancing wound cleansing without causing trauma to the wound bed. A dressing that keeps the ulcer bed continuously moist is appropriate. Wet-to-dry dressings should be used only for debridement and are not considered continuously moist saline dressings. Although no differences in pressure ulcer healing outcomes were reported in studies of different types of moist wound dressings, dressings that keep the surrounding intact skin dry while maintaining moisture in the ulcer bed and controlling the exudate without dessicating the ulcer bed should be used. Other experimental approaches supported by some evidence include electrotherapy (by applying a direct current to the wound), negative-pressure wound therapy, and hyperbaric oxygen (10).

KEY POINTS

- Standard mattresses have been consistently outperformed by a range of foam-based, low-pressure mattresses and overlays, and by "higher-tech" pressure-relieving beds in preventing pressure ulcers.
- Normal saline for cleansing most pressure ulcers is recommended rather than antiseptics.
- Dressings that keep the surrounding intact skin dry while maintaining moisture in the ulcer bed and controlling the exudate without dessicating the ulcer bed should be used.

Mild Cognitive Impairment/ Memory Loss

Memory is a complex process because there are several different types of memories of various duration involving different parts of the brain. Memory is usually classified as working, episodic, semantic, and procedural. Working memory is immediate memory and depends on a network of subcortical, frontal, prefrontal, and parietal areas and is susceptible to many neurodegenerative diseases, such as Alzheimer's, Parkinson's, and Huntington's, and can be affected by any process that disrupts the frontal lobes or their connections (11). Episodic memory involves the ability to recall personal experiences and resides in the medial temporal lobes, anterior thalamic nucleus, and prefrontal cortex. Alzheimer's disease characteristically disrupts episodic memory. Semantic memory is memory of facts, such as the name of the current president, and involves the inferolateral temporal lobes. Semantic memory also declines in patients with Alzheimer's disease, although at a different rate than episodic memory, as it does in any disorder that disrupts the inferolateral lobes, such as traumatic brain injuries, tumors, encephalitis or strokes. Procedural memory is the ability to learn skills and algorithms used at an automatic, unconscious level and involves the basal ganglia, cerebellum, and the supplementary motor areas. Parkinson's disease often impairs procedural memory, whereas Alzheimer's disease often leaves this type of memory unimpaired.

The normal aging process has many effects on memory. The ability to memorize, acquire and retain new information, and recall names diminishes with advancing age, particularly in those older than 70 years. This process is also referred to as "benign senescent forgetfulness." Memory problems in clinical practice represent a spectrum of diagnoses, from mild forgetfulness, with no objective decline in cognition or effects on functioning, to dementia, with significant deficits in various aspects of cognition and functioning (12). Mild cognitive impairment is defined as a decline in cognition that falls short of dementia, without impact on patient functioning. The criteria for this disorder include:

- problems with memory, preferably corroborated by an informant;
- essentially normal judgment, perception, and reasoning skills;
- largely normal performance of ADL;
- reduced performance on memory tests compared with people of similar age and educational background. The Mini–Mental State Examination is a good screening tool that can be used to follow the progression of cognitive impairment; and
- absence of dementia.

The prognostic implication of mild cognitive impairment is uncertain. Most studies show that up to 40% of patients with mild cognitive impairment have a full return to normality on follow-up evaluation; however, about 12% progress to dementia.

The diagnostic dilemma for clinicians who see patients with memory complaints is to differentiate the benign from the more serious forms of forgetfulness and to rule out other common and potentially reversible causes for memory decline. Laboratory studies in these patients should include a complete blood count, serum electrolyte and metabolic panels, a thyroid function test, serum vitamin B_{12} measurement, and syphilis and HIV testing (see Dementia section).

KEY POINT

- Up to 40% of patients with mild cognitive impairment have a full return to normal memory on follow-up evaluation, but the condition of approximately 12% progresses to dementia.

Falls

Falls occur in as many as 30% to 40% of older adults each year and are associated with substantial morbidity. A fracture may occur in 10% to 15% of patients who fall, with a subsequent decline in function, increased risk for nursing home placement, and increased fear of falling, which alone is associated with impaired quality of life. Risk factors for falls include age, female sex, history of falling, cognitive impairment, motor weakness, balance difficulty, psychotropic medication use, and arthritis. Age-related changes in vision, proprioception, and vestibular function predispose elderly patients to difficulties in balance that increase the risk for falling. Similarly, age-related changes in blood pressure homeostasis, cognitive function, and comorbid illnesses occur (especially those affecting motor function, such as Parkinson's disease), all of which compound the risk for falling. Falls risk assessment includes routine questioning of elderly patients about falls occurring in the past year. In those who have fallen, the following screening steps are recommended:

- musculoskeletal functional assessment, such as the "Get Up and Go" test (see Functional Assessment section);

- orthostatic evaluation;

- carotid sinus hypersensitivity assessment by monitored carotid massage and only in patients with presyncopal, fall-associated symptoms;

- review of environmental factors, such as lighting, floor covering, railings, and steps;

- hearing screening;

- visual acuity screening;

- lower-extremity sensory function testing; and

- review of medication regimen (especially for psychotropic and cardiovascular agents).

Interventions proven to reduce the risk for falls include muscle strengthening and balance retraining, home hazard assessment and modification, withdrawal of psychotropic medication, vitamin D supplementation, cardiac pacing in patients who have fallen and have carotid sinus hypersensitivity, and multidisciplinary risk-factor intervention programs (13, 14). Multifactorial falls risk-assessment and management programs and vitamin D supplementation are most effective in patients at high risk for falls, with an absolute falls risk reduction in these patients of approximately 20% compared with those who received usual care; however, these interventions have only reduced the risk for falls but not the risk for fractures or other types of morbidity.

Despite initially promising results, by-patient randomized trials (versus by-group randomization) have not found hip protectors to be efficacious in fracture prevention, although the high rate of noncompliance in the use of the hip protector may explain these findings (15).

KEY POINTS

- **Multifactorial falls risk-assessment/management programs and vitamin D supplementation are most effective in patients at high risk for falls, with a 20% risk reduction in falls compared with those who received usual care.**

- **Fall interventions reduce the risk for falls but do not reduce the risk for fractures or other types of morbidity.**

References

1. **Palmer RM.** Geriatric assessment. Med Clin North Am. 1999;83:1503-23, vii-viii. [PMID: 10584605]

2. **Sherman FT.** Functional assessment. Easy-to-use screening tools speed initial office work-up. Geriatrics. 2001;56:36-40; quiz 43. [PMID: 11505859]

3. **Hoyl MT, Alessi CA, Harker JO, Josephson KR, Pietruszka FM, Koelfgen M, et al.** Development and testing of a five-item version of the Geriatric Depression Scale. J Am Geriatr Soc. 1999;47:873-8. [PMID: 10404935]

4. **Pirozzo S, Papinczak T, Glasziou P.** Whispered voice test for screening for hearing impairment in adults and children: systematic review. BMJ. 2003 Oct 25;327(7421):967. [PMID: 14576249]

5. **Challis D, Clarkson P, Williamson J, Hughes J, Venables D, Burns A, et al.** The value of specialist clinical assessment of older people prior to entry to care homes. Age Ageing. 2004;33:25-34. [PMID: 14695860]

6. **Horn SD, Bender SA, Ferguson ML, Smout RJ, Bergstrom N, Taler G, et al.** The National Pressure Ulcer Long-Term Care Study: pressure ulcer development in long-term care residents. J Am Geriatr Soc. 2004;52:359-67. [PMID: 14962149]

7. **Brillhart B.** Pressure sore and skin tear prevention and treatment during a 10-month program. Rehabil Nurs. 2005;30:85-91. [PMID: 15912672]

8. **Cullum N, McInnes E, Bell-Syer SE, Legood R.** Support surfaces for pressure ulcer prevention. Cochrane Database Syst Rev. 2004:CD001735. [PMID: 15266452]

9. **de Laat EH, Scholte op Reimer WJ, van Achterberg T.** Pressure ulcers: diagnostics and interventions aimed at wound-related complaints: a review of the literature. J Clin Nurs. 2005;14:464-72. [PMID: 15807753]

10. **Kranke P, Bennett M, Roeckl-Wiedmann I, Debus S.** Hyperbaric oxygen therapy for chronic wounds. Cochrane Database Syst Rev. 2004:CD004123. [PMID: 15106239]

11. **Budson AE, Price BH.** Memory dysfunction. N Engl J Med. 2005;352:692-9. [PMID: 15716563]

12. **Knopman DS, Boeve BF, Petersen RC.** Essentials of the proper diagnoses of mild cognitive impairment, dementia, and major subtypes of dementia. Mayo Clin Proc. 2003;78:1290-308. [PMID: 14531488]

13. **Chang JT, Morton SC, Rubenstein LZ, Mojica WA, Maglione M, Suttorp MJ, et al.** Interventions for the prevention of falls in older adults: systematic review and meta-analysis of randomised clinical trials. BMJ. 2004;328:680. [PMID: 15031239]

14. **Bischoff-Ferrari HA, Dawson-Hughes B, Willett WC, Staehelin HB, Bazemore MG, Zee RY, et al.** Effect of Vitamin D on falls: a meta-analysis. JAMA. 2004;291:1999-2006. [PMID: 15113819]

15. **Parker MJ, Gillespie LD, Gillespie WJ.** Hip protectors for preventing hip fractures in the elderly. Cochrane Database Syst Rev. 2004:CD001255. [PMID: 15266444]

WOMEN'S HEALTH

Breast Mass

Pathophysiology

Breast tissue is naturally diffusely lobulated with glandular nodularity most pronounced in the upper outer regions of the breast and in the area of the inframammary ridge. The amount of nodularity of the breast can increase during the estrogen-stimulated proliferative phase of the menstrual period such that it is appreciable on palpation. A dominant breast mass is defined as a lump or suspicious change in the breast texture that is discrete and distinctly different from the rest of the surrounding breast tissue and the corresponding area in the contralateral breast. The differential diagnoses of a dominant breast mass include cysts, fibroadenomas, fibrocystic changes, fat necrosis, carcinoma insitu, and invasive carcinoma.

Epidemiology

Most detected breast masses are benign, but every woman who has a breast mass must undergo evaluation to exclude breast cancer. The most common causes of breast lumps and associated epidemiologic factors are presented in **Table 64**. Breast lumps are the most common symptom associated with breast cancer, with 9% to 11% of breast lumps resulting in a diagnosis of breast cancer. The prevalence of breast cancer among those presenting with a breast lump increases with age (1% in women <40 years, 9% in women aged 41 to 55 years, and 37% in women aged 55 years and older) (1). Approximately 20% to 25% of palpable breast abnormalities are simple cysts.

Risk Factors

Risk factors for breast cancer include family history of breast cancer or ovarian cancer, age of diagnosis of breast cancer in first-degree relative, parity, age at first live birth, age at menarche, late cessation of menses, use of hormone replacement therapy, previous breast biopsy, and personal history of atypical hyperplasia (ductal or lobular); however, the risk factor profile should not alter the approach to the workup of a breast mass, because 75% of women with newly diagnosed breast cancer have no identifiable risk factors.

Diagnosis and Evaluation

Patients with a breast lump must undergo a clinical breast examination to identify the presence of a dominant breast mass. After performance of bilateral diagnostic mammography, the initial focus of the workup of a dominant breast mass is to distinguish a simple cyst from a solid mass by fine-needle aspiration (FNA) or ultrasonography (2). If the fluid from FNA is bloody, the fluid should undergo cytologic evaluation.

TABLE 64 Common Causes of a Breast Mass	
Breast cyst	Occurs most often in women in their 30s
	Fluctuates with the menstrual cycle
Fibroadenoma	Presents at a median age of 30 y
	About 50% of all breast biopsies performed because of fibroadenomas; exogenous estrogen, progesterone, lactation, and pregnancy can stimulate growth
Fibrocystic changes	Occur most often in women in their 20s and 30s. Pain is a frequent complaint and can cycle with the menstrual period
Breast cancer	About 78% diagnosed after age 50 y, and 22% diagnosed before age 50 y; 7% diagnosed in women age <40 y

Women with simple cysts should undergo a breast examination 4 to 6 weeks after cyst aspiration to evaluate for cyst recurrence or a residual lump. A solid mass requires a tissue diagnosis by fine-needle aspiration biopsy (FNAB), core-needle biopsy, or excisional biopsy. Patients with benign FNAB or core-needle biopsy results and negative mammography require close clinical follow-up of the breast abnormality.

KEY POINTS

- Workup of a breast mass consists of bilateral diagnostic mammography and fine-needle aspiration or ultrasonography.
- Women with simple cysts should undergo a breast examination 4 to 6 weeks after cyst aspiration to evaluate for recurrence or a residual lump.
- A solid mass requires a tissue diagnosis by fine-needle aspiration biopsy (FNAB), core-needle biopsy, or excisional biopsy.
- Patients with benign FNAB or core-needle biopsy results and negative mammography require close clinical follow-up of the breast abnormality.

Breast Pain

Classification, Epidemiology, and Risk Factors

Breast pain is classified as cyclical mastalgia (CM) associated with the menstrual cycle or noncyclical mastalgia (NCM). Noncyclical pain is further classified as breast pain or chest wall pain. CM and NCM have a chronic-relapsing course. The cause of mastalgia is not known.

Diagnosis and Evaluation

The history of patients with breast pain should include an assessment of the location, frequency, and severity of the pain. Asking the patient to keep a record of the pain symptoms for at least 2 months may be helpful in the evaluation. A clinical breast examination and evaluation for chest wall pain are also appropriate in these patients. Patients with CM typically have bilateral symptoms, whereas those with NCM may have bilateral or unilateral symptoms. Mammography may be appropriate in patients with breast pain who are older than 30 years or in those with localized pain (3).

Treatment

The subset of women with CM who have had moderate to severe pain for more than 5 days per month for 6 months or who have pain that interferes with daily activities (<15% of women with mastalgia) requires treatment. CM is generally more responsive to treatment than NCM. Nondrug interventions that have had some benefit in women with CM include reassurance and a well-fitting support bra. Some randomized trial data have supported the efficacy of a low-fat, low-carbohydrate diet in reducing breast symptoms (4). There is a lack of consistent clinical trial evidence supporting the efficacy of evening primrose oil, vitamin E, or a methylxanthine-restricted diet (avoidance of coffee, tea, chocolate, and cola beverages) in patients with mastalgia. Evidence-supported endocrine therapies include bromocriptine, danazol, and tamoxifen, with danazol the only Food and Drug Administration–approved medication for this indication. One randomized clinical trial reported that danazol reduced symptoms of CM after 12 months compared with placebo but also increased the risk for weight gain, deepening of the voice, menorrhagia, and muscle cramps. Danazol is contraindicated in women with a history of thromboembolic disease and is teratogenic; therefore, it must be taken concurrently with nonhormonal contraception. NCM has proved to be less responsive to endocrine manipulation. For patients with moderate to severe and persistent chest wall pain, local injection of corticosteroids and a local anesthetic is another therapeutic option.

Prognosis and Follow-up

The risk of breast cancer among patients with chest pain as a sole symptom is 0.8 to 2%. Localized pain followed by the detection of a lump is the presenting symptom in up to 18% of patients with breast cancer. Breast pain secondary to cancer is usually unilateral, persistent, localized, and constant.

Cyclical breast pain resolves spontaneously within 3 months in 20% to 30% of women. Among women who undergo treatment for breast pain, up to 60% experience recurrent symptoms within 2 years. Noncyclical pain does not respond as well to treatment as does CM, but noncyclical breast pain may resolve spontaneously in up to 50% of women (5).

KEY POINTS

- **Nondrug interventions showing benefit in cyclical mastalgia (CM) are reassurance and a well-fitting support bra.**
- **Danazol is the only FDA-approved medication for CM.**
- **Localized pain followed by the detection of a lump is the presenting symptom in up to 18% of patients with breast cancer.**
- **Breast pain secondary to cancer is usually unilateral, persistent, localized, and constant.**

Contraception

Nearly half of all pregnancies in the United States, approximately 3.2 million, are unintended, and nearly half of all women ages 15 to 44 years will experience at least one unintended pregnancy. No symptoms or signs of pregnancy are diagnostic, but early findings include amenorrhea, nausea, vomiting, breast tenderness, and weight gain. Early signs of pregnancy at approximately 7 weeks gestation include cervical softening and cyanosis of the vagina and cervix. Urine pregnancy testing is accurate at the time of a missed period or soon afterwards. In a patient with amenorrhea, the differen-

tial diagnosis of pregnancy includes early menopause or hypothalamic dysfunction caused by either marked weight loss or excessive exercise.

The chance of pregnancy increases beginning 5 days before ovulation, peaks on the day of ovulation, and then drops to zero by the day after ovulation. Contraception by abstinence is therefore most effective when intercourse is limited to occurring 48 hours after ovulation through the end of the menstrual cycle (that is, when menstruation begins). Sterilization is the most effective form of contraception, with a 1.85% cumulative 10-year failure rate. Other information on nonhormonal contraceptive methods is listed in **Table 65**.

The combination estrogen-progestin oral contraceptive pills contain ethinyl estradiol and one of various progestins and are to be taken at the same dose every day (monophasic) or according to week of the cycle (biphasic or triphasic). Failure rates for this type of contraceptive range from 0.5% to 3% depending on whether women take the pills on schedule. The risk for ovarian cancer is reduced by at least half after 5 years of use of oral contraceptives, and this effect persists for 10 to 20 years after discontinuation of oral contraception (6). Women who take oral contraceptives also have a reduced risk for endometrial cancer and experience less acne (also a benefit in women who use low-dose oral contraceptives) and reduced severity of dysfunctional uterine bleeding, menstrual blood flow, and prevalence of anemia compared with those who do not take oral contraceptives.

Estimated rates of risks associated with oral contraceptive use are listed in **Table 66**. The risk for venous thromboembolism in women who take oral contraceptives is higher in patients with thrombophilias, including plasma protein C or protein S deficiency, factor V Leiden, or the prothrombin gene mutation compared with the unaffected population, although routine screening for these disorders before initiation of oral contraceptives is not currently recommended. The risks for myocardial infarction and ischemic stroke in women who take oral contraceptives are 7 to 15 times higher in patients with diabetes or hypercholesterolemia compared with persons without these diseases, and whether treatment of these conditions modifies this risk is unknown. Whether oral contraceptives contribute to the development of breast cancer remains controversial. These agents are safe in nonsmoking women older than the age of 35 years until menopause, because no studies have clearly documented that the risks far outweigh the advantages, and this group of women often benefit from noncontraceptive effects and control of erratic cycles often typical at this age (7).

Other hormonal contraceptives are the topical patch, vaginal ring, progestin-only pill, and medroxyprogesterone acetate injection. The patch containing ethinyl estradiol and norelgestromin is applied weekly for 3 concurrent weeks and then removed during the fourth week when withdrawal

TABLE 65 Nonhormonal Contraceptive Methods

Method	Percent of Unintended Pregnancies During First Year of Typical Use	Comments
No method	85	
Spermicides	29	
Cervical cap		Protects against pelvic infection and cervical dysplasia; alternative to diaphragm for women with relaxed anterior vaginal wall or diaphragm-induced, recurrent urinary tract infections
Parous women	32	
Nulliparous women	16	
Sponge		
Parous women	32	
Nulliparous women	16	
Diaphragm	16	Protects against pelvic infection and cervical dysplasia
Condom		
Female	21	
Male	15	As effective as oral contraceptives when used with spermicide
IUD		Contraindicated in women with a history of pelvic infection
Copper	0.8	Effective for 10 years. Can cause bleeding and cramping
Levonorgestrel	0.1	Effective for 5 years. Decreases period-related bleeding and cramping

Adapted from Hatcher RA. The Essentials of Contraception in Contraceptive Technology. New York: Irvington;2004:226.

IUD = intrauterine device.

TABLE 66 Age-specific Estimates of Risks from Oral Contraceptives

Excess cases/100,000 woman-years of use	Age		
	20 to 24 y	30 to 34 y	40 to 44 y
Myocardial infarction and ischemic stroke			
Nonsmokers	0.4	0.6	2
Smokers	1	2	20
Women with hypertension	4	7	29
Venous thromboembolism			
OCs with progestins: norethindrone, norethindrone acetate, levonorgestrel, ethynodiol diacetate	6	9	12
OCs with progestins: desogestrel or gestodene	16	23	30

Adapted from Petitti DB. Combination estrogen-progestin oral contraceptives. NEJM. 2003;349:1443-1450.

OCs = oral contraceptives.

bleeding should occur. Efficacy and adverse effects are similar to those of the pill, except for slightly more breast tenderness associated with the patch. Skin reactions at the application site are rare (1% to 2.4%) in patients who use the contraceptive patch, and partial or complete detachment of the patch occurs less than 5% of the time. The vaginal ring is inserted into the vagina and remains in place for 3 weeks. It releases continuous estradiol and etonogestrel until it is removed at week 4 to allow withdrawal bleeding to occur. Its efficacy and adverse effects are similar to those of the pill, except for increased incidence of vaginal infection, irritation, and discharge asso-

ciated with the vaginal ring. The progestin-only pill is taken daily, and dose timing must be very regular. The failure rate of this contraceptive is slightly higher than that of the combined estrogen–progestin pills. Medroxyprogesterone acetate injection is 99.7% effective and is administered every 3 months. It is very useful for women who cannot take estrogen because of current breast-feeding or problems with estrogen's side effects.

Two types of pills are available for emergency contraception. Both must be taken as soon as possible, or within 5 days of a risked pregnancy, and a second dose is taken 12 hours later. Levonorgestrel is the preferred formulation of emergency contraception because it is more efficacious and has fewer side effects (nausea 20% and vomiting 6%) than the second option, which is a combination of ethinyl estradiol and levonorgestrel (severe nausea and vomiting 40%); an antiemetic agent can be given 1 hour before the first dose of this formulation.

KEY POINTS

- Contraception by abstinence is most effective when intercourse is limited to the period 48 hours after ovulation and up until menstruation begins.

- Women who take oral contraceptives have a reduced risk for ovarian cancer and endometrial cancer, less acne, and reduced severity of dysfunctional uterine bleeding and menstrual blood flow and prevalence of anemia compared with those who do not take these agents.

- The risk for venous thromboembolism in women who take oral contraceptives is higher in patients with thrombophilias, including plasma protein C or protein S deficiency, factor V Leiden, or the prothrombin gene mutation compared with persons without these disorders.

- The risk for myocardial infarction and ischemic stroke in women who take oral contraceptives is 7 to 15 times higher in patients with diabetes or hypercholesterolemia compared with persons without these diseases.

- Oral contraceptives are considered safe for use in nonsmoking women older than the age of 35 years until menopause.

- Levonorgestrel is the preferred formulation of emergency contraception because it is more efficacious and has fewer side effects than combination ethinyl estradiol and levonorgestrel.

Menopause

Menopause is the period occurring after a woman experiences 6 to 12 months of amenorrhea, with the average age at menopause approximately 51 years. Perimenopause describes a period of changing pituitary gonadotropin secretion (follicle-stimulating hormone [FSH] and luteinizing hormone) and ovarian function that precedes menopause by about 2 to 8 years. The earliest laboratory finding during the perimenopausal transition is a rise in serum FSH level, but measuring this hormone level while a woman continues to menstruate is not helpful because of fluctuations in FSH levels as a function of menstruation and the perimenopausal transition. Once menstruation ceases, an FSH >30 mU/mL (30 U/L) is considered diagnostic of menopause, but this finding is not usually needed for diagnosis.

Perimenopause is marked by menstrual cycle irregularity, but approximately 30% of women experience the hallmarks of menopause, hot flushes and night sweats, prior to menstrual changes. Most women experience these vasomotor symptoms for 6 months to 2 years, and the prevalence of these symptoms varies by ethnic group. A history of premenstrual symptoms predicts occurrence of hot flushes as do several lifestyle factors, including warm air temperatures, obesity (BMI >30), lower level of physical activity (daily exercise predicts lower hot flush frequency), smoking, and higher socioeconomic status. Although no clinical trials support a relationship between frequency of hot flushes and emotional stress or consumption of hot or spicy foods or drinks, these associations have been reported anecdotally.

After menopause, higher androgen-to-estrogen ratios lead to hair loss on the scalp and increased hair growth on the upper lip and the chin. Vaginal changes include reduced production of vaginal-lubricating fluid and some loss of vaginal elasticity, leading to dyspareunia and vaginismus. Vaginal epithelial cells contain less glycogen, resulting in increased vaginal pH; increased growth of *Escherichia coli* and loss of lactobacilli leave this thin, friable tissue vulnerable to infection and ulceration, causing symptoms such as vaginal discharge, burning, itching, and bleeding. The urethra and the urinary trigone undergo atrophic changes similar to those of the vagina; dysuria, urgency, frequency, and suprapubic pain may occur in the absence of infection.

Estrogen improves menopausal symptoms, including hot flushes, night sweats, vulvar and vaginal atrophy, vaginal dryness, and itching. Improvement in vasomotor symptoms with oral conjugated equine estrogens, oral estradiol, or transdermal estradiol is clearly documented in studies, showing reduced hot flushes by approximately 16 to 22/week (8). There is no clear benefit of one estrogen-containing product over another. Evidence from a few randomized trials has shown improvement in sleep disturbances and urogenital atrophy with use of estrogen. Atypical vaginal bleeding and breast tenderness are the most common adverse effects of hormone replacement therapy. Contraindications to estrogen use include undiagnosed vaginal bleeding, breast cancer, other estrogen-sensitive cancers, current or previous history of venous or arterial thrombosis, or liver dysfunction/disease.

Estrogen can be administered orally, transdermally (patch), or vaginally; when oral or transdermal estrogen is used, it is given with progestin in women with an intact uterus to reduce the risk for endometrial cancer. Available oral forms of estrogen include conjugated equine estrogen (most commonly prescribed), estradiol (made by the premenopausal ovary), esterified estrogen, and plant-derived conjugated estrogen. Progestins include medroxyprogesterone acetate (the most common), micronized progesterone (made by the premenopausal ovary), norethindrone acetate, and norgestimate.

The Food and Drug Administration recommends use of the smallest effective dose of hormone replacement therapy for the shortest duration possible to treat menopausal symptoms only; no hormonal treatment is recommended for prevention of chronic conditions. Attempting to discontinue or decrease the estrogen dosage every 6 months to assess the continued need for hormone replacement therapy is appropriate. In women who have been taking estrogen replacement for long periods, gradual reduction of the daily dose, the days per week estrogen is taken, or a combination, is recommended (9). Women who discontinue taking hormones initially prescribed for treatment of vasomotor symptoms experience recurrence of these symptoms after discontinuation of hormonal therapy (10).

The United States Preventive Services Task Force (USPSTF) recommends against the use of estrogen or estrogen plus progestin for the prevention of chronic diseases after menopause, citing evidence from the Women's Health Initiative (WHI) study and others (11). The chronic conditions studied by the WHI investigators showed at least a trend toward an increased risk with the use of estrogen or estrogen-progestin for breast cancer, coronary heart disease, stroke, venous thromboembolism, dementia and cognitive decline (see also Reference 11), and urinary incontinence (12); quality of life measures were not clinically improved with hormone use (13).

In the initial WHI study (14) of women with an intact uterus who were taking estrogen and progestin, the risk for serious adverse events was approximately 1 in every 100 women treated for 5 years, with the average age of women enrolled in the study 63 years. Most women with vasomotor symptoms require fewer than 5 years' treatment and are often closer to 50 years of age; therefore, short-term hormone replacement therapy at this age may be an acceptable risk for some patients (see also Reference 9).

For women with disabling symptoms, there is clearly a need for alternatives to estrogen for treatment. Prescription progestins alone can be used to treat hot flushes (off-label use), including depomedroxyprogesterone acetate, oral medroxyprogesterone, and megestrol acetate. The use of these agents has been linked to breast cancer in some studies; therefore, this treatment modality is not recommended in patients with hormone-dependent tumors. In addition, progestins alone in the treatment of vasomotor symptoms have not been studied extensively, and short- and long-term benefits and harms are unknown. Perimenopausal women who need treatment of hot flushes and contraception may find low-dose oral contraceptives effective for both problems.

Many women use topical progesterone or combination estrogen–progesterone creams for treatment of hot flushes. Dosages, formulations, and additional ingredients of these agents vary widely. Results of studies of these topical agents are mixed, showing benefit or equivalent reduction in hot flushes compared with placebo. Data on the safety and side effects of these agents are lacking, including whether they are safer than conventional hormone treatment.

The North American Menopause Society (NAMS) developed an evidence-based position statement (15) detailing recommendations for the use of nonhormonal treatment of vasomotor symptoms (**Table 67**). The NAMS cautions

TABLE 67 Menopausal Treatment			
Treatment	**Mechanism***	**Dose**	**Efficacy/Safety**
Exercise	Increases β-endorphin production	Regular; not clearly specified in trials	Significant decrease in vasomotor frequency and severity
Black cohosh	Unknown	40 mg/d	Sufficient data on short-term treatment, but long-term studies lacking
Soy proteins	Selective estrogen receptor modulator (SERM)	40 to 60 g or 50 to 80 mg isoflavones/d	Mixed results from short-term treatment, but long-term studies lacking
Red clover	SERM	40 to 80 mg/d	Insufficient data
Dong quai	Unknown	Dose used in one study: 4.5 g	Insufficient data; contraindicated in patients taking warfarin
Clonidine	Reduces peripheral and central vascular activity		Sufficient data showing moderate efficacy and safety
Venlafaxine	Blocks reuptake of serotonin and norepinephrine	75 to 100 mg/d	Single RCT showing significant hot flush reduction over placebo
Paroxetine and fluoxetine	Increases serotonin and reduces luteinizing hormone	Paroxetine: 12.5 mg/d; fluoxetine: 20 mg/d	Single RCT for each treatment showing significant hot flush reduction over placebo
Gabapentin	Alters the thermoregulatory process	Initial dose of 100 mg/d, with titration up to 900 mg/d	Single RCT showing significant hot flush reduction over placebo

Reprinted with permission from Fugate SE, Church CO. Nonestrogen treatment modalities for vasomotor symptoms associated with menopause. Ann Pharmacother. 2004;38:1482-1499. Data are also from North American Menopause Society. Treatment of menopause-associated vasomotor symptoms: position statement of The North American Menopause Society. Menopause. 2004;11:11-33; and Physicians' Information and Education Resource (PIER), American College of Physicians.

RCT = randomized controlled trial.

that the placebo effect is higher in trials of hot flush treatment than for other menopausal symptoms, sometimes as high as 50%. For patients with mild hot flushes, adopting lifestyle changes, such as keeping the temperature cool and using paced respiration (slow, controlled diaphragmatic breathing), with or without the use of nonprescription treatments, such as black cohosh or soy protein, may be helpful. Regular physical activity decreases vasomotor frequency and severity. Smoking cessation might lower the number of hot flushes, but no clinical trials have specifically studied this issue. Prescription treatments that may be helpful in patients with hot flushes include gabapentin, venlafaxine, and the selective serotonin reuptake inhibitors paroxetine or fluoxetine. A recent National Institutes of Health (NIH) Conference concluded that more rigorous trials are needed to fully evaluate alternatives to estrogen, especially in diverse populations (16).

KEY POINTS

- Once menstruation ceases, a follicle-stimulating hormone level >30 mU/mL is considered diagnostic of menopause, but this finding is not usually needed for diagnosis.

- The Food and Drug Administration recommends use of the smallest effective dose of hormone replacement therapy for the shortest duration possible to treat menopausal symptoms only.

- Attempting to discontinue or decrease the estrogen dosage in menopausal therapy every 6 months to assess the continued need for hormone replacement therapy is appropriate.

- For patients with mild hot flushes, keeping the temperature cool and using paced respiration with or without the use of nonprescription treatments, such as black cohosh or soy protein, may be helpful.

- Regular physical activity decreases vasomotor frequency and severity in women with hot flushes.

Dysmenorrhea and Abnormal Uterine Bleeding

Patients with a history of menstrual pain that begins within 1 to 2 years of menarche and sometimes worsens over time usually have primary dysmenorrhea, in which no pathologic cause for the menstrual pain exists. This symptom is in contrast to secondary dysmenorrhea, defined as menstrual pain for which an organic cause exists. An underlying cause for dysmenorrhea is likely in the setting of noncyclical pain, abnormal discharge, dyspareunia, or heavy or irregular bleeding.

Primary dysmenorrhea is the result of increased prostaglandin production that occurs when estrogen and progesterone levels decrease in the luteal phase of the cycle. The prostaglandins cause elevated pressures in the uterine fundus, leading to sharp or cramp-like pains during the first days

of menstruation. The pain is generally suprapubic but might radiate to the back, inner thighs, or deep pelvis; nausea, vomiting, and diarrhea may also occur. There are no pathologic findings associated with primary dysmenorrhea on physical examination. The mainstay of treatment for this symptom is oral contraceptives or NSAIDs, with no one NSAID found to be superior to another (17). Depomedroxyprogesterone acetate (DMPA) (off-label use) can induce hypomenorrhea or amenorrhea, resulting in decreased dysmenorrhea, but only approximately 50% of patients using DMPA become completely amenorrheic in the first year of therapy. Vitamin B_1 (thiamine) is effective for dysmenorrhea (100 mg/day) based on a large randomized trial (18). Alternative therapies, including magnesium, vitamin B_6 (pyridoxine), vitamin E, and omega-3 fatty acids, have shown some benefit but have not been studied thoroughly enough to allow for a recommendation on their use (see also Reference 18).

A common cause of secondary dysmenorrhea is endometriosis, and its symptoms include dyspareunia, worsening dysmenorrhea as menses progresses, abnormal bleeding, and infertility. On physical examination, patients with endometriosis have a fixed, poorly mobile uterus and tenderness or nodularity of the uterosacral ligaments and posterior uterus. Most patients with suspected endometriosis should undergo diagnostic laparoscopy to evaluate the nature and extent of disease. The primary goal in the treatment of endometriosis is the induction of amenorrhea. The gonadotropin-releasing hormone agonist leuprolide acetate, oral contraceptives, or DMPA (off-label use) can reduce symptoms that might recur after treatment ceases.

Other causes for secondary dysmenorrhea include adenomyosis (endometriosis within the muscular layers of the uterus), pelvic inflammatory disease, presence of an intrauterine device (IUD), uterine leiomyoma, and endometrial polyps.

Abnormal uterine bleeding can take many forms, including infrequent menses, excessive flow, prolonged duration of menses, intermenstrual bleeding, and postmenopausal bleeding. Normal menstrual cycles are typically consistent in ovulating women, with duration of flow 4 + 2 days and cycle length 28 + 7 days. The differential diagnosis of abnormal bleeding varies according to age as outlined in **Table 68**.

In all cases of abnormal bleeding, physical examination should include a pelvic examination and Pap smear. In premenopausal patients, a urine pregnancy test is also appropriate. Further laboratory testing in premenopausal patients depends on the findings of the history and physical examination and may include cultures for gonorrhea and *Chlamydia trachomatis*, complete blood count, thyroid function tests, plasma glucose measurement, and coagulation studies. In patients with anovulatory bleeding as determined by irregularity of periods (that is, the cycle length falls out of the normal range or cycle length varies by more than 10 days), measurement of prolactin levels is indicated, especially in the presence of galactorrhea.

TABLE 68 Abnormal Bleeding

Age of Presentation	Common Causes	Diagnostic Clues
Menarche to teenage years	Pregnancy Anovulation Stress Bleeding disorders Infection (cervical or vaginal)	Irregular periods: Cycle length falls outside normal range or varies by 10 days or more Physical or mental Associated with other sources of bleeding (gums, nose) Postcoital bleeding and/or vaginal discharge
Teens to 40s	Pregnancy Malignancy (uterine, cervical, vaginal, or vulvar) Infection (cervical or vaginal) Cervical polyps Endometrial polyps Fibroids Adenomyosis Anovulation Hormonal contraception Bleeding disorders Endocrine abnormalities Ovarian or adrenal tumor	Postcoital bleeding and/or vaginal discharge Postcoital bleeding Dysmenorrhea Irregular periods Associated with other sources of bleeding (gums, nose) Signs of hypothyroidism, diabetes, hyperprolactinemia, polycystic ovary syndrome New-onset virilization or hirsutism
Perimenopausal	Anovulation Endometrial hyperplasia and polyps Fibroids Malignancy (uterine, cervical, vaginal, or vulvar)	Irregular periods Dysmenorrhea
Postmenopausal	Malignancy (uterine, cervical, vaginal, or vulvar) Endometrial atrophy Atrophy of vaginal mucosa Estrogen replacement therapy	Vaginal dryness, dyspareunia

TABLE 69 Tests to Assess Endometrial Lining

Procedure	Test Characteristics
Endometrial biopsy: outpatient sampling of endometrium with thin pipelle	Can miss focal lesions such as polyps and fibroids Easily completed in the outpatient setting
Transvaginal ultrasonography: ultrasonographic probe placed in vagina	Improved resolution compared with pelvic ultrasonography In premenopausal women, this test cannot reliably exclude endometrial abnormalities. Best results obtained on days 4 to 6 of menstrual cycle when endometrial lining is the thinnest In postmenopausal patients, an endometrial lining <4 to 5 mm typically rules out endometrial cancer Cannot distinguish benign from malignant endometrial thickening
Saline-infused sonography or sonohysterography: sterile saline infused into uterus, followed by pelvic ultrasonography	Better assesses presence of endometrial polyps than the above tests May be most helpful in women with negative endometrial biopsy results or with indeterminate ultrasound results
Hysteroscopy: direct visualization of the endometrial cavity	Unreliable by itself for diagnosing malignancy; usually performed with a D&C Biopsy of any suspicious areas can be performed during the test More costly and invasive than above tests

D&C = dilation and curettage.

After performing appropriate laboratory studies, an assessment of the endometrial lining is appropriate to rule out endometrial cancer or hyperplasia in patients older than 35 years of age with abnormal uterine bleeding. **Table 69** outlines available tests for assessing the endometrium. In younger patients, transvaginal or pelvic ultrasound may be appropriate to identify fibroids or structural abnormalities when no cause of bleeding is discovered by the evaluation described above, and a referral to a gynecologist may be indicated.

In premenopausal patients with no abnormal results on laboratory studies, ultrasonography, or assessment of the endometrium (or in those for whom these tests are not indicated), initial treatment depends on ovulatory status. In patients with anovulatory bleeding, initiation of oral contraceptives or cyclic progestins can help to maintain regular cycles. In patients with ovulatory bleeding, high-dose estrogens (off-label use) can stop bleeding quickly, followed by oral contraceptives to reduce the amount of bleeding at each cycle. In either case, the levonorgestrel IUD (off-label use) or NSAIDs can reduce the amount of bleeding occurring during the cycle.

Uterine fibroids are a common cause of abnormal bleeding with dysmenorrhea and can be detected by pelvic ultrasonography, although submucosal fibroids may not be visible using this method. For women with uterine fibroids, several options are available for problematic symptoms of heavy bleeding, dysmenorrhea, or pelvic pain, including uterine artery embolization, myomectomy, or hysterectomy. Interventional radiologists usually perform uterine artery embolization for treatment of uterine fibroids by injecting embolic material into the uterine artery. This procedure results in infarction and degeneration of fibroids by preferential transmission of the embolic material into the fibroids, where blood flow is higher than that in the surrounding tissue. Whether uterine artery embolization affects fertility is unknown, but this procedure does improve symptoms after causing an initial 4 to 5 days of pain and malaise (19). The perioperative risk for myomectomy is comparable to hysterectomy, but it is a second option for the treatment of fibroids in women who wish to retain fertility. Occasionally, new fibroids develop after myomectomy. Hysterectomy is reserved for patients with uterine fibroids whose bleeding does not respond to treatment and who are not planning further pregnancies. In patients who experienced abnormal uterine bleeding for a median of 4 years, hysterectomy was superior to continued medical treatment for improving health-related quality of life (20).

KEY POINTS

- Vitamin B$_1$ (thiamine) is effective for dysmenorrhea (100 mg/day) based on a large randomized trial.

- Most patients with suspected endometriosis should undergo diagnostic laparoscopy to evaluate the nature and extent of disease.

- In patients with anovulatory bleeding, measurement of prolactin levels is indicated, especially in the presence of galactorrhea.

- After appropriate laboratory studies have been performed, an assessment of the endometrial lining is appropriate to rule out endometrial cancer or hyperplasia in patients with abnormal uterine bleeding who are older than 35 years of age.

- In anovulatory bleeding, initiation of oral contraceptives or cyclic progestins can help patients to maintain regular cycles.

- In ovulatory bleeding, high-dose estrogens (off-label use) can stop bleeding quickly, and then oral contraceptives can help to reduce the amount of bleeding at each cycle.

- Uterine artery embolization improves symptoms in women with uterine fibroids after causing an initial 4 to 5 days of pain and malaise.

- Hysterectomy is reserved for patients with uterine fibroids whose bleeding does not respond to treatment and who are not planning further pregnancies.

Vaginitis

Vaginitis is characterized by vaginal irritation, pruritis, pain, or unusual discharge. Vaginal inflammation and infection occur commonly in patients with vaginitis, which may result from pathogens (bacterial vaginosis, *Trichomonas vaginalis*, *Candida albicans*, and genital warts); allergic reactions to vaginal contraceptives or other products, such as douches, tampons, or soap; coitus-induced friction; or postmenopausal atrophy. Normal vaginal secretions can increase in amount during the midcycle estrogen surge when secretions are clear, elastic, and mucoid, or during the luteal phase of the cycle or pregnancy when the secretions are thick, white, and, sometimes, adherent to the vaginal walls.

A microscopic examination of vaginal discharge with a drop of 0.9% saline solution (wet mount) can help to identify motile organisms with flagella (trichomonads) and epithelial cells covered with bacteria obscuring the cell borders (clue cells). Additional examination of the secretions with a drop of 10% potassium hydroxide is useful in identifying the fishy odor of bacterial vaginosis (whiff test) or the filaments or spores of *Candida* species. Vaginal cultures are generally not helpful in the diagnosis of vaginitis if the above evaluation has been completed.

The normal predominant vaginal organism is the *Lactobacillus* species, and this organism helps to maintain the normal vaginal pH <4.5. Bacterial vaginosis occurs because of an overgrowth of anaerobic bacteria, *Gardnerella vaginalis* and *Mycoplasma hominis*. Although this condition is usually found in sexually active women, it is not a sexually transmitted infection. Symptoms of bacterial vaginosis include increased malodorous discharge without irritation or pain. Lack of perceived odor makes this diagnosis less likely (21). On physical examination, clinical criteria for bacterial vaginosis include a homogenous, white, noninflammatory discharge that smoothly coats the vaginal walls; presence of clue cells; vaginal pH >4.5; and the presence of a fishy odor to the vaginal discharge either before or after the addition of 10% potassium hydroxide. Symptomatic patients who have at least three of these criteria should receive treatment with metronidazole or clindamycin, either orally or vaginally.

C. albicans infections occur in patients without known cause but also during pregnancy, in women with a history of diabetes, or in women who are using broad-spectrum antibiotics or corticosteroids. Heat, moisture, and occlusive clothing contribute to the likelihood for infection with this organism. Symptoms include pruritis, external and internal erythema, and nonodorous, white, curd-like discharge. Lack of pruritis makes this diagnosis less likely, and the presence of inflammation and lack of an odor make this diagnosis more likely (See also Reference 21). Because vaginal yeast is found in 10% to 20% of normal women, the identification of *Candida* species in patients without symptoms does not require treatment, which includes 1-day pills, 1-day creams, or 3- to 7-day creams or vaginal tablets. Approximately 5% of women experience recurrent vaginal infections (three or more episodes per year), and weekly oral fluconazole for 6 months reduces the recurrence of candidal vaginitis. Infections may recur after treatment is discontinued (22). *Lactobacillus* oral or vaginal tablets taken after antibiotic therapy do not prevent the occurrence of candidiasis (23).

T. vaginalis infection is sexually transmitted. Most men with this infection are asymptomatic and most women with this infection are symptomatic. A diffuse, malodorous, yellow-green vaginal discharge is common in *T. vaginalis.* The sensitivity of identifying trichomonads (characterized by a jerky motility on wet mount) is approximately 60% to 70%, whereas the specificity is almost 100% (See also Reference 21). Cultures for identifying *T. vaginalis* are more sensitive than wet-mount microscopy. All sexual partners of patients infected with *T. vaginalis* should receive treatment with a single 2-g dose of metronidazole, which is usually effective; in patients who do not respond to this regimen, a 7-day treatment course is appropriate.

> **KEY POINTS**
>
> - Lack of perceived odor makes a diagnosis of bacterial vaginosis less likely.
> - Treatment for bacterial vaginosis consists of metronidazole or clindamycin, either orally or vaginally.
> - Symptoms of *Candida albicans* include pruritis, external and internal erythema, and nonodorous white curd-like discharge.
> - Lack of pruritis makes a diagnosis of *C. albicans* less likely, and the presence of inflammation and lack of an odor make this diagnosis more likely.
> - Weekly oral fluconazole treatment for 6 months reduces the incidence of recurrent candidal vaginitis.
> - Most men infected with *Trichomonas vaginalis* are asymptomatic, and most women with this infection are symptomatic.
> - All sexual partners of patients with *T. vaginalis* infection should receive a single 2-g dose of metronidazole; in patients who do not respond to this regimen, a 7-day treatment course is appropriate.

Pelvic Pain

Pelvic pain in women is a common clinical problem with an estimated prevalence of approximately 15% in women aged 18 to 50 years. Acute pelvic pain is vastly different from chronic pelvic pain, and the two are separate entities. The focus of this section is on chronic pelvic pain.

Chronic pelvic pain is not a disease but a syndrome, thought to be a complex multifactorial entity related to neurologic, musculoskeletal, endocrine, and psychologic factors.

It is a frustrating entity for both patients and clinicians, with ill-defined symptoms and, frequently, without a definitive diagnosis, but it nevertheless is treatable. Pelvic pain is considered chronic when it persists for longer than 3 to 6 months. In addition to a thorough history and physical examination, questions concerning the nature of the pain and any cyclic variation to the symptoms are appropriate in the evaluation of patients with pelvic pain. Because mood disorders and depressive symptoms can compound any pain syndrome, the presence of these factors should be considered in these patients. Reproducing the pain during the physical examination can be valuable in determining the source of pain. The evaluation of chronic pelvic pain should include cervical cultures, a complete blood count, and urinalysis, with additional tests performed based on the patient's signs and symptoms.

The four most common disorders associated with chronic pelvic pain are endometriosis, adhesions, irritable bowel syndrome, and interstitial cystitis (24). When no definitive diagnosis is made, successful treatment usually requires pharmacologic and nonpharmacologic interventions, with the most success resulting from an integrated multidisciplinary approach to management of this syndrome.

A systematic review of the different treatment modalities of pelvic pain has focused on high-dose progesterone (medroxyprogesterone acetate), progesterone with psychotherapy, sertraline, ultrasonography as an aid to reassurance, surgical adhesiolysis, dihydroergotamine, and a multidisciplinary approach (25). Progesterone was effective in decreasing self-rated pain scores, but the benefit was not sustained 9 months after treatment, with or without psychotherapy, in patients with pelvic pain. Neither sertraline nor adhesiolysis improved pain scores in these patients. Dihydroergotamine did not produce a long-term benefit in patients with pelvic pain, with relief lasting approximately 48 hours. Reassurance combined with ultrasonography and the multidisciplinary approach led to positive outcomes in self-rating scores in patients with pelvic pain (26, 27).

> **KEY POINTS**
>
> - The four most common disorders associated with chronic pelvic pain are endometriosis, adhesions, irritable bowel syndrome, and interstitial cystitis.
> - Reassurance combined with ultrasonography and the multidisciplinary approach led to positive outcomes in self-rating scores in patients with pelvic pain.

References

1. **Sterns EE.** Age-related breast diagnosis. Can J Surg. 1992;35:41-5. [PMID: 1739898]
2. **Kerlikowske K, Smith-Bindman R, Ljung BM, Grady D.** Evaluation of abnormal mammography results and palpable breast abnormalities. Ann Intern Med. 2003;139:274-84. [PMID: 12965983]
3. **Smith RL, Pruthi S, Fitzpatrick LA.** Evaluation and management of breast pain. Mayo Clin Proc. 2004;79:353-72. [PMID: 15008609]

4. **Bundred N.** Breast pain. Clin Evid. 2002:1840-8. [PMID: 12603972]

5. **Millet AV, Dirbas FM.** Clinical management of breast pain: a review. Obstet Gynecol Surv. 2002;57:451-61. [PMID: 12172222]

6. **Petitti DB.** Clinical practice. Combination estrogen-progestin oral contraceptives. N Engl J Med. 2003;349:1443-50. [PMID: 14534338]

7. **Seibert C, Barbouche E, Fagan J, Myint E, Wetterneck T, Wittemyer M.** Prescribing oral contraceptives for women older than 35 years of age. Ann Intern Med. 2003;138:54-64. [PMID: 12513046]

8. **Nelson HD.** Commonly used types of postmenopausal estrogen for treatment of hot flashes: scientific review. JAMA. 2004;291:1610-20. [PMID: 15069049]

9. **Grady D.** Postmenopausal hormones—therapy for symptoms only. N Engl J Med. 2003;348:1835-7. [PMID: 12642636]

10. **Ockene JK, Barad DH, Cochrane BB, Larson JC, Gass M, Wassertheil-Smoller S, et al.** Symptom experience after discontinuing use of estrogen plus progestin. JAMA. 2005;294:183-93. [PMID: 16014592]

11. Hormone therapy for the prevention of chronic conditions in postmenopausal women: recommendations from the U.S. Preventive Services Task Force. Ann Intern Med. 2005;142:855-60. [PMID: 15897536]

12. **Hendrix SL, Cochrane BB, Nygaard IE, Handa VL, Barnabei VM, Iglesia C, et al.** Effects of estrogen with and without progestin on urinary incontinence. JAMA. 2005 Feb 23;293(8):935-48. [PMID: 15728164]

13. **Hays J, Ockene JK, Brunner RL, Kotchen JM, Manson JE, Patterson RE, et al.** Effects of estrogen plus progestin on health-related quality of life. N Engl J Med. 2003;348:1839-54. [PMID: 12642637]

14. **Rossouw JE, Anderson GL, Prentice RL, LaCroix AZ, Kooperberg C, Stefanick ML, et al.** Risks and benefits of estrogen plus progestin in healthy postmenopausal women: principal results From the Women's Health Initiative randomized controlled trial. JAMA. 2002;288:321-33. [PMID: 12117397]

15. Treatment of menopause-associated vasomotor symptoms: position statement of The North American Menopause Society. Menopause. 2004;11:11-33. [PMID: 14716179]

16. NIH State-of-the-Science Conference Statement on Management of Menopause-Related Symptoms. National Institutes of Health Consensus Development Program web site. Available at: http://consensus.nih.gov/2005/2005MenopausalSymptomsSOS 025html.htm. Accessed July 19, 2006.

17. **Marjoribanks J, Proctor ML, Farquhar C.** Nonsteroidal anti-inflammatory drugs for primary dysmenorrhoea. Cochrane Database Syst Rev. 2003:CD001751. [PMID: 14583938]

18. **Wilson ML, Murphy PA.** Herbal and dietary therapies for primary and secondary dysmenorrhoea. Cochrane Database Syst Rev. 2001:CD002124. [PMID: 11687013]

19. Uterine artery embolization for fibroids. Med Lett Drugs Ther. 2005;47(1206):31-32. [PMID: 15821634]

20. **Kuppermann M, Varner RE, Summitt RL Jr, Learman LA, Ireland C, Vittinghoff E, et al.** Effect of hysterectomy vs medical treatment on health-related quality of life and sexual functioning: the medicine or surgery (Ms) randomized trial. JAMA. 2004;291:1447-55. [PMID: 15039411]

21. **Anderson MR, Klink K, Cohrssen A.** Evaluation of vaginal complaints. JAMA. 2004;291:1368-79. [PMID: 15026404]

22. **Sobel JD, Wiesenfeld HC, Martens M, Danna P, Hooton TM, Rompalo A, et al.** Maintenance fluconazole therapy for recurrent vulvovaginal candidiasis. N Engl J Med. 2004;351:876-83. [PMID: 15329425]

23. **Pirotta M, Gunn J, Chondros P, Grover S, O'Malley P, Hurley S, et al.** Effect of lactobacillus in preventing post-antibiotic vulvovaginal candidiasis: a randomised controlled trial. BMJ. 2004;329:548. [PMID: 15333452]

24. **Howard FM.** Chronic pelvic pain. Obstet Gynecol. 2003;101:594-611. [PMID: 12636968]

25. **Stones RW, Mountfield J.** Interventions for treating chronic pelvic pain in women. Cochrane Database Syst Rev. 2000:CD000387. [PMID: 11034686]

26. **Bau A, Atri M.** Acute female pelvic pain: ultrasound evaluation. Semin Ultrasound CT MR. 2000;21:78-93. [PMID: 10688069]

27. **Gunter J.** Chronic pelvic pain: an integrated approach to diagnosis and treatment. Obstet Gynecol Surv. 2003;58:615-23. [PMID: 12972837]

PERIOPERATIVE MEDICINE

General Approach to Perioperative Medicine

Important aspects of perioperative care include communication with surgeons and anesthesiologists, preoperative testing, management of routine medications and herbal supplements, and strategies to prevent and manage postoperative delirium. Good communication is characterized by limiting the number of recommendations (≤5 is best), offering specific recommendations with precise "recipes" for medications (dose, route, frequency, and duration), continuing to manage and monitor the status of preexisting medical conditions, diagnosing and managing new medical problems, and providing frequent, relevant follow-up (1).

Preoperative Laboratory Testing

The evidence-based standard in preoperative laboratory testing consists of ordering fewer selective tests—rather than performing a battery of routine tests—as indicated by the medical history, medications, and physical examination (2, 3). Selective test ordering is also less expensive, resulting in fewer direct testing costs and indirect costs associated with evaluating unexpected abnormalities with little or no clinical relevance and no effect on surgical outcome. The practice of performing a routine wide battery of tests appears to persist for two reasons: 1) local hospital policies, which may vary in the extent to which they are evidence-based, and 2) physicians' fear of medical legal liability. Physicians can implement changes to promote evidence-based hospital practice by performing only selective, evidence-based preoperative tests and noting that 30% to 60% of abnormalities found on routine preoperative tests are ignored, receiving no comment in the medical record or resulting in no action taken, a practice that confers its own risks for liability. Patients whose laboratory studies were normal in the 4 months before surgery and whose clinical status has not changed do not require repeated testing (4).

Perioperative Management of Medications

Preoperative documentation of all medications and all over-the-counter drugs, vitamins, and herbal products taken is appropriate. Patients should continue to take most medicines, especially cardiovascular drugs, perioperatively, including the morning of surgery. Drugs with long half-lives can be temporarily discontinued and resumed when patients begin eating.

Aspirin, combined aspirin and dipyridamole, clopidogrel, and ticlopidine cause irreversible platelet dysfunction and should be stopped 7 days before surgery. Cilostazol and COX-1 inhibitors cause reversible platelet inhibition and must be stopped within 1 to 3 days of surgery. COX-2 inhibitors do not affect platelet function, but all NSAIDs can affect renal function and should be discontinued 1 to 3 days preoperatively (5). Selective serotonin reuptake inhibitors (SSRIs) may be associated with an increased risk for bleeding by depletion of serotonin stores. Discontinuation of these agents several days before surgery is indicated, depending on the individual drug's half-life.

Estrogen and selective estrogen receptor modulators (SERMs), such as raloxifene and tamoxifen, increase the risk for thromboembolism and should be discontinued perioperatively. An oncologist should provide consultation on how long patients can cease taking antineoplastic SERMs. Bisphosphonates, because of their risk for esophagitis, should be discontinued perioperatively until patients are fully ambulatory and have resumed normal eating patterns.

Medications for Parkinson's disease, and anticonvulsant, antipsychotic, and antidepressant agents should be continued orally up to the time of surgery and resumed as soon as possible afterwards. The anticholinergic effects of tricyclic antidepressants may increase the risk of side effects from other anticholinergics. Cessation of monoamine oxidase inhibitors, no longer commonly used, is appropriate in patients who are psychiatrically stable, with cautious continuation of these drugs reasonable in those who are psychiatrically or surgically unstable. Patients can continue taking lithium, with preoperative measurement of serum levels. Anesthetic requirements may be greater in patients taking chronic benzodiazepines than in those who do not; the risk for withdrawal syndrome on discontinuation of benzodiazepines appears higher than the risk of continuing these drugs perioperatively at a lower dose (see also Reference 5).

It is recommended that most supplements or herbal medicines be discontinued 1 week prior to surgery, although little is known of their half-lives and reversibility of effects. High-dose vitamin E, ginger, ginkgo, ginseng, garlic, and feverfew can cause bleeding. Ginseng is associated with hypoglycemia, garlic is associated with hypoglycemia and hypotension, and feverfew is associated with withdrawal symptoms, such as nervousness, insomnia, headache, and joint pain. Kava and echinacea can contribute to anesthetic-related hepatotoxicity; kava, a sedative, can increase the effects of sedative hypnotics and anesthetics, and chronic echinacea can cause immunosuppression. Valerian is also a sedative and associated with withdrawal syndrome. Ephedra (ma huang) is a sympathomimetic agent; short-term use of this supplement can cause hypertension,

tachycardia, and ventricular arrhythmia with halothane; long-term use leads to catecholamine depletion, which can cause hemodynamic instability. As with SSRIs, St. John's wort inhibits reuptake of serotonin (potentially leading to platelet dysfunction), norepinephrine, and dopamine, and it induces the cytochrome P-450 system (6, 7).

Postoperative Delirium

In the elderly, postoperative delirium is associated with poor cognitive and functional recovery and increased risk for death, complications, and institutionalization. Approximately 25% of elderly patients experience delirium during any hospitalization, with rates as high as 35% after vascular surgery and 60% after hip-fracture repair (8). Risk factors for postoperative delirium include increasing age, existing cognitive or functional impairment, cerebrovascular or neurodegenerative disease, history of delirium, alcohol abuse, preoperative use of benzodiazepines or narcotics, postoperative decreased hemoglobin or low oxygen saturation, very abnormal serum sodium potassium or plasma glucose levels, and inadequately treated pain. Delirium associated with drug toxicity is common, and multiple drugs can cause this condition. Delirium may also be the presenting sign of postoperative infection, sepsis, or myocardial ischemia or infarction.

Patients with delirium have acute, fluctuating mental status changes, with difficulty in focusing or maintaining attention, and disorganized thinking. Based on psychomotor activity, there are four types of delirium: 1) hypoactive, 2) hyperactive, 3) mixed delirium with hypo- and hyperactivity, and 4) delirium without changes in psychomotor activity. **Table 70** shows the brief Confusion Assessment Method test for identifying delirium. Nursing staff or family members can provide most, if not all, of the information needed to complete the Confusion Assessment Method test. There is also a Confusion Assessment Method test developed for patients who cannot verbalize or who are intubated in the intensive-care unit.

TABLE 70 Confusion Assessment Method Test for Delirium*	
A.	Acute onset with fluctuating course: mental status changes may last hours to days, fluctuating in presence and severity
B.	Inattention: difficulty in focusing, easily distracted, unable to follow a conversation
C.	Disorganized thinking: rambling, incoherent, irrelevant conversation, unclear or illogical flow of thoughts, unpredictably changing subjects
D.	Altered level of consciousness and psychomotor activity: hyperalert, hypervigilant, lethargic but easy to arouse, stuporous and difficult to arouse, unarouseable.

*The diagnosis of delirium requires both acute onset with fluctuating course (A) and inattention (B) plus either disorganized thinking or altered level of consciousness/psychomotor activity (C or D).

Evaluation of a patient with postoperative delirium includes a full physical examination, laboratory tests, electrocardiography, chest radiography, and medication review to determine the cause of delirium. Management of patients with delirium includes treating the precipitating causes; providing supportive care with a safe, quiet environment; offering frequent orientation cues and adequate nutrition and hydration; helping patients to maintain activity levels; and avoiding the use of physical restraints and urinary catheterization. Symptoms of postoperative delirium may be treated with haloperidol, with a low initial dose of 0.5 mg, followed by a divided maintenance dose, and a final, tapered dose administered over 3 to 5 days when delirium is resolved. New antipsychotic agents, such as risperidone and olanzapine, also appear effective in patients with postoperative delirium and have fewer extrapyramidal side effects than older antipsychotic agents have. Short-acting benzodiazepines can be useful adjunctive treatments in patients with this disorder but can cause paradoxical agitation; when used with antipsychotic drugs, lower doses of these agents are appropriate.

KEY POINTS

- The evidence-based standard in preoperative laboratory testing consists of ordering fewer selective tests as indicated by the medical history, medications, and physical examination, rather than more tests.

- Patients whose laboratory studies were normal in the 4 months before surgery and whose clinical status has not changed do not require repeated testing.

- Drugs with long half-lives can be temporarily discontinued and resumed when patients begin eating.

- Supplements or herbal medicines should be discontinued in patients prior to surgery.

- Approximately 25% of elderly patients experience delirium during any hospitalization, with rates as high as 35% after vascular surgery and 60% after hip-fracture repair.

- Patients with delirium have acute, fluctuating mental status changes, with difficulty in focusing or maintaining attention, and disorganized thinking.

- Haloperidol is appropriate for treatment of symptoms of postoperative delirium.

Cardiovascular Perioperative Medicine

Myocardial infarction after noncardiac surgery usually occurs in the first 4 days after surgery and is associated with a 15% to 25% hospital mortality rate. Nonfatal postoperative myocardial infarction is an independent risk factor for future infarction and cardiovascular death within 6 months after surgery (9). The pathophysiology of plaque rupture and thrombus formation applies to only half of cases of perioperative myocardial infarction; the other half are caused by a myocardial oxygen supply/demand imbalance in the setting of fixed, nonoccluding plaques.

Preoperative risk stratification aims to identify the degree of cardiac risk and potential benefit of noninvasive testing, angiography, and revascularization. One study evaluated four predictive indices in the same surgical population and found that the predictive accuracy of cardiac complications was poor overall (10). A more recent study found six variables that were clinically available before surgery, which were able to predict cardiac complications fairly well; these variables were 1) high-risk surgery, 2) history of ischemic heart disease, 3) history of heart failure, 4) history of cerebrovascular disease, 5) insulin treatment, and 6) serum creatinine level >2.0 mg/dL (Revised Cardiac Risk Index) (11). In the study population, rates of major cardiac complications with 0, 1, 2, or ≥3 of these variables were 0.4% to 0.5%, 0.9% to 1%, 4% to 7%, and 9% to 11%, respectively. Advanced age has been found to be an independent risk factor in some studies and a surrogate marker for medical comorbidity in others. **Table 71** shows levels of preoperative risk according to cardiac history and age; **Table 72** gives examples of surgical risk.

Two guidelines for cardiovascular risk assessment are those of the American College of Physicians (12) and the American College of Cardiology/American Heart Association (13, 14). These guidelines are similar to each other except that the ACP does not recommend the use of exertional capacity to gauge cardiovascular risk because of lack of evidence for this criterion, whereas the ACC/AHA, based on consensus, advocates the use of exertional capacity in cardiovascular risk assessment, favoring more frequent noninvasive testing for intermediate-risk patients or those of uncertain exertional capacity. Exertional capacity is classified as poor (<4 metabolic equivalents [METS]), adequate (4 to 7 METS), and excellent (>7 METS). Patients who can climb a flight of stairs, walk up a hill, do heavy housework, dance, or walk on level ground at 4 miles/hour can achieve ≥4 METS. Comparison of the accuracy of these guidelines with that of other risk indices has not occurred in well-designed prospective studies. However, evidence indicates that low-risk patients can undergo any surgery without further risk stratification. Within 5 years of revascularization or 2 years of noninvasive testing, clinically stable patients do not usually need to undergo repeated testing. For high- or intermediate-risk patients undergoing high-risk surgery, further testing may be appropriate.

Issues of uncertainty in patients with intermediate risk for cardiovascular complications include the predictive accuracy of noninvasive testing and likelihood that preoperative revascularization will reduce the risks associated with noncardiac surgery. In a recent review, dobutamine stress echocardiography and myocardial perfusion scintigraphy were found to be the most sensitive (83% and 85%, respectively), and radionuclide ventriculography and dipyridamole stress echocardiography were found to be the most specific

TABLE 71 Patient Risk Based on Clinical Cardiac Characteristics

Negligible	Low (<1%)	Moderate (1% to 5%)	High (5% to 10%)	Very High (>10%)
Normal ECG No CAD risk factors Age <75 y	Normal ECG, CAD risk factors Age >75 y	Prior CVA/TIA Peripheral vascular disease (bruits, claudication, prior vascular surgery) Diabetes Poor functional status	Known CAD Arrhythmia Systolic dysfunction	Unstable coronary syndrome Recent MI Clinical heart failure Severe aortic stenosis

ECG = electrocardiogram, CAD = coronary artery disease, CVA = cerebrovascular accident, TIA = transient ischemic attack, MI = myocardial infarction.

TABLE 72 Risk of Noncardiac Surgery

Low-Risk Surgery (<1%)	Moderate-Risk Surgery (1% to 5%)	High-Risk Surgery (>5%)
Endoscopy Superficial surgery Cataract surgery Local or breast biopsy Cystoscopy Hysterectomy Vasectomy	Carotid endarterectomy Thyroidectomy Head/neck surgery Hip/knee replacement Uncomplicated abdominal surgery Nephrectomy Prostate surgery	Emergent major surgery Aortic, major vascular surgery Peripheral vascular surgery Long procedures with large fluid shifts and/or blood loss

(91% and 86%, respectively) preoperative tests in predicting cardiac complications with vascular surgery, but the individual studies were methodologically weak (see also Reference 9). In another review, perfusion imaging and dobutamine stress echocardiography did not meet the critical criteria for accuracy, effect on decision-making, and harms–benefit ratio in cardiovascular risk assessment (15).

Until recently, there was no evidence from randomized trials that preoperative revascularization reduces surgical risk. Therefore, the decision on whether to perform preoperative revascularization was based on identifying patients with coronary disease known to benefit from this procedure (that is, three-vessel or left main disease), regardless of the planned surgery. However, a recent trial questioned this approach. After excluding patients with >50% left main arterial stenosis or a left ventricular ejection fraction <20%, patients with stable coronary disease, no prior revascularization, ≥70% stenosis of at least one major coronary artery, and those in need of elective aortic or peripheral vascular surgery were randomized to receive surgery directly or to undergo preoperative coronary revascularization (percutaneous coronary intervention or bypass graft). There was no difference in rates of postoperative myocardial infarction or death, left ventricular ejection fraction at 3 months, or mortality at 2.7 years after randomization in these patients (16). The results of this trial are generalizable to patients without unstable coronary syndromes, significant left main arterial stenosis, severe left ventricular dysfunction, or aortic stenosis. Combined with the evidence that perioperative β-blockers reduce cardiac complications in higher-risk patients and the uncertain predictive accuracy of noninvasive testing, this trial suggests that more patients than previously thought can undergo surgery while taking β-blockers with less preoperative noninvasive testing and revascularization. Because of the possible increased risk for myocardial infarction within 6

weeks of coronary stenting, elective surgery should be delayed ≥6 weeks (17). If stenting is done in anticipation of surgery, bare-metal stents should be used because they are associated with less risk of thrombosis than drug-eluting stents when antiplatelet drugs are discontinued perioperatively.

If there is no contraindication, patients with coronary artery disease or significant risk factors should receive perioperative β-blockers, titrated to a resting heart rate of 60/minute. Patients not already taking β-blockers may also meet the criteria for long-term use of these agents. β-Blockers should be titrated over 7 to 10 days before surgery; if this approach is not feasible, quick titration can occur preoperatively and intraoperatively. Recent studies suggest that the benefit of β-blockers is not yet fully elucidated in perioperative management. Although several small meta-analyses of 5 to 11 trials consistently found β-blockers to be of benefit in this setting, a recent meta-analysis of 22 trials found no benefit in total mortality, cardiovascular mortality, or nonfatal myocardial infarction, and found benefit only in a composite outcome of major perioperative cardiac complications (risk reduction 0.44, 95% CI 0.20 to 0.97) (18). Additionally, a large retrospective cohort study of patients undergoing major noncardiac surgery found β-blockers to be associated with reduced hospital mortality in patients with Revised Cardiac Index scores ≥2, no benefit in patients with a score of 1, and increased mortality in patients with a score of 0 (19).

Heart failure is as significant a cardiac risk factor as is ischemic disease. Patients with compensated, asymptomatic heart failure can generally undergo surgery if other risk factors are acceptable. The condition of patients who are decompensated or symptomatic should be stabilized before elective surgery. Noninvasive testing may be necessary to fully characterize systolic function. The risk for cardiac complications appears increased within 1 week of an episode of pulmonary edema; therefore, elective procedures should be delayed at least that long in these patients. The role of B-type natriuretic peptide in preoperative risk assessment is currently undefined (20, 21).

Hypertension is not an independent predictor of postoperative cardiac complications. Blood pressure ≤180/110 mm Hg does not appear to increase the risk for complications unless it is associated with undiagnosed coronary disease (for example, silent Q waves on electrocardiography), heart failure, left ventricular hyperplasia, renal insufficiency, or cerebrovascular disease (22). The blood pressure of patients with a diastolic reading >110 should be gradually controlled over 6 to 8 weeks before elective surgery is performed.

Patients with chronic mitral or aortic regurgitation or mitral stenosis and asymptomatic heart failure generally tolerate noncardiac surgery well if tachycardia and volume overload are avoided. Patients with severe pulmonary hypertension and significant aortic stenosis are at risk for cardiac complications because of sudden changes in hemodynamics or volume status. Valve replacement should be considered in patients with severe or symptomatic aortic stenosis before elective major noncardiac surgery is performed. Asymptomatic patients with moderate to severe aortic stenosis but good exercise tolerance have an acceptable risk profile for most noncardiac surgery but should receive careful hemodynamic monitoring. Patients with valvular disease need endocarditis prophylaxis for contaminated or clean-contaminated procedures but not for clean procedures (for example, elective total joint replacement).

Patients should continue taking β-blockers, oral nitrates, and most antihypertensive medications until the morning of surgery, and resume taking them when they begin to eat after surgery. Abrupt discontinuation of these agents appears to increase postoperative cardiac risk. ACE inhibitors and angiotensin receptor blockers have been associated with intraoperative hypotension; they should be withheld on the morning of surgery, with management of blood pressure by parenteral drug administration. Transdermal nitrates are variably absorbed; therefore, oral formulations should be substituted for transdermal formulations preoperatively. Intravenous nitroglycerin can be used intraoperatively and postoperatively until patients can take oral medications. Most antiarrhythmic agents and long-acting drugs (for example, digoxin and amiodarone) can be briefly withheld, with intravenous forms or substitutes given to patients in whom arrhythmias occur. Three observational studies and one small trial suggest that the anti-inflammatory and plaque-stabilizing effects of statins reduce cardiac complications (23). A statin should be considered for perioperative use in patients with coronary disease or cardiac risk factors, although the results of large trials on the efficacy of these agents in perioperative management are not yet known.

Patients at high risk for postoperative cardiac complications should receive surveillance electrocardiography in the recovery room and on postoperative days 1 and 2. Cardiac enzyme measurement in these patients is appropriate to identify signs or symptoms of ischemia, pulmonary edema, or hemodynamic instability. Close monitoring and control of plasma glucose in patients in the intensive care unit reduces morbidity and mortality (24). Telemetry or Holter monitoring should be considered in patients at high risk for postoperative cardiac complications who are facing high-risk surgery. Right heart catheterization does not reduce cardiac complications or mortality in high-risk surgical patients (25).

KEY POINTS

- **Myocardial infarction usually occurs in the first 4 days after noncardiac surgery and is associated with a 15% to 25% hospital mortality rate.**
- **Six predictors of cardiovascular complications are high-risk surgery; history of ischemic heart disease, heart failure, and cerebrovascular disease; insulin treatment; and serum creatinine level >2.0 mg/dL.**
- **Patients should continue taking β-blockers, oral nitrates, and most antihypertensive medications until the morning of surgery, and resume taking them when they begin to eat after surgery.**
- **Patients at high risk for postoperative cardiac complications should receive surveillance electrocardiography in the recovery room and on postoperative days 1 and 2, and cardiac enzyme measurement and tight control of plasma glucose postoperatively.**

Pulmonary Perioperative Medicine

Postoperative pulmonary complications are as common as cardiac complications and equally important clinically in terms of mortality, morbidity, and length of stay. However, perioperative pulmonary risk management has been less well studied than perioperative cardiac risk management; the first systematic reviews of evidence regarding risk factors and preventive strategies for pulmonary complications have only recently been published (26, 27, 28). **Table 73** shows postoperative pulmonary complication risk factors supported by good and fair evidence. Importantly, there is good evidence that obesity, controlled asthma, or hip and gynecologic surgery do not increase the risk for postoperative pulmonary complications. Fair evidence exists indicating that diabetes does not increase this risk, but there is insufficient evidence to determine whether obstructive sleep apnea, corticosteroid use, HIV infection, arrhythmia, or poor exercise capacity do. Although spirometry is a useful tool in the diagnosis of obstructive pulmonary disease, it does not predict the risk for postoperative pulmonary complications better than clinical evaluation alone.

In addition, two recent analyses from a large Veterans Affairs cohort study derived and validated separate predictive indices for postoperative pneumonia and respiratory failure

TABLE 73 Summary of Overall Evidence Regarding Factors Associated with Increased Risk of Postoperative Pulmonary Complications

Factor	Strength of Evidence
Advanced age	Good
ASA class ≥2	Good
Functional dependence	Good
COPD	Good
Heart failure	Good
Emergency surgery or prolonged surgery	Good
Aortic aneurysm repair, thoracic surgery, abdominal surgery, neurosurgery, head and neck surgery, vascular surgery	Good
Serum albumin <3.5 g/dL	Good
Impaired sensorium	Fair
Abnormal chest examination or radiograph	Fair
Cigarette or alcohol use	Fair
Weight loss	Fair
BUN >21 mg/dL	Fair

ASA = American Society of Anesthesiologists; COPD = chronic obstructive pulmonary disease; BUN = blood urea nitrogen.

TABLE 74 Variables Increasing Risk in Predictive Indices for Postoperative Pneumonia and Respiratory Failure from Veterans Affairs Cohort Study

Variables Common to Risk Index for Pneumonia and Risk Index for Respiratory Failure

Type of surgery: abdominal aortic aneurysm repair, thoracic surgery, upper abdominal surgery, vascular surgery, neck surgery, neurosurgery

Emergency surgery

Advanced age

Functional status: totally dependent > partially dependent > independent

History of COPD

BUN >30 mg/dL

Additional Variables Unique to the Individual Indices

Pneumonia Risk Index	Respiratory Failure Index
General anesthesia versus spinal/epidural	Albumin <3 g/dL
Weight loss >10% in prior 6 months	
Chronic steroid use	
Alcohol >2 drinks/d in prior 2 wk	
Smoker within prior year	
Impaired sensorium	
History of cerebrovascular accident	
Preoperative transfusion >4 units	

COPD = chronic obstructive pulmonary disease; BUN = blood urea nitrogen.

Data are from Arozullah AM, Khuri SF, Henderson WG, et al. Development and validation of a multifactorial risk index for predicting postoperative pneumonia after major noncardiac surgery. Ann Intern Med. 2001;135:847-57; and Arozullah AM, Daley J, Henderson WG, Khuri SF. Multifactorial risk index for predicting postoperative respiratory failure in men after major noncardiac surgery. The National Veterans Administration Surgical Quality Improvement Program. Ann Surg 2000;232:242-253.

(29, 30). As shown in **Table 74**, the two indices have six variables in common, but at least five of these are not modifiable with any intervention. The respiratory failure index included one additional significant factor, hypoalbuminemia, a marker for malnutrition. However, evidence from randomized trials indicates that the use of parenteral or enteral preoperative hyperalimentation does not reduce this risk, except perhaps in the settings of severe malnutrition and prolonged postoperative periods with inadequate nutritional intake. Eight additional risk factors were significant in the pneumonia risk index, but many of these are not modifiable, and evidence from randomized trials indicates that transfusions do not increase the risk for postoperative pulmonary infection.

There is good evidence supporting selective nasogastric decompression after abdominal surgery in patients with nausea, vomiting, or abdominal distension only (versus routine nasogastric decompression after abdominal surgery until bowel function returns) and supporting routine lung expansion with incentive spirometry and deep-breathing exercises to prevent postoperative pulmonary complications. No one pulmonary-expansion modality has been found to be clearly superior to the other.

Fair evidence suggests that at least 2 months of smoking cessation and short-acting neuromuscular blockade with agents other than pancuronium reduce postoperative pulmonary risk. Enteral formulations fortified with arginine, 3-omega fatty acids, and nucleotides appear to enhance immune status and prevent postoperative infection, including

pneumonia, and reduce hospital stay after elective surgery, but this research is still in the preliminary stages.

Several meta-analyses indicate that epidural anesthesia or analgesia, compared with general anesthesia and other routes of analgesia, reduce postoperative pulmonary complications, but recent large trials do not show such benefit. Right heart catheterization, routine nutritional support for malnutrition, and limiting transfusions or using leukocyte-depleted blood in transfusions have not been found to prevent postoperative pulmonary complications.

Evidence on prophylactic corticosteroids, transverse versus open abdominal incisions, and laparoscopic versus open operations in the prevention of postoperative pulmonary complications is insufficient. It is clear that laparoscopic, compared with open, surgery, compromises pulmonary function less, but the evidence does not confirm that laparoscopic procedures reduce postoperative pulmonary complications.

Reasonable, but untested, indications for preoperative spirometry include dyspnea of unclear etiology and chronic obstructive pulmonary disease or asthma in patients in whom it is uncertain that airflow limitation has been maximally reduced. Maximization of pulmonary function and control of asthma should occur before surgery. Patients should use inhalers, β-agonists, anticholinergic agents, and corticosteroids until immediately before surgery and as soon as possible postoperatively, especially if they are at high risk for postoperative pulmonary complications or are undergoing high-risk surgery. The addition of intravenous corticosteroids and aminophylline is appropriate in patients with refractory bronchospasm if needed. Patients can continue to take leukotriene inhibitors through the morning of surgery; there is no known risk to temporarily stopping them.

KEY POINTS

- Obesity, controlled asthma, or hip and gynecologic surgeries do not increase the risk for postoperative pulmonary complications.
- Although spirometry is a useful tool in diagnosing obstructive pulmonary disease, it does not predict the risk for postoperative pulmonary complications better than clinical evaluation alone.
- Blood transfusions do not increase the risk for postoperative pulmonary infection.
- Selective nasogastric decompression after abdominal surgery in patients with nausea, vomiting, or abdominal distension only, as well as routine lung expansion with incentive spirometry and deep-breathing exercises, are effective in preventing postoperative pulmonary complications.
- Patients should use inhalers, β-agonists, anticholinergic agents, and corticosteroids until immediately before surgery and as soon as possible postoperatively, especially those at high risk for postoperative pulmonary complications or undergoing high-risk surgery.

Hematologic Perioperative Medicine

Surgery is clearly associated with an increased risk for venous thromboembolism. Without prophylaxis, rates vary from 0.4% and 0.2% for proximal deep venous thrombosis (DVT) and pulmonary embolism, respectively, in low-risk surgery, and 10% to 30% and 4% to 10%, respectively, in high-risk surgery. **Table 75** summarizes perioperative risk factors for venous thromboembolism.

Prophylaxis prevents 50% to 80% of cases of venous thromboembolism (31). Besides drugs, mechanical prophylactic devices include sequential compression leg devices (SCDs) or intermittent pneumatic compression and gradient compression stockings. SCDs are an appealing option because they do not increase bleeding, but their efficacy in preventing venous thromboembolism has been less well studied than

TABLE 75 Perioperative Risk Factors for Venous Thromboembolism*

Patient Factors
  Age
  Obesity
  Chronic venous stasis
  Reduced mobility
  Pregnancy
  Estrogen use

Surgical factors
  Type of surgery: risks higher in major vs. minor surgery; high risk = intracranial surgery, orthopedic surgery, major vascular surgery, bowel resection, gastric bypass, radical cystectomy, renal transplantation
  Trauma, especially pelvic, femur, lower-extremity fractures

Medical comorbidities
  Malignancy
  Heart failure
  Chronic obstructive pulmonary disease
  Stroke
  Hematologic disease
  Polycythemia vera
  Essential thrombocytosis
  Thrombophilic disorders
  Paroxysmal nocturnal hemoglobinuria

Specific medical diseases
  Nephrotic syndrome
  Inflammatory bowel disease
  Systemic lupus erythematosus

*Asian ethnicity is associated with lower risk of perioperative venous thromboembolism.

that of anticoagulants. Patient compliance with SCDs varies; these devices are effective only if worn by patients continuously while they are not ambulating. SCDs vary in compression patterns and length (foot, knee-length, and thigh-length); it is not clear if length affects efficacy. Current evidence-based guidelines recommend SCDs primarily for use in patients at high risk for bleeding or in conjunction with anticoagulants in those at high risk for venous thromboembolism (32).

Lower-gradient, standard-issue support hose offer some protection to patients while they are supine, but the elastic does not have a sufficient pressure gradient to override gravity once patients are sitting or ambulating. Tighter, more expensive, custom-fitted hose provide protection when legs are dependent, but poorly fitting stockings that are too tight proximally (the "garter" effect) may increase venous pressure below the knees and increase the risk for DVT.

Low-molecular-weight heparin (LMWH) is more expensive than unfractionated heparin but confers less risk for heparin-induced thrombocytopenia and bleeding (except in patients with perispinal hematoma; see below) and is more effective than unfractionated heparin in thromboembolism prophylaxis before major orthopedic surgery. Patients who take warfarin require monitoring, but this drug is as effective as unfractionated heparin, LMWH, and SCD in this setting. Warfarin administration should begin 10 to 14 days before surgery, with titration to an INR of <1.5; however, administration of this anticoagulant can also be started the night before or immediately after surgery. The target postoperative INR is 2.5. Patients are at increased risk for venous thromboembolism for months after hip-replacement surgery or hip-fracture repair, and prophylaxis should be continued after discharge. The pentasaccharide fondaparinux, an indirect thrombin inhibitor, appears more effective than enoxaparin in patients undergoing elective hip and knee surgery or hip-fracture repair but is associated with more bleeding complications and is more expensive. The new direct thrombin inhibitors ximelagatran, desirudin, and lepirudin appear as effective and safe as enoxaparin in thromboembolism prophylaxis but are also more expensive.

The choice of prophylactic agent depends on the surgery-associated risk for DVT; bleeding risk; history of heparin-induced thrombocytopenia; and presence of high-risk hypercoagulable states, such as the lupus anticoagulant and plasma protein C and S and antithrombin deficiency. Use of multiple prophylactic modalities is recommended in patients undergoing high-risk surgery. Combined pre- and postoperative prophylaxis is more effective than postoperative prophylaxis alone. Even in patients in whom pharmacologic or mechanical prophylaxis is used, aggressive ambulation remains an important adjunct to prophylaxis. A 25% increase in dose of LMWH may be appropriate DVT prophylaxis in the setting of significant obesity. **Table 76** summarizes current prophylactic recommendations for patients undergoing nonorthopedic surgery (33). The approach to DVT prophylaxis for orthopedic surgery includes consideration of low-dose warfarin and fondaparinux and possible extension of prophylaxis after discharge; recommendations are summarized in **Table 77**.

Epidural anesthesia and analgesia increase the postoperative risk for perispinal hematomas. Patients in whom perispinal hematomas develop usually have multiple risk factors, including coagulopathy, taking drugs that increase bleeding, vertebral bony or vascular abnormalities, traumatic or repeated catheter insertion, older age, and female sex. Epidural anesthesia or analgesia and venous thromboembolism prophylaxis

TABLE 76 Summary of Recommendations for Perioperative Prophylaxis of Venous Thromboembolism

Aggressive ambulation	Low-risk general surgery: minor procedure plus age <40 y and no additional risk factor Vascular surgery, no additional risk factor (usually given antithrombotics to protect the surgical site) Gynecologic surgery ≤30 min plus benign disease Low-risk urologic surgery Laparoscopic surgery and no additional risk factor Elective spine surgery and no additional risk factor
Low-dose UH or low-dose LMWH	Moderate-risk general surgery: nonmajor procedure plus age 40 to 60 y or additional risk factor; or major surgery plus age <40 y, and no additional risk factor Major vascular surgery plus additional risk factor Laparoscopic gynecologic surgery plus additional risk factor
Low dose UH or low-dose LMWH or SCD	Major gynecologic surgery for benign disease and no additional risk factor Laparoscopic surgery plus additional risk factor Elective spine surgery plus additional risk factor or neurologic deficit or anterior approach Intracranial neurosurgery and no additional risk factor
Low-dose UH or low-dose LMWH plus SCD and/or graduated compression stockings	Elective spine surgery and multiple risk factors Intracranial neurosurgery plus additional risk factor
Low- or high-dose UH or low- or high-dose LMWH or SCD	Major open urologic procedures
High-dose UH or high-dose LMWH	High-risk general surgery: nonmajor surgery plus age >60 y, or additional risk factor; or major surgery plus age >40 y, or additional risk factor (high- or very-high-risk general surgery or major cancer resection requires postdischarge LMWH for 2 to 4 w)
High-dose UH or high-dose LMWH plus SCD and/or graduated compression stockings	Very-high-risk general surgery: major surgery plus multiple risk factors Major gynecologic surgery for malignancy plus other risk factors (very high risk: above plus age >60 y or prior venous thromboembolism requires postdischarge LMWH for 2 to 4 w) Major open urologic surgery plus multiple risk factors
SCD or graduated compression stockings	General surgery, increased risk for bleeding Major urologic surgery with bleeding or increased risk for bleeding

Data are from Geerts WJ, Pineo GF, Heit JA et al. Prevention of venous thromboembolism. The Seventh ACCP Conference on Antithrombotic and Thrombolytic Therapy. Chest 2004;126(3):338S-400S.

UH = unfractionated heparin, LMWH = low-molecular-weight heparin, SCD = sequential compression device or intermittent pneumatic compression, graduated compression stockings.

Low-dose: UH 5000 U subcutaneously twice daily, LMWH <3400 U daily (enoxaparin 40 mg subcutaneously once daily).

High-dose = 5000 U subcutaneously three times daily, LMWH >3400 U daily (enoxaparin 30 mg subcutaneously twice daily).

TABLE 77 Orthopedic Surgery and Summary of Recommendations for Perioperative Prophylaxis of Venous Thromboembolism

Knee arthroscopy and no additional risk factor	Aggressive ambulation
Knee arthroscopy plus long or complicated procedure or other additional risk factors	Low- or high-dose LMWH
Elective knee arthroplasty	High-dose LMWH or fondaparinux 2.5 mg begun 6 to 8 h after surgery; or adjusted-dose warfarin begun before or evening after surgery, with target INR of 2.5; or continuous SCD Hospital duration: at least 10 days Postdischarge duration: none No single-modality use of UH or foot SCD or stockings
Elective hip arthroplasty	High-dose LMWH 12 h before or 12 to 24 h after, or 4 to 6 h after surgery at half dose, then full dose next day; or fondaparinux 2.5 mg begun 6 to 8 h after surgery; or adjusted-dose warfarin begun before or evening after surgery, with target INR of 2.5 Hospital duration: at least 10 d Postdischarge duration: 28 to 35 d with low-dose LMWH, fondaparinux, or warfarin No single-modality use of UH, SCD, foot SCD, or graduated compression stockings
Hip-fracture repair	High-dose LMWH or fondaparinux 2.5 mg begun 6 to 8 h after surgery, or adjusted-dose warfarin with target INR of 2.5, or low-dose UH Hospital duration: at least 10 d Extended duration: 28 to 35 d with low-dose LMWH, fondaparinux, or warfarin If surgery is delayed: low-dose UH or low-dose LMWH until surgery If high risk of bleeding: SCD, otherwise no single-modality use of UH, foot SCD, or graduated compression stockings after surgery

Data are from Geerts WJ, Pineo GF, Heit JA et al. Prevention of venous thromboembolism. The Seventh ACCP Conference on Antithrombotic and Thrombolytic Therapy. Chest 2004;126(3):338S-400S.

UH = unfractionated heparin, LMWH = low-molecular-weight heparin, SCD = sequential compression device or intermittent pneumatic compression, graduated compression stockings.

Low-dose = UH 5000 U subcutaneously twice daily, LMWH <3400 U daily (enoxaparin 40 mg subcutaneously once daily).

High-dose = 5000 U subcutaneously three times daily, LMWH >3400 U daily (enoxaparin 30 mg subcutaneously twice daily).

generally can be used together with caution except in patients with bleeding disorders or in those who take chronic antithrombotics. LMWH may confer higher risks than unfractionated heparin for perispinal hematomas. NSAIDs and aspirin do not appear to increase the risk for this complication, but other antiplatelet agents should be stopped 7 days before surgery to avoid increasing this risk. The epidural catheter should be inserted 8 to 12 hours after subcutaneous unfractionated heparin administration or ≥18 hours after once-daily LMWH administration, and it should be removed at the time of trough concentration level before administration of the next dose. Unfractionated heparin and LMWH should be delayed until at least 2 hours after epidural catheter/spinal needle removal; in patients taking warfarin, epidural catheters should be used ≤2 days, and the INR should be <1.5 at catheter removal. Patients should be monitored frequently for signs of spinal cord compression in this setting (see also Reference 33). When epidural anesthesia/analgesia is used and single-modality venous thromboembolism prophylaxis is indicated, SCDs may be the safest choice in preventing development of perispinal hematomas.

Management of patients receiving chronic warfarin varies by planned surgery and reason for anticoagulation. Patients undergoing dermatologic, cataract, and dental surgery can usually continue receiving warfarin; bleeding risks may actually be higher in those continuing antiplatelet medications.

Tranexamic acid or epsilon aminocaproic acid mouthwashes can control bleeding in patients undergoing dental procedures. For major procedures, physicians must decide if discontinuing warfarin requires short-term bridging with therapeutic unfractionated heparin or LMWH. **Table 78** summarizes current perioperative recommendations for patients receiving chronic anticoagulation therapy (see also Reference 32).

Hematologic problems commonly encountered perioperatively include coagulopathy, thrombocytopenia, and anemia (34). History of bleeding problems (for example, bleeding for >1 day after tooth extraction, epistaxis, hematuria, hemarthrosis, gastrointestinal bleeding, or prolonged bleeding after delivery) and family bleeding should documented. Patients with a negative history for bleeding and normal physical examination undergoing low-risk procedures do not need screening for coagulopathy. The prothrombin time (PT)/INR, partial thromboplastin time (PTT), and platelet count should be performed in the setting of a positive history of bleeding difficulties, surgery associated with a high risk for bleeding, coagulopathy-associated diseases (for example, malabsorption syndromes or liver disease), or chronic anticoagulation therapy. In addition, plasma fibrinogen measurement and von Willebrand factor testing are recommended in patients with a history of bleeding problems. Although the bleeding time may be prolonged in patients with von Willebrand's disease, thrombocytopenia, and platelet disorders, this test is notoriously imprecise and does not correlate

TABLE 78 Perioperative Management of Chronic Anticoagulation

Risk of Thromboembolism	Management
Surgery with Moderate or High Risk of Bleeding	
Low risk: atrial fibrillation without history of stroke or CHADS2 score = 0	Stop warfarin ~4 d preop, monitor INR return to near normal; venous thromboembolism prophylaxis (UH low-dose or LMWH low-dose pre- and postop as indicated); restart warfarin when hemostasis achieved
Intermediate risk: CHADS2 score = 1 to 2	Stop warfarin ~4 d preop, monitor INR fall; UH (low-dose or high-dose) or LMWH (low- or high-dose) ~2 d preop and continue postop; restart warfarin when hemostasis achieved
High risk: venous thromboembolism <3 months, arterial thromboembolism 4 to 6 wk, mechanical valve in mitral position, old technology ball/cage mechanical valve, CHADS2 score ≥3	Stop warfarin ~4 d preop, monitor INR return to normal; ~2 d preop start full therapeutic subcutaneous dose of UH or LMWH; when admitted, give therapeutic intravenous UH, and discontinue 5 h preop or therapeutic subcutaneous UH or LMWH and discontinue 12 to 24 h before surgery; restart full-dose intravenous or subcutaneous heparin or subcutaneous LMWH postop; restart warfarin when hemostasis adequate, continue full-dose UH or LMWH until INR at target
Surgery with Low Risk of Bleeding (some gynecologic and orthopedic surgery procedures)	
	Continue, but lower dose of warfarin ~4-5 d before surgery; perform surgery when target INR of 1.3-1.5 is achieved; return to usual dose when hemostasis adequate; venous thromboembolism prophylaxis with UH or LMWH as indicated
Superficial Dermatologic Procedures	
	Continue usual warfarin dose
Dental Procedures	
	Continue usual warfarin dose, tranexamic acid mouthwash or epsilon aminocaproic acid mouthwash for local hemostasis

UH = unfractionated heparin; LMWH = low-molecular-weight heparin. Preop = preoperatively; postop = postoperatively.

UH low-dose = 5000 U subcutaneously daily, high-dose = 5000 U subcutaneously twice daily.

LMWH low-dose = <3400 U daily (enoxaparin 40 mg daily), high-dose = >3400 U daily (enoxaparin 30 mg twice daily).

CHADS2 score = 1 point each for heart failure, hypertension, age ≥75 y, and diabetes mellitus; 2 points for prior stroke needing secondary prevention (these data are from Gage BF, Waterman AD, Shannon W et al. Validation of clinical classification schemes for predicting stroke. Results from the National Registry of Atrial Fibrillation. JAMA 2001;285;(22):2864-2870). Note that CHADS2 score is for long-term risk of thromboembolism and may not be generalizable to the setting of short-term discontinuation of anticoagulation for surgery.

with bleeding problems or add information to more specific tests, such as mixing studies, and need never be done.

Liver disease and vitamin deficiency are the usual causes of a prolonged PT and can be treated with vitamin K; the differential diagnosis is broader for defects in the intrinsic coagulation pathway that cause a prolonged PTT or disorders causing prolongation of both PT and PTT. Patients with factor deficiencies require consultation with a hematologist, adequate laboratory support, timing of elective surgery to factor replacement with recombinant or plasma concentrates, and factor replacement with immunosuppression for acquired factor inhibitors. The presence of lupus anticoagulant antibodies confers an increased risk for thrombosis and requires aggressive venous thromboembolism prophylaxis.

Platelet dysfunction may be quantitative (underproduction, consumptive coagulopathy, or hypersplenism) or qualitative (caused by aspirin and clopidogrel [irreversible platelet dysfunction, drugs should be stopped 7 days preoperatively] or NSAIDs [reversible dysfunction, drug should be stopped 1 to 3 days before surgery]). Surgery is usually safe in patients with a platelet count >100,000/µL. Decisions about surgery and transfusion must be individualized in patients with platelet counts of 50,000 to 100,000/µL; transfusion and/or delay of surgery is indicated in patients with platelet counts <50,000/µL.

In patients with perioperative anemia, the cause must be determined and when to provide blood transfusion established. This condition occurs commonly and should be evaluated diagnostically as it would be in any other setting. Nutritional deficiencies should be addressed in patients with perioperative anemia; iron supplementation for deficiency due to surgical bleeding in these patients is often forgotten, especially on discharge. The appropriate hemoglobin level necessitating transfusion depends on several patient variables besides the extent of active bleeding. Morbidity and mortality increase as hemoglobin falls to <10 g/dL, especially in patients with cardiovascular disease, and especially in those with a hemoglobin <6 g/dL. However, the available trials of transfusion at different hemoglobin levels do not clarify what is the best "trigger" for hemoglobin transfusion. Current guidelines, pending further evidence, are to initiate transfusion in patients who have 1) a hemoglobin level of 9 to 10 g/dL with cardiovascular disease; 2) acute symptoms of anemia; and 3) active bleeding if it occurs rapidly or is expected to lower the hemoglobin level below a clinically determined threshold. Transfusion should be considered in stable asymptomatic patients if the hemoglobin level is <7g/dL.

KEY POINTS

- Sequential compression devices (SCDs) are recommended primarily for patients at high risk for bleeding or in conjunction with anticoagulants for those at high risk for venous thromboembolism.

- Low-molecular-weight heparin is more expensive than unfractionated heparin but confers less risk for heparin-induced thrombocytopenia and bleeding and is more effective than unfractionated heparin in thromboembolism prophylaxis before major orthopedic surgery.

- Initiating deep venous thromboembolism (DVT) prophylaxis preoperatively is more effective than using postoperative prophylaxis alone.

- The approach to DVT prophylaxis for orthopedic surgery includes low-dose warfarin and fondaparinux and possible extension of prophylaxis after discharge.

- When epidural anesthesia/analgesia is used and single-modality venous thromboembolism prophylaxis is indicated, SCDs may be the safest choice in avoiding perispinal hematomas.

- Patients with a negative history for bleeding and normal physical examination undergoing low-risk procedures do not need coagulopathy screening.

- The prothrombin time/INR, partial thromboplastin time, and platelet count should be performed in the setting of a positive history of bleeding, surgery associated with a high risk for bleeding, coagulopathy-associated diseases, or chronic anticoagulation therapy.

- Surgery is usually safe in patients with a platelet count >100,000/μL.

- Transfusion should be initiated in patients who have a hemoglobin level of 9 to 10 g/dL with cardiovascular disease; acute symptoms of anemia; and active bleeding if it occurs rapidly or is expected to lower the hemoglobin level below a clinically determined threshold.

Endocrine Perioperative Medicine

The physiologic stress of anesthesia and surgery increases hyperglycemia, protein catabolism, risk of ketoacidosis, and osmotic diuresis through increased gluconeogenesis and levels of the insulin antagonists epinephrine, norepinephrine, cortisol, and growth hormone; epinephrine also decreases

insulin secretion. Patients with diabetes mellitus have a higher risk for perioperative cardiac complications caused by macrovascular disease, microvascular disease–related renal failure, and aspiration and delay of oral intake with gastroparesis. Autonomic neuropathy increases the risk for cardiac arrest, ileus, and urinary retention. Wound healing is impaired and risk of infection increased in patients with diabetes because of hyperglycemia-induced impaired granulocyte function and collagen synthesis, plus associated vascular and renal disease (35). Several retrospective studies have indicated reduced postoperative wound infection in patients in whom plasma glucose was monitored and controlled closely.

A large landmark trial of 1548 critically ill surgical patients studied conventional versus tight glucose control. Patients randomized to conventional control and with plasma glucose >215 mg/dL received insulin infusion adjusted to maintain plasma glucose levels between 180 and 200 mg/dL. Patients randomized to intensive control with plasma glucose levels >110 mg/dL received insulin infusion adjusted to maintain plasma glucose levels between 80 and 110 mg/dL. The tight-control group had significantly lower hospitalization and 1-year mortality rates, sepsis, acute renal failure, critical-illness polyneuropathy, and days of intensive care and ventilatory support compared with the conventional glucose control group (36). Benefit was greatest in patients requiring >5 days of intensive care and in those with sepsis and multiorgan failure.

Patients with type 1 diabetes mellitus who are undergoing minor, brief, or day surgery procedures should receive a third to half of their usual intermediate- or long-acting insulin the morning of surgery, supplemental short-acting insulin as needed every 4 to 6 hours, intravenous fluids with 0.45% saline and 5% dextrose in water with potassium chloride 20 meq/L (unless there is hyperkalemia or chronic renal insufficiency) at 100 mL/hour, and monitoring of plasma glucose every 1 to 2 hours. For major, long or complex, or emergency surgery, patients with type 1 diabetes, unstable type 2 diabetes, or diabetic ketoacidosis should receive similar management. These patients should receive no subcutaneous insulin the morning of surgery and should begin receiving an insulin infusion 2 to 3 hours before surgery (for example, 25 U regular insulin in 250 mL normal saline at 1 to 3 U/hour; tubing should be flushed first with 50 mL of insulin to saturate insulin-binding sites). These patients should also receive intravenous fluids with 0.45% saline and 5% dextrose in water with potassium chloride 20 meq/L (unless there is hyperkalemia or renal insufficiency). Monitoring of plasma glucose and serum electrolyte levels should occur hourly; monitoring of serum ketones for an increase >350 mg/dL or consecutive increases >250 mg/dL is also indicated. Insulin infusion should continue until patients begin eating; subcutaneous regular insulin should be initiated 30 minutes before the insulin infusion is stopped (37).

Patients receiving insulin administered by pump should receive care guided by an endocrinologist. Those with stable type 2 diabetes should receive intravenous fluids with 0.45% saline and 5% dextrose in water with management specific to their usual regimen. The last dose of insulin before surgery in patients receiving basal insulin (glargine), morning or evening dosing, should be decreased by half. Patients receiving NPH insulin should receive no insulin before morning surgery and half the usual morning dose if receiving nothing by mouth for afternoon surgery. Patients who take oral agents to control their diabetes should not receive short-acting drugs the morning of surgery and while receiving nothing by mouth. Metformin should be discontinued in patients 48 hours before surgery or for 48 hours after receiving contrast dye. Any long-acting oral agents should be discontinued 48 to 72 hours before surgery. Patients should not receive any thiazolidinediones while receiving nothing by mouth.

Patients with mild or moderate hypothyroidism can safely undergo surgery but may have problems with intraoperative hypotension, delirium, and afebrile infection. Mildly hypothyroid or euthyroid patients can stop taking their usual thyroid-replacement medication for several days if they are not eating because of levothyroxine's half-life of 5 to 9 days (38, see also Reference 35). Elective surgery should be delayed in patients with severe disease until thyroid hormone levels can be partly or fully replaced. Patients with severe hypothyroidism needing urgent/emergent surgery should receive endocrinologic consultation, intravenous T3 and T4, and empirical corticosteroids for possible adrenal insufficiency.

Surgery need not be delayed in patients with mild hyperthyroidism. Elective surgery should be delayed in those with moderate or severe disease if they become euthyroid, and β-blockers should be administered in these patients. Patients with moderate or severe disease needing urgent/emergent surgery should receive β-blockers, thyroid antagonists (for example, iodine, thionamides, methimazole, propylthiouracil, or iopanoic acid), corticosteroids for possible hypoadrenalism due to hyperthyroidism, and endocrinologic consultation. Perioperative thyroid storm is a critical situation requiring multiple thyroid antagonists, β-blockers, corticosteroids, and treatment in the intensive-care unit (39; see also Reference 35).

The primary issue of perioperative corticosteroid coverage is determining when stress-dose coverage is appropriate if there is not time for a cosyntropin stimulation test (40). Previous recommendations are now considered overreactive and to have erred on the side of unnecessary coverage. Current recommendations, summarized in **Table 79**, favor corticosteroid stress-dose coverage in fewer patients (see also Reference 35).

KEY POINTS

- Critically ill surgical patients who received tight glucose control with insulin infusion to maintain plasma glucose levels between 80 and 110 mg/dL experienced reduced postoperative wound infection compared with patients whose glucose levels were maintained between 180 and 200 mg/dL.

- Mildly hypothyroid or euthyroid patients can stop taking their usual thyroid-replacement medication for several days if they are not eating.

- Patients with severe hypothyroidism needing urgent/emergent surgery should receive endocrinologic consultation, intravenous T3 and T4, and empirical corticosteroids.

- Elective surgery should be delayed and β-blockers should be administered to patients with moderate or severe hyperthyroidism until they become euthyroid.

- Patients with moderate or severe hyperthyroidism needing urgent surgery should receive β-blockers, thyroid antagonists, corticosteroids, and endocrinologic consultation.

- Perioperative thyroid storm is a critical situation requiring multiple thyroid antagonists, β-blockers, corticosteroids, and intensive-care treatment.

Renal and Hepatic Perioperative Medicine

In patients undergoing noncardiac surgery, renal insufficiency is an independent predictor of postoperative cardiac (serum creatinine >2.0 mg/dL) and pulmonary (blood urea nitrogen >22 mg/dL) complications. Preoperative kidney disease also increases the risk for postoperative deterioration of renal function. Acute postoperative renal failure independently predicts mortality in patients undergoing cardiac surgery (41).

Perioperative acute renal failure is evaluated as it would be in any setting, with attention to volume status, perioperative hypotension, sepsis, intra-abdominal abscess with third-spacing and immune complex–mediated glomerulonephritis, heart failure, and exposure to nephrotoxic drugs. Elective surgery should be delayed in patients who are volume depleted until volume repletion occurs. Traditional management of postoperative renal failure with furosemide or dopamine has not been supported by evidence in randomized trials and does not appear beneficial (see also Reference 41).

Patients with end-stage renal disease receiving chronic dialysis have increased perioperative morbidity and mortality because of immunosuppression, associated cardiovascular disease, uremic platelet dysfunction, and inability to handle fluid and electrolyte flux. Metabolism of benzodiazepines,

TABLE 79 Stress-Dose Corticosteroid Coverage in Patients Taking Chronic Oral Corticosteroids

Stress-Dose Coverage Not Needed	Perioperative Management
<5 mg prednisone equivalent for any period Every-other-day, short-acting, morning-dose corticosteroid, any dose or duration Any dose corticosteroid for <3 weeks	Usual daily morning dose or every-other-day dose if currently taking
Stress-Dose Coverage Needed	**Perioperative Management**
>20 mg prednisone equivalent daily for ≥3 wk Cushingoid	Minor procedure: usual daily morning dose preop Moderate-risk surgery: usual daily morning dose preop plus 50 mg intravenous hydrocortisone preop, then 25 mg intravenously every 8 h for 24 to 48 h postop, then usual daily oral dose or equivalent intravenous dose if stable Major/high-risk operation: usual daily morning dose preop plus 100 mg intravenous hydrocortisone preop, then 50 mg intravenously every 8 h for 48 to 72 h postop, then usual daily oral dose or equivalent intravenous dose if stable
Adrenal Status Uncertain	**Perioperative Management**
Currently taking 5 to 20 mg prednisone equivalent for ≥3 wk ≥5 mg prednisone equivalent* for ≥3 wk in past year	Minor procedure: usual daily morning dose preop Moderate- or high-risk surgery: cosyntropin standard (250 μ) stimulation test or empiric stress-dose coverage as above for moderate-risk surgery or major/high-risk surgery

*Prednisone equivalent = prednisone or equipotent dose of other corticosteroid. Preop = preoperatively; postop = postoperatively

meperidine, and morphine are especially problematic in patients with end-stage renal disease, whereas fentanyl, which is hepatically metabolized, has been found to be safer in these patients. Because the condition of patients with end-stage renal disease is complex, collaborative care by an internist with expertise in perioperative medicine, a nephrologist, and a cardiologist may be the most appropriate management approach. For patients undergoing emergent or elective surgery, decisions about timing of dialysis are critical.

Patients with acute hepatitis or cirrhosis have increased anesthetic and surgical risks because of impaired hepatic blood flow and metabolism in addition to sequelae of chronic cirrhosis, such as malnutrition, hypoalbuminemia, coagulopathy, thrombocytopenia, and risk for hepatic encephalopathy. Elective surgery for patients with acute hepatitis should be delayed until liver function is normalized. The Child-Pugh score appears to predict the risk for patients with cirrhosis; mortality rates approximate 10%, 30%, and 80% for Child's class A, B, and C liver disease, respectively. Preoperative treatment to improve encephalopathy, ascites, and coagulopathy appears to reduce risk in these patients (42).

Patients with mild chronic viral or nonalcoholic steatosis hepatitis have a lower risk for postoperative renal complications than those with alcoholic hepatitis and can generally proceed to surgery. Alcoholic hepatitis is associated with increased risk for wound complications, infection, bleeding, complications occurring with hepatically metabolized drugs, and alcohol withdrawal syndromes. Elective surgery should be delayed at a minimum until the high-risk period of 3 to 5 days has passed in patients at risk for delirium tremens (see also Reference 42).

KEY POINTS

- Elective surgery should be delayed in patients who are volume depleted until volume repletion occurs.
- Fentanyl is safer for use in patients with end-stage renal disease compared with benzodiazepines, meperidine, and morphine.
- Elective surgery for patients with acute hepatitis should be delayed until liver function is normalized.
- Elective surgery should be delayed until the high-risk period of 3 to 5 days has passed in patients at risk for delirium tremens.

References

1. **Cohn SL.** The role of the medical consultant. Med Clin North Am. 2003;87:1-6. [PMID: 12575881]

2. **Smetana GW, Macpherson DS.** The case against routine preoperative laboratory testing. Med Clin North Am. 2003;87:7-40. [PMID: 12575882]

3. Practice advisory for preanesthesia evaluation: a report by the American Society of Anesthesiologists Task Force on Preanesthesia Evaluation. Anesthesiology. 2002;96:485-96. [PMID: 11818784]

4. **Macpherson DS, Snow R, Lofgren RP.** Preoperative screening: value of previous tests. Ann Intern Med. 1990;113:969-73. [PMID: 2240920]

5. **Mercado DL, Petty BG.** Perioperative medication management. Med Clin North Am. 2003;87:41-57. [PMID: 12575883]

6. **Ang-Lee MK, Moss J, Yuan CS.** Herbal medicines and perioperative care. JAMA. 2001;286:208-16. [PMID: 11448284]

7. **Ciocon JO, Ciocon DG, Galindo DJ.** Dietary supplements in primary care. Botanicals can affect surgical outcomes and follow-up. Geriatrics. 2004;59:20-4. [PMID: 15461234]

8. **Amador LF, Goodwin JS.** Postoperative delirium in the older patient. J Am Coll Surg. 2005;200:767-73. [PMID: 15848371]

9. **Devereaux PJ, Goldman L, Cook DJ, Gilbert K, Leslie K, Guyatt GH.** Perioperative cardiac events in patients undergoing noncardiac surgery: a review of the magnitude of the problem, the pathophysiology of the events and methods to estimate and communicate risk. CMAJ. 2005;173:627-34. [PMID: 16157727]

10. **Gilbert K, Larocque BJ, Patrick LT.** Prospective evaluation of cardiac risk indices for patients undergoing noncardiac surgery. Ann Intern Med. 2000;133:356-9. [PMID: 10979880]

11. **Lee TH, Marcantonio ER, Mangione CM, Thomas EJ, Polanczyk CA, Cook EF, et al.** Derivation and prospective validation of a simple index for prediction of cardiac risk of major noncardiac surgery. Circulation. 1999;100:1043-9. [PMID: 10477528]

12. Guidelines for assessing and managing the perioperative risk from coronary artery disease associated with major noncardiac surgery. American College of Physicians. Ann Intern Med. 1997;127:309-12. [PMID: 9265433]

13. **Eagle KA, Berger PB, Calkins H, Chaitman BR, Ewy GA, Fleischmann KE, et al.** ACC/AHA guideline update for perioperative cardiovascular evaluation for noncardiac surgery—executive summary: a report of the American College of Cardiology/American Heart Association Task Force on Practice Guidelines (Committee to Update the 1996 Guidelines on Perioperative Cardiovascular Evaluation for Noncardiac Surgery). J Am Coll Cardiol. 2002;39:542-53. [PMID: 11823097]

14. **Palda VA, Detsky AS.** Perioperative assessment and management of risk from coronary artery disease. Ann Intern Med. 1997 Aug 15;127(4):313-28. [PMID: 9265434]

15. **Grayburn PA, Hillis LD.** Cardiac events in patients undergoing noncardiac surgery: shifting the paradigm from noninvasive risk stratification to therapy. Ann Intern Med. 2003;138:506-11. [PMID: 12639086]

16. **McFalls EO, Ward HB, Moritz TE, Goldman S, Krupski WC, Littooy F, et al.** Coronary-artery revascularization before elective major vascular surgery. N Engl J Med. 2004;351:2795-804. [PMID: 15625331]

17. **Wilson SH, Fasseas P, Orford JL, Lennon RJ, Horlocker T, Charnoff NE, et al.** Clinical outcome of patients undergoing noncardiac surgery in the two months following coronary stenting. J Am Coll Cardiol. 2003;42:234-40. [PMID: 12875757]

18. **Devereaux PJ, Beattie WS, Choi PT, Badner NH, Guyatt GH, Villar JC, et al.** How strong is the evidence for the use of perioperative beta blockers in non-cardiac surgery? Systematic review and meta-analysis of randomised controlled trials. BMJ. 2005;331:313-21. [PMID: 15996966]

19. **Lindenauer PK, Pekow P, Wang K, Mamidi DK, Gutierrez B, Benjamin EM.** Perioperative beta-blocker therapy and mortality after major noncardiac surgery. N Engl J Med. 2005;353:349-61. [PMID: 16049209]

20. **Hernandez AF, Newby LK, O'Connor CM.** Preoperative evaluation for major noncardiac surgery: focusing on heart failure. Arch Intern Med. 2004;164:1729-36. [PMID: 15364665]

21. **Shammash JB, Ghali WA.** Preoperative assessment and perioperative management of the patient with nonischemic heart disease. Med Clin North Am. 2003;87:137-52. [PMID: 12575887]

22. **Fleisher LA.** Preoperative evaluation of the patient with hypertension. JAMA. 2002;287:2043-6. [PMID: 11966361]

23. **Devereaux PJ, Goldman L, Yusuf S, Gilbert K, Leslie K, Guyatt GH.** Surveillance and prevention of major perioperative ischemic cardiac events in patients undergoing noncardiac surgery: a review. CMAJ. 2005;173:779-88. [PMID: 16186585]

24. **van den Berghe G, Wouters P, Weekers F, Verwaest C, Bruyninckx F, Schetz M, et al.** Intensive insulin therapy in the critically ill patients. N Engl J Med. 2001;345:1359-67. [PMID: 11794168]

25. **Sandham JD, Hull RD, Brant RF, Knox L, Pineo GF, Doig CJ, et al.** A randomized, controlled trial of the use of pulmonary-artery catheters in high-risk surgical patients. N Engl J Med. 2003;348:5-14. [PMID: 12510037]

26. **Smetana GW, Lawrence VA, Cornell JE.** Preoperative pulmonary risk stratification for noncardiothoracic surgery: systematic review for the American College of Physicians. Ann Intern Med. 2006;144:581-95. [PMID: 16618956]

27. **Lawrence VA, Cornell JE, Smetana GW.** Strategies to reduce postoperative pulmonary complications after noncardiothoracic surgery: systematic review for the American College of Physicians. Ann Intern Med. 2006;144:596-608. [PMID: 16618957]

28. **Qaseem A, Snow V, Fitterman N, Hornbake ER, Lawrence VA, Smetana GW, et al.** Risk assessment for and strategies to reduce perioperative pulmonary complications for patients undergoing noncardiothoracic surgery: a guideline from the American College of Physicians. Ann Intern Med. 2006;144:575-80. [PMID: 16618955]

29. **Arozullah AM, Khuri SF, Henderson WG, Daley J.** Development and validation of a multifactorial risk index for predicting postoperative pneumonia after major noncardiac surgery. Ann Intern Med. 2001;135:847-57. [PMID: 11712875]

30. **Arozullah AM, Daley J, Henderson WG, Khuri SF.** Multifactorial risk index for predicting postoperative respiratory failure in men after major noncardiac surgery. The National Veterans Administration Surgical Quality Improvement Program. Ann Surg. 2000;232:242-53. [PMID: 10903604]

31. **Kaboli P, Henderson MC, White RH.** DVT prophylaxis and anticoagulation in the surgical patient. Medical Clinics of North America 2003;87;77-110.

32. **Ansell J, Hirsh J, Poller L, Bussey H, Jacobson A, Hylek E.** The pharmacology and management of the vitamin K antagonists: the Seventh ACCP Conference on Antithrombotic and Thrombolytic Therapy. Chest. 2004;126:204S-233S. [PMID: 15383473]

33. **Geerts WH, Pineo GF, Heit JA, Bergqvist D, Lassen MR, Colwell CW, et al.** Prevention of venous thromboembolism: the Seventh ACCP Conference on Antithrombotic and Thrombolytic Therapy. Chest. 2004;126:338S-400S. [PMID: 15383478]

34. **Armas-Loughran B, Kalra R, Carson JL.** Evaluation and management of anemia and bleeding disorders in surgical patients. Med Clin North Am. 2003;87:229-42. [PMID: 12575892]

35. **Schiff RL, Welsh GA.** Perioperative evaluation and management of the patient with endocrine dysfunction. Med Clin North Am. 2003;87:175-92. [PMID: 12575889]

36. **van den Berghe G, Wouters P, Weekers F, Verwaest C, Bruyninckx F, Schetz M, et al.** Intensive insulin therapy in the critically ill patients. N Engl J Med. 2001;345:1359-67. [PMID: 11794168]

37. **Glister BC, Vigersky RA.** Perioperative management of type 1 diabetes mellitus. Endocrinol Metab Clin North Am. 2003;32:411-36. [PMID: 12800539]

38. **Stathatos N, Wartofsky L.** Perioperative management of patients with hypothyroidism. Endocrinol Metab Clin North Am. 2003;32:503-18. [PMID: 12800543]

39. **Langley RW, Burch HB.** Perioperative management of the thyrotoxic patient. Endocrinol Metab Clin North Am. 2003;32:519-34. [PMID: 12800544]

40. **Axelrod L.** Perioperative management of patients treated with glucocorticoids. Endocrinol Metab Clin North Am. 2003;32:367-83. [PMID: 12800537]

41. **Joseph AJ, Cohn SL.** Perioperative care of the patient with renal failure. Med Clin North Am. 2003;87:193-210. [PMID: 12575890]

42. **Rizvon MK, Chou CL.** Surgery in the patient with liver disease. Med Clin North Am. 2003;87:211-27. [PMID: 12575891]

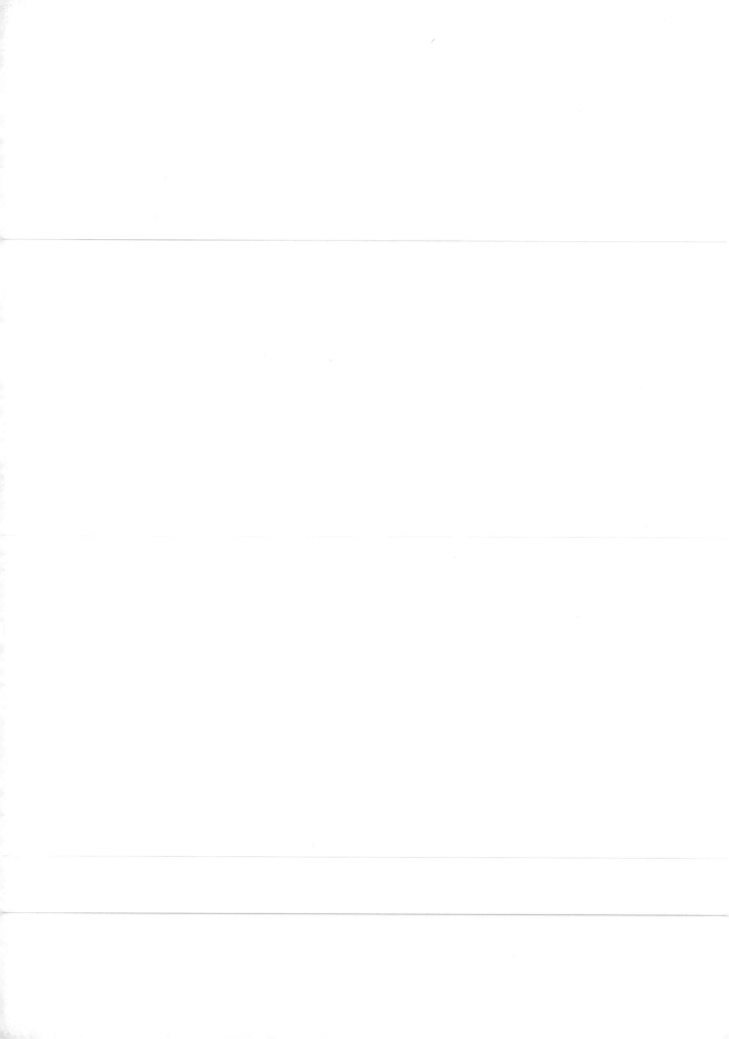

Self-Assessment Test

This self-assessment test contains one-best-answer multiple-choice questions. Please read these directions carefully before answering the questions. Answers, critiques, and bibliographies immediately follow these multiple-choice questions.

The American College of Physicians is accredited by the Accreditation Council for Continuing Medical Education (ACCME) to provide continuing medical education for physicians.

The American College of Physicians designates MKSAP 14® General Internal Medicine for a maximum of 19 *AMA PRA Category 1 Credits*™. Physicians should only claim credit commensurate with the extent of their participation in the activity.

Separate answer sheets are provided for each book of the MKSAP program. Please use one of these answer sheets to complete the General Internal Medicine self-assessment test. Indicate in Section H on the answer sheet the actual number of credits you earned, up to the maximum of 19, in ¼-credit increments. (One credit equals one hour of time spent on this educational activity.)

Credit is available from the publication date of December 29, 2006, until July 31, 2009. You may submit your answer sheets at any time during this period.

Self-scoring Instructions:
General Internal Medicine

Compute your percent correct score as follows:

Step 1: Give yourself 1 point for each correct response to a question.

Step 2: Divide your total points by the total number of questions: 145.

The result, expressed as a percentage, is your percent correct score.

	Example	Your Calculations
Step 1	125	
Step 2	125 ÷ 145	÷ 145
% Correct	86%	%

Item 1

A 51-year-old woman with chronic low back pain is evaluated for a 2-week history of moderate low back pain radiating down her right leg to her right foot following a paroxysm of sneezing. She has no leg weakness or numbness. She takes no prescription medications. Her medical history is notable for a hysterectomy.

On physical examination, the temperature is 36.9 °C (98.5 °F). The lumbar paraspinal muscles are tender to palpation. A straight-leg-raising test is positive on the right. Her perineal sensation and rectal sphincter tone are intact. She has difficulty extending her right great toe against resistance, but lower-extremity strength, sensation, and reflexes are otherwise normal. Radiography of the spine shows some degenerative changes in the lower lumbar spine but no disc narrowing or vertebral collapse.

Which of the following is the most appropriate initial management of this patient?

(A) Referral to orthopedic surgeon
(B) Bed rest for 7 days
(C) MRI of the lumbar spine
(D) NSAIDs
(E) Back exercises

Item 2

A 62-year-old man is evaluated for a 2-week history of dizziness. Episodes of dizziness occur several times per day, usually in the morning and at bedtime, and typically last about 15 to 30 seconds, particularly when he rolls over in bed. The dizziness is described as a spinning sensation and is associated with mild nausea but no vomiting. He had one previous episode of dizziness at the age of 28 years for which he went to the emergency department and received meclizine; that episode resolved in 3 days. The patient has hypertension and diabetes mellitus, and his current medications are hydrochlorothiazide, 50 mg daily, and glipizide, 10 mg daily.

On physical examination, supine pulse rate and blood pressure are 72/min and 120/80 mm Hg and values on standing are 76/min and 116/84 mm Hg. The head-hanging test (Hallpike maneuver) results in dizziness and mild nystagmus when the patient is recumbent with the left ear down but not with the right ear down. There are no focal neurologic findings, and the remainder of the physical examination is normal.

Laboratory studies indicate a hemoglobin A_{1C} of 9.6%, nonfasting plasma glucose level of 170 mg/dL (9.44 mmol/L), serum potassium level of 3.6 meq/L (3.6 mmol/L), and serum sodium concentration of 136 meq/L (136 mmol/L).

Which of the following is most appropriate for managing this patient's disorder?

(A) CT scan of the head
(B) Electronystagmography
(C) Meclizine
(D) Habituation exercises
(E) Decreased hydrochlorothiazide dose

Item 3

A 35-year-old man is evaluated for acute epistaxis. He denies any trauma, intranasal drug use, insertion of foreign bodies in the nose, symptoms of recent allergic or viral rhinitis, or recent use of aspirin or NSAIDs, and has not previously had bleeding difficulties. He is otherwise healthy.

On physical examination, the blood pressure is 150/90 mm Hg. There are several nasal blood clots that are easily removed and no obvious sources of bleeding. Bleeding stops with external pressure but then recurs in 30 minutes.

Which of the following is the best management approach in this patient?

(A) Anterior packing
(B) Posterior packing
(C) Topical oxymetazoline
(D) Silver nitrate cautery

Item 4

A 60-year-old man is evaluated for a 3-month history of persistent left lower facial pain in the mandibular region that has worsened and been unresponsive to treatment with acetaminophen, 4 g four times daily, over the past 3 weeks. He describes the pain as "electrical" in nature, often triggered by dental manipulation or extreme temperature exposure. His dentist found no oral or dental cause for the pain but treated him with a 14-day course of amoxicillin for presumptive sinusitis without improvement.

The physical examination, including a complete neurologic evaluation, is normal. Laboratory studies and CT of the sinuses are normal.

Which of the following is the most cost-effective and efficacious treatment for this patient?

(A) Narcotic analgesia
(B) Gabapentin
(C) Tricyclic antidepressants
(D) Carbamazepine
(E) Tetrahydrocannabinol analogs

Item 5

A 75-year-old woman is evaluated for symptoms of urinary incontinence that have increased gradually over the past several months. She notes the frequent urge to urinate and has difficulty controlling her urine flow. She now wears pads in the daytime and at night. She lives alone and is able to care for herself. A few months ago, she was diagnosed with depression and began taking nortriptyline. Her medical history is significant for a hysterectomy for uterine fibroids, and hypertension well controlled with nifedipine and atenolol for several years.

On physical examination, the pulse rate is 65/min, and blood pressure is 125/82 mm Hg. The pelvic examination reveals atrophy of the vaginal tissues and the absence of a uterus and cervix. Results of urinalysis are normal.

Which of the following is the most appropriate next step in the management of this patient?

(A) Replace nortriptyline with another class of antidepressant
(B) Replace atenolol with another class of antihypertensive agent
(C) Replace nifedipine with another class of antihypertensive agent
(D) Begin oxybutynin
(E) Begin oral estrogen therapy

Item 6

A 22-year-old woman is evaluated during a routine physical examination. She has mild exercise-induced asthma. She does not smoke, drinks alcohol only socially, and does not use illicit drugs. She has had a total of four sexual partners, and currently is in a monogamous relationship with a serious boyfriend. She has no history of sexually transmitted infections and takes an oral contraceptive to prevent pregnancy. A recent HIV test was negative. She is due for a Pap smear. She has had baseline pulmonary function tests.

In addition to the Pap smear, which of the following is most appropriate for this patient?

(A) Encourage use of sunscreen
(B) Prescribe a multivitamin with folic acid daily
(C) Screen for *Chlamydia trachomatis*
(D) Measure fasting plasma glucose

Item 7

A 37-year-old woman is evaluated for major depression that was diagnosed 1 month ago and treated with fluoxetine. Two weeks after treatment, she had no suicidal ideation, and her depressive symptoms had improved, with a 5-point decrease in her PHQ-9 score. During today's visit, she reports that her depressive symptoms have continued to improve, although she has experienced sexual dysfunction manifested by anorgasmia. Her medical history includes hypertension, for which she takes hydrochlorothiazide and lisinopril.

On physical examination, the BMI is 29, and blood pressure is 146/90 mm Hg. The remainder of the examination is normal.

Which of the following is the most appropriate alternative treatment option for this patient's depression?

(A) Citalopram
(B) Mirtazapine
(C) Venlafaxine
(D) Bupropion
(E) Sertraline

Item 8

A 41-year-old woman is evaluated for a 3-week history of red, itchy eyelids. She wears contact lenses daily. She has not used any new cosmetics, soaps, or laundry detergents. She has no history of asthma or atopy.

Physical examination shows erythema and mild edema of the upper eyelids only. There is no blurred vision, purulent eye discharge, or dry skin around the eyes or lashes. The rest of her skin examination is normal. There is no lymphadenopathy or muscle weakness.

Which of the following is the most likely diagnosis?

(A) Seborrheic blepharitis
(B) Rosacea
(C) Dermatomyositis
(D) Lichen simplex
(E) Contact dermatitis

Item 9

A 75-year-old man undergoes postoperative evaluation after right hip-fracture surgical repair. His history includes mild dementia, coronary artery disease treated with intracoronary stenting to the left anterior descending artery 2 years ago, hypertension, hyperlipidemia, and type 2 diabetes mellitus. Preoperative medications included atenolol, fosinopril, hydrochlorothiazide, simvastatin, glipizide, lorazepam as needed for sleep, and daily aspirin. Preoperatively, the physical examination was notable for normal vital signs, distress due to pain, full orientation, nonfocal neurologic findings, and normal cardiopulmonary and abdominal examinations. Laboratory studies were remarkable for a hematocrit of 38%. A chest radiograph was normal, and an electrocardiogram showed an old inferior infarction.

On postoperative day 1, he is acutely confused, agitated, rambling, illogical in speech, and unable to focus attention on conversation. The temperature is normal, pulse rate is 80 to 100/min depending on state of agitation, and blood pressure is 130/76 mm Hg. The remainder of the examination, including neurologic examination, is unremarkable.

Which of the following is the optimal postoperative management strategy for this patient?

(A) Haloperidol, patient restraints for safety, and CT of the head
(B) Olanzapine and MRI of the head

(C) Risperidone, empiric antibiotics, and lumbar puncture

(D) Chest radiography, electrocardiography, metabolic profile, and haloperidol

Item 10

A 24-year-old man requests antibiotics during an evaluation for symptoms he has attributed to a sinus infection. He reports sinus congestion and clear nasal drainage that has persisted for 1 month after he developed a cold; he has no fever, sinus pain, purulent nasal drainage, sneezing, or nasal itching. Since the onset of his symptoms, he has been using a nasal decongestant spray with only short-term symptomatic relief, but he states that antibiotics have been effective in the past for treating his sinus infections. His history includes allergic rhinitis, but his primary allergens are not in season.

Nasal examination shows congested nasal mucosa with a profuse watery discharge. The nasal septum appears normal, the turbinates are pale, and there are no polyps. The remainder of the physical examination is normal.

Which of the following is the most likely reason for this patient's symptoms?

(A) Allergic rhinitis

(B) Bacterial sinusitis

(C) Nonallergic rhinitis

(D) Rhinitis medicamentosa

(E) Viral upper respiratory infection

Item 11

A 40-year-old woman is evaluated during a 6-month follow-up visit for episodes of abnormal uterine bleeding. Prior to these abnormal bleeding episodes, she had heavy 5-day menstrual periods, with dysmenorrhea for the first 3 days of menstruation. Examination findings from 6 months ago included a normal pelvic examination, negative transvaginal ultrasonographic scan, and a negative Pap smear. She also had a normal complete blood count and serum thyroid-stimulating hormone level. Since that evaluation, she has had three episodes of bleeding between periods, with the last occurring 1 month ago.

Which of the following is the most appropriate next step in the management of this patient?

(A) Placement of a progesterone intrauterine device

(B) Uterine artery embolization

(C) Endometrial biopsy

(D) Repeated transvaginal ultrasonography

Item 12

A 20-year-old college wrestler is evaluated for a painful lesion on his upper back. He first noted a small painful area 7 days ago, and the lesion enlarged and became more red and painful during the next several days. The patient states that other members of his wrestling team have developed similar lesions. His history is otherwise uneventful. Examination of the upper back reveals a 1 × 1-cm red, raised pustule that is tender to palpation, with a 4 × 4-cm area of surrounding erythema. The remainder of the physical examination, including vital signs, is normal.

The lesion is incised and drained. A culture is sent to the laboratory.

Which of the following is the most appropriate empiric treatment pending culture results?

(A) Levofloxacin

(B) Doxycycline

(C) Dicloxacillin

(D) Cephalexin

Item 13

A 60-year-old man undergoes preoperative evaluation before total hip-replacement surgery. His history includes asthma and obstructive sleep apnea (OSA) but no known coronary artery disease. He also has osteoarthritis of the knee, which does not allow him to walk far without pain, although he is able to perform yard activities that do not require much walking, such as weeding, pruning trees, and splitting wood. His medications include flunisolide, salmeterol, and albuterol as needed. He also uses positive continuous airway pressure at night.

On physical examination, the BMI is 31. Blood pressure is normal, and oxygen saturation is 90% on room air. Scattered wheezes are heard on pulmonary examination. The remainder of the examination is unremarkable.

Which of the following preoperative strategies will most reduce this patient's risk for postoperative pulmonary complications?

(A) Five percent weight loss

(B) Improved asthma control

(C) Surgical correction of OSA

(D) Preoperative spirometry

Item 14

A 32-year-old woman is evaluated for chronic headaches that have increased in frequency from severe headaches occurring monthly and milder headaches occurring weekly to daily headaches. The headaches have no prodrome or aura, are located mostly on the right side of the head, and are associated with nausea, rare emesis, and photophobia. Occasionally, the headaches are bad enough that she must spend the day in bed. The patient has had migraine headaches since she was 19 years old. Her mother also had migraine headaches.

Her severe headaches have responded well to sumatriptan and her mild headaches to acetaminophen or naproxen; however, because her daily headaches have become unresponsive to these agents, she has been taking butalbital-aspirin-caffeine three to four times daily over the past month. She is otherwise healthy and reports that her stressors are unchanged. There is no fever, chills, neck stiffness, parasthesias or weakness, or other constitutional symptoms associated with her headaches, and she has had no known tick exposures. Her only other daily medication is the oral contraceptive ethinyl estradiol norethindrone, which she has been taking for 5 years.

The physical examination, including vital signs and neurologic evaluation, is normal.

Which of the following is the most likely cause of this patient's daily headaches?

(A) Cerebral artery aneurysm
(B) Butalbital-aspirin-caffeine
(C) Status migrainosus
(D) Medication seeking

Item 15

A 37-year-old woman is evaluated for a 6-week history of gradually progressive aching right heel pain. The pain is worse in the morning, especially when she first steps out of bed. She has no numbness or tingling in her feet. She is overweight and began jogging several months ago to lose weight. She was carefully fitted for comfortable running shoes before she began running. Her only medical problem is hypothyroidism for which she takes levothyroxine.

On physical examination, she has no bony abnormalities, swelling, or skin changes over the feet and ankles. There is tenderness to palpation only over the medial aspect of the right calcaneus; dorsiflexion of the toes increases the heel pain. Ankle range of motion is intact; she has no pain with inversion or eversion and dorsiflexion of the foot. She also has no discomfort with reflex hammer tapping over the medial aspect of the heel just below and behind the medial malleolus or with compression of the calcaneus.

Which of the following is the most likely diagnosis in this patient?

(A) Achilles tendonitis
(B) Calcaneal stress fracture
(C) Plantar fasciitis
(D) Tarsal tunnel syndrome

Item 16

A 60-year-old woman is evaluated for dry eyes, which have bothered her for several years and initially responded to treatment with methylcellulose drops, but have become recalcitrant to this therapy. She reports no environmental or occupational exposures affecting her eye moisture. Her medical history and review of symptoms are noncontributory, and she takes no medications. Her physical examination is unremarkable. Laboratory studies, including erythrocyte sedimentation rate and antinuclear antibody assay, are unremarkable.

Which of the following is the most appropriate treatment for this patient at this time?

(A) Cevimeline
(B) Guaifenesin
(C) Cyclosporine
(D) Topical corticosteroid
(E) Topical NSAID

Item 17

A 38-year-old woman is evaluated for a 4-week history of episodes of frequent awakening in the middle of the night, although she falls asleep without difficulty. During the day, she notes a feeling of hyperarousal and irritability, which is interfering with her effectiveness at work. The patient works as a lawyer in a competitive and stressful environment and often feels anxious regarding her job performance. She is in excellent health and runs competitively. She does not smoke or drink alcohol. She has had similar symptoms in the past and has used over-the-counter antihistamines to help her sleep, but they are no longer effective.

On physical examination, pulse rate is 60/min, and blood pressure is 120/75 mm Hg. The BMI is 20. The remainder of the examination is normal. A diagnosis of acute insomnia is established, and a recommendation is given to the patient to avoid strenuous exercise or alcohol within a few hours of bedtime, develop a relaxing evening routine, and avoid afternoon caffeine. The patient follows this advice but continues to have difficulty sleeping.

Which of the following is the most appropriate treatment for this patient?

(A) Kava
(B) Zolpidem
(C) Selective serotonin reuptake inhibitor
(D) Diphenhydramine
(E) Triazolam

Item 18

A 55-year-old woman is evaluated for what she believes is toenail fungus. Embarrassed by the appearance of her toenails, she is interested in an oral treatment that she read about in a magazine. She is otherwise healthy and takes no medications.

On physical examination, thickened and dystrophic nails are noted on each of her largest toes. The remainder of the examination is normal.

Which of the following is the most appropriate next step in management?

(A) Oral terbinafine
(B) Topical ciclopirox
(C) Aggressive nail debridement
(D) Culture of debris under nail

Item 19

An 87-year-old wheelchair-bound woman is evaluated during a routine examination. She is accompanied by her son. The patient lives in a residential living setting in her own apartment and has recently become socially isolated, no longer visiting with friends, eating in the common dining room, or finding enjoyment from watching television. Her medical history includes hypertension, coronary artery disease, and osteoporosis, for which she takes hydrochlorothiazide, metoprolol, aspirin, calcium carbonate, and alendronate.

On physical examination, the patient appears well-groomed and has a friendly demeanor. The pulse rate is 70/min, and the blood pressure is 125/75 mm Hg. The BMI is 18.3. She is oriented to person, place, and time and is able to ambulate with assistance. Neurologic examination is significant for a resting tremor in the right hand but no other focal findings. Laboratory studies, including complete blood count, basic serum chemistries, and serum thyroid-stimulating hormone level, are normal. Results of the Five-Item Geriatric Depression screen are 1/5.

Which of the following is the most appropriate management option in addressing the current symptom?

(A) Assess hearing and vision
(B) Discontinue hydrochlorothiazide
(C) Initiate sertraline
(D) Schedule neuropsychologic testing

Item 20

A 35-year-old man is evaluated during a routine examination. He does not smoke and has no family history of early coronary artery disease.

On examination, BMI is 35.2, and waist circumference is 114 cm (45 in). Blood pressure is 142/88 mm Hg. The remainder of the physical examination is normal. Laboratory studies indicate borderline hyperglycemia (fasting plasma glucose, 121 mg/dL [6.7 mmol/L]). Serum total cholesterol level is 246 mg/dL (6.36 mmol/L), high-density lipoprotein level is 31 mg/dL (0.8 mmol/L), and low-density lipoprotein level is 158 mg/dL (4.05 mmol/L).

Which of the following recommendations is most appropriate for this patient?

(A) Electron-beam CT
(B) Exercise treadmill test
(C) Hydrochlorothiazide
(D) Intensive lifestyle modification
(E) Intake of red wine

Item 21

A 45-year-old man is evaluated for a 6-month history of midabdominal pain, fatigue, and a 2.26-kg (5-lb) weight loss. He has a long-standing history of constipation-predominant irritable bowel syndrome (IBS) but reports the current abdominal pain is different from that associated with his previous IBS symptoms. He has no diarrhea, hematochezia, melena, or genitourinary complaints. He denies alcohol or drug use and has undergone no previous surgical procedures.

Physical examination is normal except for moderate obesity (weight of 118 kg [260 lb]) and some mild, mid-abdominal tenderness but no hepatosplenomegaly, masses, guarding, or rebound tenderness. Laboratory studies, including hemoglobin, serum creatinine level, liver chemistry tests, serum lipase level, and urinalysis, are normal. Results of colonoscopy are also normal.

Which of the following is the most appropriate next radiologic imaging test for this patient?

(A) MRI of the abdomen
(B) Magnetic resonance cholangiopancreatography
(C) CT of the abdomen
(D) CT colonography
(E) Abdominal ultrasonography

Item 22

A 77-year-old man is evaluated for a 7-month history of urinary frequency and nocturia. He denies dysuria and hematuria. His medical history is notable for oxygen-dependent emphysema, coronary artery disease, and hypothyroidism. His medications include inhaled bronchodilators, inhaled corticosteroids, an ACE inhibitor, a statin, aspirin, and a multivitamin.

On physical examination, the temperature is normal, pulse rate is 62/min, and blood pressure is 144/84 mm Hg. On cardiopulmonary examination, decreased breath sounds and a prolonged expiratory phase are audible in the lungs, and the heart rate is regular with normal heart sounds. The abdomen is soft and nontender to palpation, and there are normally active bowel sounds. His bladder cannot be percussed, and he has no flank tenderness. Rectal sphincter tone is intact, and the prostate is smooth, symmetric, and moderately enlarged. His AUA symptom index score is 13 (moderate lower urinary tract symptoms).

Which of the following is the most appropriate next diagnostic step for this patient?

(A) Intravenous pyelogram
(B) Postvoid residual measurement
(C) Prostate-specific antigen measurement
(D) Urinalysis
(E) Urine flow-rate studies

Item 23

A 45-year-old male warehouse worker is evaluated for a back injury he experienced 4 months ago when lifting a heavy box; he has been bedridden intermittently since then. Today he is asking for a disability form to be completed so that he can be reassigned to a desk job. His back pain does not radiate and he has no lower-extremity weakness; however, he reports that both legs are completely numb. He takes over-the-counter NSAIDs but no prescription medications. He has no history of injection drug use and is otherwise healthy.

On physical examination, the temperature is normal, pulse rate is 74/min, and blood pressure is 126/82 mm Hg. The patient has exquisite diffuse lumbar and paraspinal tenderness to light palpation, with no areas of erythema or warmth; his spinal range of motion is decreased. Pressing downward on his head elicits lower back pain. Although he is able to passively extend his legs without pain when sitting down, he has back pain radiating down his right leg with a supine straight-leg-raising test. Lower-extremity motor strength is intact, and patellar and ankle reflexes are symmetric.

Which of the following is the most appropriate next step in the management of this patient's back pain?

(A) Cyclobenzaprine
(B) Psychologic evaluation
(C) Epidural corticosteroid injection
(D) Radiography of the lumbar spine
(E) MRI of the lumbar spine

Item 24

A 37-year-old male Army reservist is evaluated for generalized muscle aches and persistent fatigue 3 months after returning to the United States from a 1-year deployment in Iraq. He also reports that his joints are somewhat stiff and painful, particularly in the back, knees, and hips. He has not had fever, chills, weight loss, cough, or headaches. The patient is accompanied by his wife, who says that her husband has been having problems sleeping and concentrating, and that they have been having problems with intimacy. Although he says he is having some problems adjusting to being home, he denies feeling depressed; however, he admits he is not as involved in pleasurable activities as he was before his deployment because he has not felt well since his return. He also describes having nightmares about a roadside bomb that killed several friends.

The patient is hesitant to return to his job as a cross-country truck driver, stating that he feels uncomfortable driving, particularly in heavy traffic, and he is not ready to leave his family. His medical history is noncontributory, and the physical examination is unremarkable.

Laboratory studies, including complete blood count, tuberculin skin testing, renal function and liver chemistry tests, serum electrolyte and calcium levels, and urinalysis, are normal.

In addition to cognitive behavioral therapy, which of the following is the best treatment option for this patient?

(A) Chlordiazepoxide
(B) Lithium
(C) Divalproex
(D) Sertraline

Item 25

A 76-year-old man is evaluated for a syncopal episode that occurred last night after a coughing paroxysm following a fit of laughter. The patient is accompanied by his wife, who found him unconscious and slumped against the wall in the bathroom but reported that he regained consciousness quickly when she laid him fully on the floor and raised his legs. On regaining consciousness, he was fully oriented, spoke clearly, and had no difficulty standing up or walking. He reports having felt lightheaded and faint several times recently while trying to urinate but had not passed out

before. His history includes coronary artery disease, stable angina, hypertension, chronic obstructive pulmonary disease with paroxysmal coughing, and benign prostatic hyperplasia with increasing difficulty urinating. He also has a seizure disorder caused by a remote head injury, with seizures occurring every 1 to 2 months, and the most recent one occurring 2 months ago. Physical examination, including complete neurologic evaluation, is normal.

Which of the following is the most likely diagnosis?

(A) Vertebrobasilar transient ischemic accident
(B) Situational syncope
(C) Carotid sinus syncope
(D) Grand mal seizure

Item 26

A 48-year-old woman is evaluated for a 1-week history of right ear pain, pruritus, purulent discharge, and pain on manipulation of the ear. Her medical history is noncontributory.

On physical examination, she is afebrile. There is prominent swelling and erythema of the ear canal. Evacuation of the canal with curettage yields purulent detritus.

Which of the following interventions is associated with the best outcomes in patients with this condition?

(A) Cerumenolytics
(B) Topical neomycin/polymyxin
(C) Topical corticosteroid drops plus acetic acid drops
(D) Oral antibiotics
(E) Topical acetic acid drops

Item 27

A 62-year-old man is evaluated for left anterior hip pain that began 3 days earlier. He was recently hospitalized for kidney stone extraction and was discharged 4 days ago. The pain is worse with activity and disturbs his sleep. He has chills, but no rash, palpitations, or back pain. He has a history of degenerative joint disease in his hips and knees and has gout attacks in his first metatarsophalangeal joints about three times annually. There is no history of tick exposure.

On physical examination, temperature is 38.7 °C (101.7 °F), pulse rate is 110/min, and blood pressure is 142/72 mm Hg. There is markedly decreased range of motion and pain in his left hip and some warmth over the lateral aspect. All other joints are normal on palpation. Plain radiography of the hip shows an effusion.

Which of the following tests is most appropriate?

(A) Serology for *Borrelia burgdorferi*
(B) Urethral swab for *Neisseria gonorrhoeae*
(C) Antinuclear antibody and rheumatoid factor titers
(D) Hip joint aspiration
(E) Bone scan

Item 28

A 68-year-old woman is evaluated for gradual vision loss in the left eye. She notes that colors appear faded, it is difficult to recognize faces, and it is difficult to see in rooms without good lighting. She denies eye pain. Her medical history is significant for a 15-pack-year smoking history, hypertension, and type 2 diabetes mellitus.

On physical examination, the pulse rate is 70/min, and blood pressure is 125/85 mm Hg. The ophthalmoscopic examination shows soft drusen clustered within the central macula and well-defined areas of retinal pigment epithelium loss.

Which of the following is the most likely diagnosis?

(A) Cataracts
(B) Proliferative diabetic retinopathy
(C) Dry age-related macular degeneration
(D) Wet age-related macular degeneration
(E) Open-angle glaucoma

Item 29

A 48-year-old woman is evaluated for frequent hot flushes and night sweats that interfere with her work and sleep. She has not menstruated for 8 months. She is speaking at a conference in 3 weeks and desires immediate resolution to the embarrassing sweats associated with her hot flushes. Her medical history is noncontributory, and she takes no medications. Physical examination, including vital signs, is normal.

Which of the following is the most appropriate next step in the treatment of this patient's symptoms?

(A) Short-term, low-dose hormone replacement therapy
(B) Duloxetine
(C) Cognitive behavioral therapy
(D) Red clover

Item 30

A 30-year-old woman is evaluated for a common wart on her right thumb that she first noticed 6 months ago. She began treating the wart with over-the-counter salicylic acid 1 month ago when writing with the affected hand became painful. She has noticed a reduction in the size and pain of the wart, but she wants a more effective treatment. The medical history is noncontributory. On physical examination, the common wart is found to be directly adjacent to the thumb nail bed and is 4 × 4 mm in size. The rest of the examination is unremarkable.

Which of the following is the most appropriate next step in management?

(A) Continuation of salicylic acid therapy
(B) Cryotherapy
(C) Topical imiquimod
(D) Candida antigen injection

Item 31

A 23-year-old woman is evaluated for worsening discomfort and severe pelvic pain just prior to and during menses for the past 3 to 4 months. Her cycle has been 2 to 3 days longer than usual. Previously, her cycles were normal, with no pain. She has a 4-year history of dyspareunia, which is now worsening. She recently married and is monogamous. History includes eight previous sexual partners, with whom she used barrier contraception. She takes no medications and has never been pregnant. She has no known history of abnormal Pap smears, sexually transmitted disease, or pelvic inflammatory disease. Her last Pap smear was 7 months ago. She has no fever, chills, or vaginal discharge. Her weight has been stable.

On examination, she is in no acute distress. The temperature is normal, pulse rate is 88/min, and blood pressure is 104/72 mm Hg. There is no costovertebral tenderness to palpation. The abdomen is tender to palpation in lower quadrants, with no rebound or guarding. External genitalia are normal, and the cervix appears healthy. There is no cervical motion tenderness, but there is tenderness with deep palpation of the uterus.

Polymerase chain reaction assay for *Neisseria gonorrhoeae* and *Chlamydia trachomatis* is negative.

Which of the following is the most appropriate next step in diagnosis?

(A) Laparotomy
(B) Colonoscopy
(C) Transvaginal ultrasonography
(D) Cystoscopy
(E) Hysterosalpingography

Item 32

A 65-year-old man is evaluated for a facial lesion on his upper cheek bone just below his right eye. The medical history is noncontributory.

On physical examination, a flesh-colored, dome-shaped nodule is noted. It has adjacent telangiectasia and a pearly, translucent surface. The remainder of the examination is normal.

Which of the following is the most likely diagnosis?

(A) Basal cell cancer
(B) Squamous cell cancer
(C) Keratoacanthoma
(D) Sebaceous hyperplasia

Item 33

A 55-year-old woman undergoes preoperative evaluation before elective laparoscopic cholecystectomy. The medical history includes three pregnancies and full-term deliveries with no complications or health problems in the mother or the neonate. She also has an allergy to trimethoprim–sulfamethoxazole. She has had no previous surgeries, problems with prolonged bleeding after tooth extractions, or episodes of epistaxis. Her last menstrual period was 18 months ago. She does not smoke and drinks 1 to 2 glasses of wine with dinner a few times weekly. The physical examination is normal.

Which of the following is the best approach to preoperative laboratory screening in this patient?

(A) Complete blood count (CBC)
(B) CBC and INR
(C) CBC, INR, prothrombin time (PT), and partial thromboplastin time (PTT)
(D) CBC, INR, PT, PTT, and bleeding test

Item 34

A 70-year-old woman with hypothyroidism fell and fractured her hip. During preoperative evaluation for hip-fracture repair, she mentions recent mild fatigue, which has not significantly limited performance of her daily activities, and ongoing right upper-quadrant abdominal pain after eating. She takes levothyroxine 0.075 mg daily.

Physical examination is normal except for moderate obesity.

Laboratory results show mild anemia (hemoglobin 11 g/dL [6.83 mmol/L], and hematocrit 34% [0.34]). Serum thyroid-stimulating hormone level is 11.2 µU/mL (11.2 mU/L), thyroxine level is 7.2 µg/dL (92.67 nmol/L), and triiodothyronine uptake is 45% (0.45). Liver chemistry tests are normal.

Which of the following management options is most appropriate?

(A) Proceed with surgery
(B) Increase levothyroxine dosage and delay surgery until thyroid levels are normal
(C) Administer intravenous thyroid hormone and proceed with surgery
(D) Administer intravenous thyroid hormone plus hydrocortisone and proceed with surgery

Item 35

A 43-year-old woman is evaluated for a 1-week history of acute left knee pain that began when she stepped down from a dock onto a sailboat and experienced a "popping sensation" and a gradual onset of knee joint swelling over the next 4 to 6 hours. She immediately applied ice to her knee and took ibuprofen with some pain relief. Over the past few days, she has continued to have moderate pain, particularly when walking up or down stairs, which has responded to ibuprofen. She reports no locking or giving way of the knee nor any previous knee injury, fever, chills, pain in other joints, dry eyes or mouth, rash, sun sensitivity, known tick exposure, back pain, diarrhea, or abdominal pain. Her medical history includes hypertension, well controlled with lisinopril and hydrochlorothiazide. She has a monogamous relationship with her husband of 21 years. Her mother has rheumatoid arthritis.

On physical examination, the left knee has minimal effusion, without warmth or erythema, with full range of motion. Palpation of the medial aspect of the joint line is

tender. Maximally flexing the hip and knee and applying abduction to the knee while externally rotating the foot and passively extending the knee result in some tenderness but no crepitance. There is no palpable snap or pain.

Which of the following is the most appropriate next step in management of this patient?

(A) MRI of the knee
(B) Arthrocentesis
(C) Exercise on "stair-stepper"
(D) Straight-leg-raising exercise without weights
(E) Orthopedic surgery

Item 36

A 23-year-old woman is evaluated because her mother, who has accompanied her, is concerned that she is too thin. The patient reports that she has lost 8.6 kg (19 lb) in the past 6 months from her baseline of 48.08 kg (106 lb). Her current BMI is 14.9. Her daily dietary intake usually consists of a yogurt for breakfast and a salad or bagel with a "double-espresso coffee" for dinner. She says that she feels full and bloated after eating anything, and she thinks her stomach looks big. Although she feels tired, she drinks two to three caffeinated diet beverages per day to maintain her energy level. Sometimes, when she stands up quickly, she feels lightheaded. Her last menstrual period was 2 months ago. She denies bingeing, laxative use, vomiting, depression, or anhedonia.

On physical examination, she is a very thin, well-groomed woman, in no apparent distress. She is orthostatic and tachycardic, but her other vital signs are normal. Her hair is thin and brittle, and her integument dry. The remainder of the physical examination is unremarkable. Laboratory studies include a serum potassium level of 3.1 meq/L (3.1 mmol/L), and a serum phosphorus level of 2.2 mg/dL (0.71 mmol/L).

Which of the following is the best initial management option for this patient?

(A) Citalopram
(B) Immediate hospitalization
(C) Outpatient psychiatric referral
(D) Olanzapine
(E) Nutrition consultation

Item 37

A 45-year-old black man is evaluated for concerns about prostate cancer. A good friend was recently diagnosed with extensive disease and has a poor prognosis. The patient asks if he should have a screening test for this disease. He reports once-nightly nocturia but has no hesitancy, urinary frequency, or dribbling.

Which of the following is the most appropriate course of action for this patient?

(A) Prostate-specific antigen (PSA) measurement
(B) PSA measurement and digital rectal examination
(C) Transrectal ultrasonography

(D) Transrectal ultrasonography with random biopsies

(E) Discussion of benefits and harms of PSA testing

Item 38

A 19-year-old college student is evaluated for left testicle pain that began 3 to 4 days earlier. He is newly sexually active. The symptoms started slowly, but now the left testicle is painful even when he walks. He has had no dysuria, urinary frequency, penile discharge, or ulcerations. He reports no fever or chills.

On examination, temperature is normal. He has an area of tenderness at the superior pole of the left testicle, with normal-sized testes, smooth surface, and negative transillumination. There is no evidence of urethral discharge. Urinalysis in the office shows leukocytes (7/hpf) and erythrocytes (5/hpf). DNA amplification is performed. Urethral swabs are sent for culture.

Which of the following is the best empiric treatment for this patient?

(A) Doxycycline

(B) Ceftriaxone and doxycycline

(C) Amoxicillin

(D) Trimethoprim—sulfamethoxazole

Item 39

An 81-year-old man is evaluated for a 3-month history of difficulty controlling his urine; he is accompanied by his daughter. The patient notes a frequent urge to urinate that requires him to wear pads during the day and at night. After a trial of oxybutynin, the patient experienced dry mouth, and the drug was discontinued. The medical history includes Alzheimer's disease, cerebral vascular disease, and hypertension.

On physical examination, the prostate is normal, and neurologic findings are nonfocal. The Mini–Mental State Examination Score is 20/30. Laboratory studies, including serum chemistries and urinalysis, are normal.

Which of the following is the most appropriate treatment in this patient?

(A) Tolterodine

(B) Doxepin

(C) Midodrine

(D) Duloxetine

Item 40

A 36-year-old woman is evaluated for a 7-month history of mild, bilateral breast pain, which occurs cyclically and is associated with her menstrual period. The patient is otherwise healthy, and the medical history is unremarkable. She is sexually active and takes oral progestin-estrogen contraceptives.

On physical examination, the breasts are noted to have glandular tissue that is bilaterally symmetric, with no appreciable dominant breast mass. There is no pain on palpation of the breasts. Results of a bilateral diagnostic mammogram are negative, with a Breast Imaging Reporting and Data System (BIRADS)-1 reading.

Which of the following is the most appropriate next step in the management of this patient?

(A) Reassurance

(B) Trial of vitamin E and evening primrose oil

(C) Avoidance of coffee, tea, chocolate, and cola beverages

(D) Initiation of danazol after a negative pregnancy test

(E) Breast ultrasonography

Item 41

A 45-year-old woman is evaluated for a 1-year history of almost-daily exhaustion and difficulty performing her daily functions. Her symptoms are exacerbated by physical effort and performing complex cognitive tasks she was normally fully capable of doing. Although she reports chronic low levels of energy, she has not had any sleep disturbances, daytime somnolence, spousal reports of her snoring, depressed mood, anhedonia, or excessive life stressors, and she takes no medications except for the periodic use of psyllium. Her medical history is significant for irritable bowel syndrome. She has been evaluated by several other physicians since the onset of her fatigue and has undergone extensive work-ups to rule out malignancy, including colonoscopy, mammography, Papanicolaou testing, and cardiopulmonary evaluation, the results of which have all been normal.

On physical examination, her vital signs are normal, and BMI is 26. Cardiopulmonary examination is unremarkable, and laboratory studies, including complete blood count, erythrocyte sedimentation rate, and serum thyroid-stimulating hormone level, are normal.

Which of the following is the most appropriate next step in the management of this patient?

(A) Cognitive behavioral therapy

(B) Fluoxetine

(C) Galantamine

(D) Hydrocortisone plus fludrocortisone

Item 42

A 70-year-old woman undergoes preoperative evaluation before cataract surgery and excision of a 0.75-cm basal cell carcinoma on the right lateral thigh. Her history includes coronary artery disease, with no angina since she has been adhering to her current medical regimen, and nonvalvular atrial fibrillation for which she takes chronic anticoagulation therapy. She has not had a stroke or transient ischemic attack. Her functional capacity is good.

Which of the following is the best management approach to anticoagulation for these procedures?

(A) Continue warfarin at usual dose and target INR for both procedures

(B) Reduce warfarin dose to achieve a lower target INR of 1.3 to 1.5

(C) Stop the warfarin and perform surgery when the INR is normal for both procedures

(D) Stop warfarin and use therapeutic enoxaparin until 12 hours before surgery

Item 43

A 55-year-old man experiences blunt abdominal trauma and multiple fractures in a car accident. He has a history of type 2 diabetes well controlled with metformin and glipizide. After emergency exploratory surgery, repair of a hepatic laceration, and initial stabilization of bilateral femur fractures, he has a myocardial infarction. Pneumonia and sepsis develop, and renal function deteriorates.

He is given enteral feeding with oral liquid nutrition.

Which of the following offers the best management of his diabetes in the surgical intensive care unit?

(A) Regular insulin every 6 hours to maintain blood glucose <250 mg/dL (13.88 mmol/L)

(B) Regular insulin every 6 hours to maintain blood glucose <200 mg/dL (11.1 mmol/L)

(C) Basal glargine plus regular insulin every 6 hours to maintain glucose <150 mg/dL (8.32 mmol/L)

(D) Regular insulin by continuous infusion to maintain blood glucose <110 mg/dL (6.11 mmol/L)

Item 44

A 24-year-old woman is evaluated for a severe, pulsating headache located on the left side of the head. The headache began 2 hours ago, is 8/10 in severity, and is associated with photophobia and fatigue. She also has diffuse pain to the slightest touch of the skin on the left side of her face, which occurs commonly with her severe headaches. She has a headache two to three times monthly, lasting all day, and severe headaches three to four times yearly. She denies any aura or other warning of headache onset. Although her headaches have frequently responded to a combination of acetaminophen-isometheptene-dichloralphenazone and naproxen, her current episode is refractory to these agents, and she experienced emesis on her attempt at taking the naproxen. Her history is significant for two visits in the past year to a local urgent care clinic for severe headaches that were treated with sumatriptan and intravenous metoclopramide, respectively, with good relief of symptoms. She takes no other medications.

On physical examination, temperature is 36.6 °C (97.9 °F), and blood pressure is 147/93 mm Hg. The remainder of the examination is normal except for the presence of hyperalgia over the left cheek.

Which of the following is the most appropriate treatment for this patient?

(A) Rizatriptan

(B) Sumatriptan

(C) Ketorolac

(D) Metoclopramide

Item 45

A 69-year-old man is evaluated for chronic leg heaviness and aching. His medical history is notable for hypertension treated with hydrochlorothiazide.

On physical examination, pulse rate is 72/min, and blood pressure is 112/66 mm Hg. The BMI is 30. Examination of the lower extremities is notable for tortuous, large (>4 mm), dilated veins over the thighs and calves. There is no warmth, erythema, ulceration, or hyperpigmentation over his legs, but there is symmetric 1-mm pitting edema of the ankles.

Which of the following is the most appropriate initial management for this patient's symptoms?

(A) Compression stockings

(B) Furosemide

(C) Laser therapy

(D) Injection sclerotherapy

(E) Vein stripping

Item 46

A 17-year-old female basketball player is evaluated after experiencing an inversion sprain (supination injury) of her right ankle when she landed awkwardly after jumping for a rebound. She is able to bear weight on her ankle and hobble over to the examination table without assistance.

On physical examination, she has moderate ankle swelling and ecchymosis over the lateral ankle. She has mild joint instability with restricted range of motion. Passive inversion causes lateral ankle pain and tenderness to palpation over the anterior talofibular ligament but not over the lateral malleolus or the base of the fifth metatarsal bone.

Which of the following is the most appropriate next step in the management of this patient's injury?

(A) MRI of the ankle

(B) Radiography of the ankle

(C) Cast immobilization

(D) Compression bandage

(E) Surgical repair

Item 47

A 68-year-old man recently diagnosed with adenocarcinoma of the cecum undergoes preoperative evaluation before surgical resection. His medical history includes inoperable coronary artery disease, heart failure with a left ventricular ejection fraction (LVEF) of 35%, hypertension, and hyperlipidemia. Angina is stable, occurring approximately monthly, and he has no orthopnea or paroxysmal nocturnal dyspnea. Medications include lisinopril, carvedilol, furosemide, simvastatin, and daily aspirin. He plays golf weekly, using a cart, walks 2 miles three to four times weekly, and carries groceries up a flight of stairs to his apartment.

On physical examination, the pulse rate is 64/min, and blood pressure is 120/64 mm Hg. Jugular venous pressure is 6 cm. On cardiopulmonary examination, the lungs are clear to auscultation, and the heart is regular without an S₃. There is no peripheral edema. Laboratory studies, including complete blood count, serum electrolyte levels, and renal function, are normal. The electrocardiogram is unchanged, with a normal sinus rhythm and evidence of an old inferior infarction.

Which of the following is the most appropriate next step in the preoperative evaluation of this patient?

(A) Plasma B-type natriuretic peptide measurement
(B) Echocardiography
(C) Exercise stress testing
(D) Nuclear imaging for LVEF
(E) No further evaluation

Item 48

A 54-year-old man is evaluated for a 3-day history of nasal congestion, rhinorrhea, scratchy throat, and non-productive cough. He has had no obvious contact with ill patients and does not have a history of allergic rhinitis. He is otherwise healthy except for a history of hypertension well controlled with hydrochlorothiazide and lisinopril.

On physical examination, the temperature is 37.3 °C (99.2 °F). There is no conjunctival erythema, pharyngeal exudate, cervical lymphadenopathy, or adventitious lung sounds.

Which of the following treatments is supported by evidence for improving symptoms in patients with this syndrome?

(A) Echinacea
(B) Antihistamines
(C) Pseudoephedrine
(D) Zinc
(E) Vitamin C

Item 49

A 50-year-old woman is evaluated for a rash on the back of her elbows and knees. A similar rash has occurred in the past, with her first episode as a young adult. She has used over-the-counter hydrocortisone cream without relief. She does not smoke or drink and is otherwise healthy.

The skin examination of the back of the patient's elbows is **shown**.

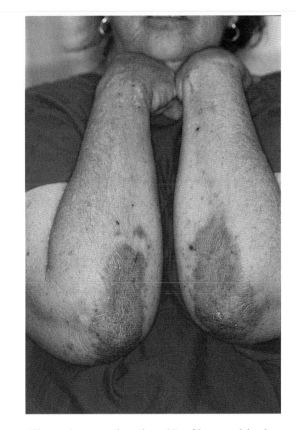

The rash covers less than 3% of her total body area. Laboratory studies, including complete blood count and differential, basic serum chemistries, and urinalysis, are normal.

Which of the following is the most appropriate next step in the management of this patient?

(A) Topical coal tar
(B) High-potency topical corticosteroids
(C) Topical tacrolimus
(D) Phototherapy
(E) Methotrexate

Item 50

A 65-year-old woman is admitted to the hospital with unstable angina. Cardiac catheterization shows stable coronary artery disease, which does not require coronary artery bypass graft. Her history includes coronary artery disease and stable angina controlled with medications. She has also followed a low-fat diet. Her medications include metoprolol, 50 mg twice daily; aspirin, 81 mg daily; and isosorbide dinitrate, 20 mg three times daily. She is not experiencing any further chest pain.

Laboratory studies:

Serum troponin	Normal
Serum total cholesterol	164 mg/dL (4.24 mmol/L)

Serum triglycerides	120 mg/dL (1.35 mmol/L)
Serum high-density lipoprotein cholesterol	50 mg/dL (1.29 mmol/L)
Serum low-density lipoprotein cholesterol	90 mg/dL (2.33 mmol/L)

Which of the following is the most appropriate next step in the management of this patient?

(A) Low-cholesterol diet
(B) Exercise program
(C) Niacin therapy
(D) Statin therapy

Item 51

A 35-year-old woman is evaluated for dysmenorrhea. The bleeding has improved since she began taking an oral contraceptive 6 months ago, but she continually forgets to take the pill daily, despite the use of behavioral techniques. As a result, she experiences bothersome episodes of breakthrough bleeding, and she has frequently worried over the uncertainty of possibly being pregnant. She is otherwise healthy.

Physical examination, including vital signs, is normal.

Which of the following is the most appropriate next step in the management of this patient?

(A) Condoms plus contraceptive pill
(B) Copper intrauterine device
(C) Progestin-only contraceptive pill
(D) Topical contraceptive patch

Item 52

A 45-year-old man undergoes preoperative evaluation before elective arthroscopic knee repair of a sports-related injury. His medical history includes hypertension treated with atenolol, hydrochlorothiazide, and daily aspirin. He has no bleeding problems associated with prior tooth extractions or an appendectomy he underwent as a teenager or any other medical problems. He usually drinks one to two glasses of wine with dinner, does not smoke, and does not use illicit drugs. Results of laboratory studies performed 6 months ago, including serum electrolyte levels, creatinine level, and lipid profile, were normal.

On physical examination, pulse rate is 64/min, and blood pressure is 120/72 mm Hg. The remainder of the examination is normal.

Which of the following is the most appropriate approach to preoperative laboratory testing in this patient?

(A) Electrocardiography and serum electrolyte and creatinine measurement
(B) Chest radiography, complete blood count, and serum electrolyte measurement
(C) Electrocardiography, serum electrolyte measurement, complete blood count, and urinalysis
(D) Complete blood count, prothrombin time/INR, and urinalysis

Item 53

A 34-year-old woman from Arkansas is evaluated because she is concerned she may have been bitten by a brown recluse spider on the lateral aspect of her right forearm. She describes the bite as feeling "like a pinprick" and states that it is beginning to sting. The patient reports that the spider was brown, with a "violin-shaped" pattern on its back. She has seasonal allergies well controlled with fexofenadine during the fall and is otherwise healthy.

On physical examination, the lesion is warm and erythematous.

Which of the following is the most appropriate management option for this patient?

(A) Fexofenadine
(B) Ice application, wound elevation, and avoidance of use of arm muscles
(C) Intralesional triamcinolone
(D) Hyperbaric oxygen therapy
(E) Incision and suctioning of venom

Item 54

A 72-year-old man is evaluated during a routine examination. His history includes chronic obstructive pulmonary disease and hypertension. He has used oxygen, 2 L/min, for the past year, mostly at night. He snores loudly but does not stop breathing and has no daytime somnolence. Since reporting erectile dysfunction 3 months earlier, he has received testosterone cypionate injections, 200 mg, every 3 weeks. His other medications include bronchodilator inhalers, hydrochlorothiazide, and aspirin.

On physical examination, oxygen saturation on room air is 90%, and lung sounds are diminished but clear. He has atrophic testes and minimal bilateral gynecomastia. Laboratory studies include a hematocrit of 51%, leukocyte count of 6500/μL (6.5×10^9/L), and platelet count of 220,000/μL (220×10^9/L). His values from 6 months ago included a hematocrit of 44%, leukocyte count of 6700/μL (6.7×10^9/L), and platelet count of 230,000/μL (230×10^9/L).

Which of the following is the most appropriate management of this patient's erythrocytosis?

(A) Increase supplemental oxygen
(B) Refer for polysomnography
(C) Initiate phlebotomy
(D) Measure leukocyte alkaline phosphatase level
(E) Decrease testosterone dosage

Item 55

A 65-year-old man is evaluated during a routine visit. His medical history includes hypertension controlled with hydrochlorothiazide. He is otherwise healthy.

On physical examination, the blood pressure is 125/85 mm Hg, the BMI is 30, and the remainder of the examination is unremarkable.

Laboratory studies:

Serum total cholesterol (fasting)	179 mg/dL (4.63 mmol/L)
Serum triglycerides (fasting)	200 mg/dL (2.26 mmol/L)
Serum high-density lipoprotein cholesterol (fasting)	39 mg/dL (1.01 mmol/L)
Serum low-density lipoprotein cholesterol (fasting)	100 mg/dL (2.59 mmo/L)

Which of the following is the most appropriate next step in the management of this patient?

(A) Statin therapy

(B) Fibric acid derivative

(C) Serum low-density lipoprotein cholesterol particle-size measurement

(D) Diet and exercise

Item 56

A 73-year-old woman who lives in a nursing home is evaluated for a 6-month history of frequent awakening during the night, although she falls asleep without difficulty. The patient is distressed because she is fatigued throughout the day. Her medical history is significant for dementia secondary to cerebral vascular disease and hypertension. She does not have urinary incontinence. Her Mini–Mental State Examination score is 20/30. A diagnosis of primary insomnia is established, and a recommendation is given to the patient to avoid drinking caffeinated beverages and eating before bedtime, as well as to minimize nighttime disturbances. When nighttime awakening persists, the patient begins taking triazolam before bedtime. After a few days of treatment, the patient is noted by the nursing home staff to be confused.

On physical examination, she is afebrile. The pulse rate is 63/min, respiration rate is 12/min, and blood pressure is 120/72 mm Hg. The neurologic examination indicates no new focal findings. She is oriented to person but not to place or time. Laboratory studies, including complete blood count, serum chemistries, and urinalysis, are normal.

Which of the following is the most appropriate next step in management?

(A) Discontinue triazolam

(B) Decrease triazolam dose

(C) Perform CT of the head and blood and urine cultures

(D) Substitute diphenhydramine for triazolam

(E) Initiate cognitive behavioral therapy

Item 57

A 56-year-old woman is evaluated during a routine annual visit. The patient would like to lose weight. She works as a teacher and is physically active, walking briskly 2 or 3 times a week for 20 or 30 minutes. She does not smoke and drinks alcohol only on occasion. Her medical history includes hypertension and hyperlipidemia, both well controlled with medications.

On physical examination, the blood pressure is 135/88 mm Hg. The BMI is 36. The remainder of the physical examination is normal. Laboratory studies include a fasting plasma glucose level of 105 mg/dL (5.83 mmol/L) and a serum thyroid-stimulating hormone level of 2.5 µU/mL (2.5 mU/L). A diagnosis of class II obesity is established. A goal is set for a 5% to 15% reduction in weight.

Which of the following diets should be advised for this patient?

(A) A balanced low-calorie diet (1200 to 1500 Kcal/day)

(B) A very-low-calorie diet (<1000 Kcal/day)

(C) A reduced-fat diet (fat constitutes <30% of total caloric intake/day)

(D) A low-carbohydrate diet (<35 g of carbohydrates/day)

Item 58

A 27-year-old man is evaluated for left lower-extremity pain with episodic swelling and skin discoloration 6 months after a motor vehicle accident. His current medications include acetaminophen, oxycodone as needed, and nortriptyline. The remainder of the medical history is noncontributory.

The physical examination, including examination of the joints, is unremarkable except for an inability to flex the knee without inducing pain. The neurologic examination is normal. Radiographs of the knee, femur, hip, and lumbar spine are unremarkable except for patchy demineralization of the femur. MRI of the lumbar spine is normal. A bone scan shows increased uptake in the left tibia.

In addition to analgesics, which of the following is the most efficacious treatment for improving this patient's pain?

(A) Bisphosphonates

(B) Transcutaneous electrical stimulation

(C) Tricyclic antidepressants

(D) Corticosteroids

(E) Fluoxetine

Item 59

A 76-year-old man is evaluated for a syncopal episode that occurred as he was stepping into his truck; he is accompanied by his wife. He reports experiencing palpitations before the episode occurred. His wife states he looked suddenly sweaty and ashen before passing out. On regaining consciousness approximately 1 minute later, he appeared slightly dazed but was oriented and mentating normally. He reports remembering nothing prior to the syncope except for a sense of his heart racing. There was no bowel or bladder incontinence. His medical history is significant for coronary artery disease and stable angina, diabetes mellitus, hypertension, and hyperlipidemia, for which he takes atenolol, fosinopril, metformin, simvastatin, and aspirin.

On physical examination, pulse rate is 64/min, and blood pressure is 126/74 mm Hg. The remainder of the examination, including cardiac and neurologic evaluation, is unremarkable. Results of electrocardiography are consistent with his most recent electrocardiogram, with evidence of an old bifascicular block. Results from 24-hour ambulatory electrocardiography, exercise stress testing, and echocardiography are normal.

Which of the following is the most appropriate next step in diagnosis?

(A) Electrophysiologic testing
(B) 72-Hour ambulatory electrocardiography
(C) Cardiac catheterization
(D) Tilt-table testing
(E) External or implanted continuous loop recorder

Item 60

A 35-year-old man is evaluated for red eye and acute onset of right eye pain. He wears contact lenses daily. Fluorescein staining is positive for corneal abrasion without a dendritic, or branching, pattern. He is instructed to stop wearing the contact lenses until the abrasion is healed. He calls the next day to report that the pain has worsened, even though he has not worn his contact lenses.

On examination, compared with the previous day's findings, the patient appears to be in more pain, visual acuity of the right eye is worse with Snellen's test, and the abrasion is larger on fluorescein staining. The eye remains red, and there is a mucopurulent discharge.

Which of the following is the most likely diagnosis?

(A) Hypopyon
(B) Infectious keratitis
(C) Herpetic keratitis
(D) Anterior uveitis

Item 61

A 67-year-old man undergoes urgent evaluation for a 2-month history of low back pain radiating down his right leg that has worsened over the past 3 days, causing him difficulty with walking due to leg weakness. He has also been unable to urinate for the past 24 hours. His medical history is notable for chronic obstructive pulmonary disease, diabetes mellitus, prostate cancer, and hyperlipidemia. Medications include bronchodilator inhalers, insulin, leuprolide, simvastatin, and aspirin.

On physical examination, he is in obvious discomfort. The temperature is normal, pulse rate is 88/min, and blood pressure is 148/72 mm Hg. He has severe lower-

lumbar tenderness to palpation, with no bony abnormalities. Lower-extremity strength is 4/5 bilaterally, and the straight-leg-raising test is positive on the right. On rectal examination, there is decreased rectal sphincter tone and diminished sensation over the perineal region and buttocks. His prostate is asymmetric and hard.

Which of the following is the most appropriate diagnostic imaging evaluation for this patient?

(A) CT of the lumbar spine
(B) MRI of the lumbar spine
(C) Radiography of the lumbar spine
(D) Positron emission tomography
(E) Radionuclide bone scan

Item 62

A 54-year-old woman is evaluated for a 4-day history of an acute headache that has been gradually worsening and is located diffusely on the left side of her head. The patient is nauseous but does not have photophobia, fever, chills, history of tick exposures, trauma, stiff neck, muscle weakness, parasthesias, or bowel or bladder problems. She awakens with the headache and it gradually worsens during the day, and she experiences slight relief with acetaminophen and ibuprofen. She has a family history of migraines and, as a teenager and in her mid-30s, had a few migraine headaches that were more severe than her current episode and were associated with photophobia and severe fatigue. However, since those episodes, she had been headache free until now.

Her medical history includes hypertension, diabetes mellitus, breast cancer for which she underwent lumpectomy 4 years ago, and osteoarthritis. Current medications include atenolol, metformin, tamoxifen, and enteric-coated aspirin.

On physical examination, the patient appears to be in mild distress, but vital signs are normal. The neurologic evaluation is significant for decreased vibratory and monofilament perception in the bilateral lower extremities in a stocking distribution.

Which of the following is the most appropriate management option for this patient?

(A) MRI of the head
(B) Lumbar puncture and cerebrospinal fluid analysis
(C) Bone scan
(D) Enzyme-linked immunosorbent assay for *Borrelia burgdorferi*
(E) Sumatriptan therapy

Item 63

A 22-year-old nursing school graduate is evaluated during a pre-employment physical examination for a job at a children's hospital. She has systemic lupus erythematosus, which is well controlled with prednisone, 10 mg daily. She has no recollection of having had chickenpox as a child; results of a varicella titer are negative.

Which of the following is the most appropriate recommendation?

(A) No vaccination

(B) Single vaccination (shortened series), clear for work

(C) Single vaccination (shortened series), delay work for 4 weeks

(D) Two-dose vaccination series over 6 weeks, clear for work

(E) Two-dose vaccination series over 6 weeks, delay work for 4 weeks

Item 64

A 25-year-old man requests a second opinion for evaluation of episodes of large, raised red welts and intense itching all over his body. The lesions usually last at least 24 hours and then disappear. He has at least two to three episodes every week, and he cannot identify any specific trigger for the attacks. He was told his condition was hives and was given hydroxyzine and then fexofenadine, neither of which significantly controlled his symptoms. He reports no mouth or lip swelling, no difficulty breathing, and no gastrointestinal symptoms. His weight has been stable.

On examination, temperature is 38.1 °C (100.7 °F). There are discrete dark wheal and flare lesions consistent with urticaria on both arms and legs and the trunk and back. Some lesions look like purpura. Urinalysis shows erythrocytes and erythrocyte casts.

Which of the following is most likely to help establish the diagnosis?

(A) C1 esterase inhibitor measurement

(B) Urine eosinophil count

(C) Skin biopsy

(D) Antigenic skin testing

(E) Thyroid-stimulating hormone measurement

Item 65

A 40-year-old woman is evaluated during a routine visit. She has had two uneventful pregnancies and deliveries, one 4 years ago and the other 6 years ago, and now wishes to discuss contraceptive options. She and her husband have been using condoms, but they have had some problems with condom breakage and inconsistent use. The patient does not want additional children, but her husband is undecided on the issue. She has regular, very heavy periods that last 6 days, including dysmenorrhea for the first 3 days. Her history is significant for a deep vein thrombosis after a long car ride 2 years ago. No further evaluation was completed at that time. She is otherwise healthy and does not smoke. Physical examination, including vital signs, is normal.

Which of the following is the safest and most effective way to prevent pregnancy in this patient?

(A) Oral contraceptive pill

(B) Topical contraceptive patch

(C) Diaphragm

(D) Levonorgestrel intrauterine device

Item 66

A 70-year-old man is evaluated for an episode of herpes zoster. Two months ago, he developed a painful rash over the right trunk and was examined after symptoms persisted for 1 week. He was advised to use acetaminophen for pain and was given a prescription for acetaminophen with codeine. He continues to experience sharp pain, particularly when trying to sleep, and he has not found the pain medications to be effective. His history is significant for benign prostatic hyperplasia and hypertension for which he takes doxazosin and hydrochlorothiazide. On physical examination, vital signs are normal. Examination of the right posterior trunk reveals scattered areas of hypopigmentation in a dermatomal distribution. The patient notes tingling and pain with light touch.

Which of the following is the most appropriate treatment for this patient's condition?

(A) Oral famciclovir

(B) Oral prednisone

(C) Oral gabapentin

(D) Oral oxycodone

Item 67

A 50-year-old man is evaluated for chronic, intermittent chest pain, unrelated to exertion. After being hospitalized 6 months ago with a suspected acute coronary syndrome for the same symptoms, a coronary catheterization showed normal coronary arteries. Subsequent testing for gastroesophageal disease was normal, and results of echocardiography and CT of the chest were unremarkable. He does not use cocaine. The patient continues to have chronic, daily, bothersome chest pain. Although he is anxious and distressed by his pain, he is not experiencing significant anxiety, stress, or episodes of overwhelming panic.

The physical examination is normal. Results of electrocardiography performed today are normal and are unchanged from his recent hospitalization.

Which of the following treatments has been shown to be helpful for this condition?

(A) Colchicine

(B) NSAIDs

(C) Tricyclic antidepressants

(D) Fluoxetine

(E) Tramadol

Item 68

An 82-year-old woman is evaluated for a 4.5-kg (10-lb) weight loss from baseline over the past 6 months. Her medical history includes hypertension, depression, and osteoarthritis of the knee, treated with hydrochlorothiazide, sertraline, and occasional ibuprofen as needed. She has never smoked. She states that her mood is good and has a score of 1 on the Five-Item Geriatric Depression Scale. She shops on her own at the grocery store and sometimes finds it difficult to do so more than once weekly. The review of systems, including for anorexia, abdominal pain, and change in bowel habits, is negative.

On physical examination, vital signs are normal. The BMI is 18.6. The lungs are clear to auscultation, and the cardiac, abdominal, and rectal examinations are normal. There is no pedal edema. Laboratory studies, including complete blood count and serum thyroid-stimulating hormone level, are normal. Results of a recent series of fecal occult blood testing and chest radiography were normal.

Which of the following is the most appropriate next step in the management of this patient?

(A) CT of the abdomen
(B) Shopping or meal preparation assistance
(C) Colonoscopy
(D) Substitution of mirtazapine for sertraline
(E) Discontinuation of ibuprofen

Item 69

A 74-year-old woman is evaluated for a 5-year history of chronic dizziness. She describes her dizziness as a mixture of vertigo, light-headedness, and unsteadiness when walking. She also reports chronic fatigue and trouble falling asleep but denies depressed mood, anhedonia, or symptoms of anxiety. Her medical history includes osteoarthritis, noninsulin-dependent diabetes mellitus, and mild hearing loss.

Physical examination is normal except for bony enlargement in both knees, decreased vibratory sense in the feet, and unsteadiness with tandem gait but no falling or other neurologic abnormalities. An audiogram discloses a bilateral sensorineural hearing loss consistent with presbycusis (that is, the degenerative hearing loss most commonly occurring with aging). MRI of the head shows mild cortical atrophy and scattered white-matter abnormalities but no evidence of space-occupying lesions or prior infarcts. Laboratory studies, including hemoglobin and serum electrolyte levels, are normal. Results of electrocardiography are unremarkable.

Which of the following is the most appropriate treatment for this patient?

(A) Vestibular rehabilitation exercises
(B) Habituation exercises
(C) Paroxetine and cognitive behavioral therapy
(D) Vestibular nerve ablation
(E) Meclizine and an antiemetic

Item 70

A 32-year-old man is evaluated during a follow-up examination. Last night, he visited the emergency department with acute chest heaviness, palpitations, dyspnea, and a tingling in the tips of both fingers and in the perioral region. He also had mild abdominal discomfort and a subsequent bout of diarrhea consisting of loose stools without blood. His symptoms began while he was leisurely walking his dog. He reports having had similar symptoms three times over the past 2 months, including a previous admission to the emergency department, the examination results of which were unremarkable and the symptoms of which were attributed to stress. The patient used to run 3 to 5 miles two to three times weekly but has ceased because of concern over his heart, although he never experienced these symptoms while running. He also has been reluctant to leave home except to go to work because he is afraid that he might have another episode in public. He does not drink or use illicit drugs. He takes no dietary supplements, weight-loss pills, or medications. He denies depression and anhedonia, nervousness, anxiety, or feeling on edge during the past month. He also states that he was not feeling stressed last night. His father died of a myocardial infarction at age 73 years.

On physical examination, the patient is alert and oriented. The heart rate is 93/min, and the blood pressure is 132/78 mm Hg. The remainder of the examination, including cardiopulmonary evaluation, is normal.

Laboratory studies from last evening's emergency department visit, including serum electrolyte, calcium, creatinine and blood urea nitrogen levels and cardiac enzymes and urinalysis, were normal. The urine drug screen was negative, and the electrocardiogram taken while the patient was symptomatic was unremarkable.

Which of the following is the most appropriate initial management option for this patient?

(A) Adenosine stress testing
(B) Serum thyroid-stimulating hormone and 24-hour urine catecholamine and metanephrine measurement
(C) Paroxetine
(D) Quetiapine

Item 71

A 23-year-old woman is evaluated for abdominal pain of several years' duration and a 5.4-kg (12-lb) weight loss occurring over the past few months. The pain is diffuse, although mostly occurring in the lower abdomen, and is crampy in nature and so severe at times that it "doubles her over." She does not experience an increase or relief of pain with oral intake. The pain is frequently associated with diarrhea, especially when she is under stress, or intermittent constipation, although on most days she has a normal, formed bowel movement. Currently, she reports having up to six bowel movements daily, consisting of loose, watery, and foul-smelling stools, but without blood or mucous. She gets some relief of pain with defecation but denies fecal urgency. She has taken loperamide, with relief, for her diarrhea. She has never sought care for her abdominal problems in the past but seeks help now because the pain has become more severe and is interfering with her activities of daily living. Her family history is remarkable for irritable bowel syndrome.

Recent laboratory studies indicated that she has mild anemia, for which she takes a daily iron supplement.

On physical examination, she is a thin-appearing, fatigued woman in mild distress. Temperature is 36.9 °C (98.4 °F), respiration rate is 12/min, and blood pressure is 114/53 mm Hg. The height is 162.56 cm (64 in), and weight is 57.6 kg (127 lb).

The abdominal examination reveals normal bowel sounds and no hepatosplenomegaly, and the abdomen is diffusely tender without guarding, rebound, or rigidity. No palpable masses are appreciated. The remainder of the examination, including pelvic and rectal examination, is unremarkable.

Which of the following is the best diagnostic option for this patient?

(A) CT of the abdomen
(B) Colonoscopy
(C) Flexible sigmoidoscopy
(D) Abdominal ultrasonography
(E) Fecal calprotectin analysis

Item 72

A 47-year-old man is evaluated for right lateral shoulder pain. He has been pitching during batting practice for his son's little league baseball team for the past 2 months. He has shoulder pain when lifting his arm overhead and also when lying on the shoulder while sleeping. Acetaminophen has not been helpful. The history is noncontributory.

On physical examination, he has no shoulder deformities or swelling. Range of motion is normal. He has subacromial tenderness to palpation, with shoulder pain elicited at 60 degrees of passive abduction. He also has pain with resisted midarc abduction but no pain with resisted elbow flexion or forearm supination. He is able to smoothly lower his right arm from a fully abducted position, and his arm strength for abduction and external rotation against resistance is normal.

Which of the following is the most likely diagnosis in this patient?

(A) Adhesive capsulitis
(B) Bicipital tendonitis
(C) Glenohumeral arthritis
(D) Rotator cuff tear
(E) Rotator cuff tendonitis

Item 73

A 21-year-old man is evaluated for painful sores in his mouth. Episodes of these sores have occurred two to three times yearly since he was 16 years old, and he believes they are associated with stress. They usually appear on the inside of his mouth as a single, round, painful lesion, lasting for 5 to 10 days and resolving without scarring. He now has concerns about whether he might have herpes.

He has had no fever, chills, arthralgias, genital ulcers, rashes, eye problems, diarrhea, abdominal pain, or weight loss. He is sexually active and has had only a few sexual partners, although he is currently monogamous. All of his sexual interactions have been heterosexual. He does not use illicit drugs. Results of HIV testing for his sexual partner and him from 3 months ago were negative. The remainder of the history is noncontributory.

On physical examination, the vital signs are normal. The oral examination is significant for the lesion **shown**.

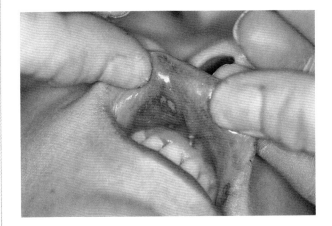

The remainder of the physical examination is unremarkable.

Which of the following is the most appropriate management option for this patient?

(A) Thalidomide
(B) Herpes simplex testing
(C) HIV testing
(D) Reassurance
(E) Candidiasis culture

Item 74

A 68-year-old man undergoes preoperative evaluation before abdominal aortic aneurysm repair. His history is significant for coronary artery disease, hypertension, and hyperlipidemia. His medications include lisinopril, hydrochlorothiazide, simvastatin, and daily aspirin. He has not had angina since undergoing three-vessel coronary artery bypass graft 4 years ago. He plays golf weekly, walking and carrying his clubs on a hilly course, walks 2 miles in 35 to 40 minutes three to four times weekly, and vacuums the house.

On physical examination, the pulse rate is 78/min, and the blood pressure is 140/87 mm Hg. The remainder of the examination is unremarkable. Results of electrocardiography are consistent with his most recent electrocardiogram, with evidence of an old inferior infarction. Laboratory studies, including complete blood count, serum electrolyte level, and renal function, are normal.

Which of the following is the most appropriate perioperative management in this patient?

(A) Atenolol
(B) Exercise stress testing
(C) Echocardiography
(D) Intraoperative right heart catheterization

Item 75

A 36-year-old day-care provider is evaluated in the emergency department after sustaining an injury to her head and neck. On the previous day, a large box of toys slipped off a high shelf as she was taking it down; the box landed on the back of her head and neck. She estimates the weight of the box to have been between 6.8 to 9 kg (15 to 20 lb). She now has persistent neck and shoulder pain and had difficulty sleeping last night. She reports no hand or arm numbness or weakness, or persistent headache. She sustained no other injuries from the accident.

On physical examination, pulse rate is 108/min, respiration rate is 14/min, and blood pressure is 128/72 mm Hg. Her neck is tender over the shoulder blades and trapezius, but there is no midline tenderness on palpation. She has full range of motion of the cervical spine with flexion, extension, and rotation, although rotation is painful at the extremes. She is anxious, but alert and oriented; neurologic findings are normal.

Which of the following is the best management option for this patient?

(A) Symptomatic treatment
(B) MRI of the cervical spine
(C) CT of the cervical spine
(D) Radiography of the cervical spine

Item 76

A 69-year-old woman is evaluated for persistent fatigue. Her weight is stable, she is sleeping well, and her mood is good. The medical history is notable for hypothyroidism, diabetes mellitus, recently diagnosed glaucoma, and osteoporosis. Prescription medications include alendronate, glyburide, levothyroxine, and timolol and latanoprost eye drops.

On physical examination, the temperature is 36.9 °C (98.4 °F), pulse rate is 58/min, and blood pressure is 108/62 mmHg. The remainder of the physical examination is unremarkable. Laboratory studies include a hemoglobin A_{1c} of 7.5%, and a serum thyroid-stimulating hormone level of 6.4 µU/L (6.4 mU/mL). Renal function and liver chemistry tests are normal.

Which of the following medications is the most likely cause for this patient's fatigue?

(A) Alendronate
(B) Glyburide
(C) Latanoprost eye drops
(D) Levothyroxine
(E) Timolol eye drops

Item 77

A 38-year-old woman is evaluated because she thinks she might be depressed. She reports feeling tired all the time and sometimes cries with little provocation. She denies anhedonia, problems with sleeping or appetite, suicidal ideation, psychomotor retardation, or problems with concentration. She has two children, ages 4 and 2 years, and finds motherhood frustrating and challenging, but also rewarding. She sometimes feels guilty because she works part-time and believes that she has failed to meet her end

of the family's financial responsibilities. Her medical history is noncontributory. She takes no medications except for a multivitamin. She drinks 1 glass of wine on most evenings and does not use illicit drugs.

On physical examination, she appears well groomed, alert, and oriented. The remainder of the physical examination is unremarkable. Laboratory studies, including complete blood count, serum electrolyte, creatinine, blood urea nitrogen, and thyroid-stimulating hormone levels and urinalysis, are normal.

Which of the following is the most appropriate management option for this patient?

(A) Paroxetine
(B) Follow-up monitoring
(C) Psychotherapy
(D) Clonazepam
(E) Quetiapine

Item 78

A 60-year-old woman undergoes preoperative evaluation for abdominal hysterectomy and bilateral oophorectomy. Her medical history is significant for depression, breast cancer with no evidence of malignancy after lumpectomy, osteopenia, and seizure disorder. Medications include fluoxetine, tamoxifen, alendronate, carbamazepine, and as-needed naproxen for pain; she also takes the herbal supplements ginkgo, garlic, and valerian. Her depression and seizure disorder are well controlled.

Physical examination, including blood pressure, is normal.

In addition to stopping the herbal supplements 1 week and naproxen 2 to 3 days before surgery, which of the following is the most appropriate approach to the perioperative management of the fluoxetine, tamoxifen, and alendronate in this patient?

(A) Stop fluoxetine and tamoxifen 1 week before surgery; continue alendronate
(B) Stop fluoxetine and alendronate 1 week before surgery; continue tamoxifen
(C) Continue all three drugs perioperatively
(D) Stop all three drugs 1 week before surgery

Item 79

A 55-year-old woman is evaluated for severe, intolerable hot flushes that began shortly after she stopped estrogen and progesterone hormone replacement therapy 2 weeks ago. She reports that her current hot flushes are as severe as the symptoms that prompted her to begin hormone replacement therapy 3 years ago. She is otherwise healthy and exercises daily. Physical examination, including vital signs, is normal.

Which of the following is the most appropriate management strategy at this time?

(A) Increased exercise
(B) Bupropion

(C) Gradual reduction of hormone replacement therapy

(D) Reinstitution of progesterone alone

Item 80

A 45-year-old obese woman undergoes evaluation after learning her nonfasting serum total cholesterol level, which was measured at a health screening fair 1 month ago, was 260 mg/dL (6.72 mmol/L). The review of systems indicates increasingly heavy menstruation and constipation. Her family history is negative for coronary artery disease. The patient is otherwise healthy and does not smoke.

On physical examination, blood pressure is 120/80 mm Hg. The remainder of the examination is normal.

Laboratory studies:

Serum total cholesterol	256 mg/dL (6.62 mmol/L)
Serum triglycerides	205 mg/dL (2.31 mmol/L)
Serum high-density lipoprotein cholesterol	40 mg/dL (1.03 mmol/L)
Serum low-density lipoprotein cholesterol	175 mg/dL (4.53 mmol/L)

Which of the following is the most appropriate next step in the management of this patient?

(A) Fibric acid derivative

(B) Statin

(C) Fish oil supplement

(D) Serum thyroid-stimulating hormone measurement

Item 81

A 67-year-old man is evaluated for pain in his knees with ambulation. He smokes 1 pack of cigarettes per day and drinks alcohol occasionally. His medical history includes hypertension controlled with metoprolol, and hyperlipidemia controlled with simvastatin.

On physical examination, the pulse rate is 65/min, respiration rate is 14/min, and blood pressure is 145/92 mm Hg. The BMI is 36, and the abdominal circumference is 130 cm (51 in). The musculoskeletal examination reveals crepitus on knee flexion and extension but no synovial joint effusions or signs of inflammation. Laboratory studies indicate a fasting plasma glucose level of 110 mg/dL (6.11 mmol/L).

A moderate 5% weight loss will be associated with which of the following outcomes in this patient?

(A) Decreased risk in cardiovascular mortality

(B) Decreased risk in overall mortality

(C) Decreased risk of progression to type 2 diabetes mellitus

(D) Improvement in symptoms of osteoarthritis

(E) Social and economic benefits from weight loss

Item 82

A 55-year-old man is evaluated for a 2-week history of nasal congestion and cough. The cough was initially nonproductive but over the past week has become productive of greenish-yellow sputum that he believes is coming from his chest. He also states that his anterior chest is sore, especially when he coughs. He has not had fevers, chills, or dyspnea. The patient is otherwise healthy.

The physical examination, including vital signs, is normal.

The presence of which of the following comorbid medical conditions would be an indication for antibiotics in the treatment of this condition?

(A) Heart failure

(B) Diabetes mellitus

(C) Asthma

(D) Renal failure

(E) Chronic obstructive pulmonary disease

Item 83

A 45-year-old woman with known fibromyalgia for the past year is evaluated for persistent musculoskeletal symptoms and fatigue and an inability to function in her job at her premorbid level. Compared with her initial presentation, several of her symptoms, including sleep disturbances and mood problems, have improved with the initiation of fluoxetine, 40 mg, in the morning and nortriptyline, 10 mg, at night; however, her fatigue and diffuse musculoskeletal pain continue to be bothersome. She takes no other medications.

The physical examination is remarkable for tender points over numerous muscles in all four quadrants of the body. Laboratory studies, including complete blood count, erythrocyte sedimentation rate, serum B_{12} level, and thyroid-stimulating hormone level, are normal.

Which of the following nonpharmacologic therapies is most appropriate in this patient at this time?

(A) Relaxation and flexibility training

(B) Ultrasonography

(C) Massage therapy

(D) Graded exercise therapy

Item 84

A 19-year-old woman is evaluated for a 2-year history of lower abdominal pain. She is particularly bothered by the pain in the first few days of her menstrual period. She has tried acetaminophen and cimetidine without clear benefit. She has mild constipation but no diarrhea or genitourinary symptoms and is currently not sexually active.

On physical examination, there is some mild, lower abdominal tenderness but no hepatosplenomegaly, masses, or guarding. Bilateral lower-abdominal tenderness is detected on pelvic examination, but the findings are otherwise normal.

Laboratory studies, including hemoglobin and urinalysis, are normal. Results of abdominal-pelvic ultrasonography are normal.

Which of the following is the most appropriate treatment for alleviating this patient's pain?

(A) Psyllium
(B) Naproxen
(C) Oral contraceptives
(D) Anesthetic/corticosteroid injection
(E) Tegaserod

Item 85

An 81-year-old man is evaluated for a 6-month history of a constant buzzing sound in both ears. The noise interferes with reading, watching television, and sleep. He denies headache, vertigo, or sinus pain. His medical history includes diabetes mellitus, hypertension, coronary artery disease, and emphysema for which he takes glyburide metformin, metoprolol, clopidogrel, and an albuterol inhaler. Depression screening results are negative.

On physical examination, the pulse rate is 62/min, and blood pressure is 137/84 mm Hg. Cardiopulmonary examination is normal. No sounds are audible over his carotid arteries or periaural region, and there are no pulsatile neck masses. On cranial nerve examination, the patient only faintly hears finger rubbing next to both ear canals.

Which of the following is the most appropriate initial management step in this patient?

(A) Audiometric testing
(B) MRI of the head
(C) Magnetic resonance angiography
(D) Institution of sertraline
(E) Cessation of clopidogrel

Item 86

A 67-year-old man is evaluated during a routine visit. His history is significant for coronary artery disease, hypertension, hyperlipidemia, and benign prostatic hyperplasia. He mentions that, although he is still interested in sexual activity, he has had difficulty during the past year maintaining an erection. He is happily married, enjoying retirement, and denies being depressed or anxious. His medications include metformin, terazosin, simvastatin, lisinopril, sublingual nitroglycerin, and aspirin.

His pulse rate is 64/min, and blood pressure is 128/76 mm Hg. Genitourinary examination shows an enlarged, smooth prostate without nodules or asymmetry; his testicles are of normal size and consistency, and there are no fibrous penile plaques.

Which of the following is the most appropriate initial treatment in this patient?

(A) Intracavernous alprostadil
(B) Penile implant
(C) Sildenafil

(D) Testosterone
(E) Trazodone

Item 87

An 83-year-old man is evaluated for left shoulder pain he experienced after falling from a ladder and landing on his outstretched left arm. He reports shoulder weakness and pain over his shoulder and upper back that is worse at night when lying on the shoulder.

On physical examination, he has subacromial tenderness and decreased strength with external rotation and abduction of the shoulder. He is not fully able to abduct his right shoulder and cannot smoothly lower his raised, abducted right arm to his side. He has some right bicipital groove tenderness and minimal pain caused by elbow flexion, but the biceps muscle strength and contour is normal. Radiography of the shoulder shows some degenerative changes of the glenohumeral joint but no fractures or dislocation.

Which of the following is the most likely diagnosis in this patient?

(A) Adhesive capsulitis
(B) Glenohumeral arthritis
(C) Rotator cuff tear
(D) Rotator cuff tendonitis
(E) Ruptured biceps tendon

Item 88

A 67-year-old man is evaluated for a painful right lower-extremity ulceration that developed over the past week. He reports some clear weeping drainage from the wound but no streaking or redness, and he has not had a fever. His medical history is notable for venous insufficiency, hypertension, peripheral vascular disease, and hyperlipidemia. Daily medications include lisinopril, aspirin, felodipine, furosemide, and a statin.

On physical examination, the temperature is normal, pulse rate is 76/min, and blood pressure is 104/73 mm Hg. On examination of the lower extremities, there is a shallow, red-based, 3-cm ulceration with a moderate serosanguinous exudate above the right medial malleolus, with no surrounding erythema or warmth. Bilateral symmetric 2-mm pitting pretibial edema and hyperpigmentation of the anterior shins are also noted. His lower legs and feet are hairless, and the pedal pulses are not palpable. The ankle-brachial index on the right is 0.7.

Laboratory studies include a leukocyte count of 7300/mL (7.3×10^9/L) with a normal differential, blood urea nitrogen level of 30 mg/dL (10.71 mmol/L), and a serum creatinine level of 1.7 mg/dL (150.31 µmol/L).

Which of the following is the most appropriate treatment for this patient's condition?

(A) Oral antibiotic with skin flora coverage
(B) Elastic compression stockings
(C) Increased oral diuretic dosage

(D) Intermittent pneumatic compression pump

(E) Occlusive hydrocolloid dressing

Item 89

A 42-year-old woman is evaluated for occasional episodes of severe vertigo with nausea, vomiting, tinnitus, and a feeling of ear fullness. Her first episode occurred 3 years ago, and since then, she has had approximately six episodes, each of which may last from a few hours to 1 or 2 days. Meclizine and diazepam taken at the onset of symptoms provide partial relief, but she often must resort to bed rest during these episodes, missing 1 to 2 days of work. She has a family history of migraine headache, although the patient does not experience headache or visual symptoms with her episodes of dizziness.

Physical examination, including vital signs, is normal. An audiogram discloses a bilateral low-frequency sensorineural hearing loss. MRI of the head is normal.

Which of the following is the most likely diagnosis in this patient?

(A) Acephalgic migraine

(B) Meniere's disease

(C) Acoustic neuroma

(D) Benign positional vertigo

(E) Vestibular neuritis

Item 90

A 72-year-old woman undergoes preoperative evaluation 1 week before elective total hip-replacement surgery. Her history is significant for stable coronary artery disease, occasional angina, hypertension, and hyperlipidemia. Medications include metoprolol, daily aspirin, isosorbide dinitrate, amlodipine, and atorvastatin. She lives alone, is fully independent, and does all her own household chores. She had been walking 2 miles in 45 minutes 5 to 6 days weekly until her hip pain became too severe 3 months ago.

On physical examination, the pulse rate is 66/min, and blood pressure is 130/65 mm Hg. The remainder of the examination is unremarkable. The electrocardiogram is normal.

Besides stopping the aspirin 1 week before surgery and continuing the metoprolol and atorvastatin until the morning of surgery, which of the following is the best approach to perioperative management of her amlodipine and nitrates?

(A) Stop amlodipine and oral nitrates

(B) Stop amlodipine; give oral nitrates morning of surgery

(C) Stop amlodipine and oral nitrates; give transdermal nitrate the morning of surgery

(D) Give amlodipine and oral nitrates the morning of surgery

Item 91

A 72-year-old man is evaluated during a routine examination. He has a 45-pack-year history of smoking but quit smoking 10 years ago. He is fit and exercises aggressively. He has no known coronary artery disease and no medical problems.

On physical examination, BMI is 26.4. Pulse rate is 62/min, and blood pressure is 118/64 mm Hg.

Laboratory studies:

Serum total cholesterol	175 mg/dL (4.53 mmol/L)
Serum high-density lipoprotein cholesterol	52 mg/dL (1.34 mmol/L)
Serum low-density lipoprotein cholesterol	102 mg/dL (2.64 mmol/L)
Serum triglycerides	105 mg/dL (1.19 mmol/L)

Which of the following is most appropriate next step in the management of this patient?

(A) Electron-beam CT for calcium score

(B) Carotid artery ultrasonography

(C) Ultrasound to evaluate for abdominal aortic aneurysm

(D) Statin therapy

Item 92

A 58-year-old man is evaluated for an enlarging dark mole on his hand. One of its borders bleeds occasionally. He feels well and has no history of rash, trauma to that area, or skin cancer. The skin examination findings are **shown**.

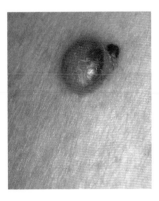

Which of the following is the most appropriate next step in management?

(A) Superficial shave biopsy

(B) Excisional biopsy

(C) Application of liquid nitrogen

(D) Electrodessication

Item 93

A 22-year-old woman is evaluated for dysmenorrhea, which has worsened over the past 3 years. Although the frequency of her periods is regular, her menstrual period lasts for 5 to 7 days. When menstruating, she sometimes misses work because of pain. Ibuprofen and naproxen do not resolve her symptoms and upset her stomach. She is not currently sexually active. Her medical history is unremarkable. Pelvic examination is normal.

Which of the following is the most appropriate treatment for this patient?

(A) Oral contraceptives
(B) Depot-medroxyprogesterone acetate (DMPA)
(C) Meclofenamate
(D) Magnesium
(E) Tramadol

Item 94

A 47-year-old man is evaluated for difficulty falling asleep and resulting daytime fatigue occurring at least 3 to 4 times per week for the past several months. He denies snoring or sleepwalking, shortness of breath, and chest pain. He is employed as an accountant and recently went through a divorce. The divorce has caused some personal and financial stress in his life. He smokes one-half pack per day of cigarettes.

On physical examination, pulse rate is 72/min, and blood pressure is 138/85 mm Hg. The BMI is 26. The remainder of the examination is normal.

Laboratory studies include a hematocrit of 42%, a leukocyte count of 4200/μL (4.2 x10^9/L), a fasting plasma glucose of 100 mg/dL (5.55 mmol/L), and a serum thyroid-stimulating hormone level of 2.5 μU/mL (2.5 mU/L). Results of a chest radiograph and electrocardiogram are normal.

Which of the following is the most appropriate next diagnostic step?

(A) Polysomnography
(B) Spirometry
(C) Cardiac stress testing
(D) Depression screening

Item 95

A 55-year-old woman is evaluated during a routine visit. Her medical history includes osteopenia. She does not smoke, have any other medical problems, or take any medications. Her mother had a myocardial infarction at age 70 years.

On physical examination, the blood pressure is 132/80 mm Hg, fairly typical for this patient during previous office visits. The remainder of the examination is unremarkable.

Laboratory studies:

Serum total cholesterol (fasting)	220 mg/dL (5.69 mmol/L)
Serum triglycerides (fasting)	140 mg/dL (1.58 mmol/L)
Serum high-density lipoprotein cholesterol (fasting)	42 mg/dL (1.09 mmol/L)
Serum low-density lipoprotein cholesterol (fasting)	150 mg/dL (3.88 mmol/L)

Which the following is the most appropriate next step in the management of this patient?

(A) Diet rich in plant stanols or sterols
(B) Statin therapy
(C) Niacin therapy
(D) Repeated serum cholesterol measurement in 5 years

Item 96

A 28-year-old woman is evaluated for a 2-week history of cough productive of yellowish sputum, sneezing, tearing and gritty sensation in the eyes, nasal and sinus congestion, and postnasal drainage. Her medical history includes seasonal allergies. She has not had any recent contacts with sick or febrile persons. She is requesting antibiotics because her previous doctor prescribed them during allergy season to prevent bacterial sinusitis.

On physical examination, temperature is 37.0 °C (98.6 °F). The conjunctivae are mildly injected without drainage, and the oropharynx is clear except for the presence of clear postnasal discharge.

Sinus examination by transillumination and percussion is negative. There is no cervical lymphadenopathy, and the lungs are clear to auscultation except for end-expiratory wheezes.

Which of the following is the most appropriate management?

(A) Oral antibiotics, nasal decongestant, and cough suppressant
(B) Oral antibiotics, nasal decongestant, and inhaled β-agonist
(C) Inhaled β-agonist, oral antihistamine, and cough suppressant
(D) Oral antihistamine, nasal corticosteroid, and inhaled β-agonist

Item 97

A 48-year-old man is evaluated for left knee pain that occurred after he slipped while shoveling snow yesterday. Although he did not strike his knee, he experienced the gradual onset of swelling and pain in his left knee over the next few hours, and he applied ice to the knee and took ibuprofen for pain relief. His normal activities include jogging 2 to 3 miles, three times weekly, without knee pain. He has not had problems with standing or walking on his left knee either immediately after his fall or currently, although it is sore. His medical history includes hypertension and hyperlipidemia, well controlled with lisinopril, hydrochlorothiazide, and atorvastatin.

On physical examination, there is mild effusion without erythema or warmth of the left knee. The patella is ballottable, but without pain. Palpation around the knee does not produce pain at the pes anserine, on the patella, or on the head of the fibula. He has full range of motion in both knees, although his left knee is slightly painful. He is able to bear weight with either leg. Specific maneuvers for meniscal tears were negative, and there is no evidence of laxity of the anterior cruciate, the posterior cruciate, or the medial or lateral collateral ligaments.

Which of the following is the most appropriate next step in management?

(A) Radiography of the knee
(B) Arthrocentesis
(C) MRI of the knee
(D) Reassurance and symptomatic treatment

Item 98

A 45-year-old man is evaluated for acute onset of nearly complete hearing loss in the left ear since awakening this morning. He has no ear pain and feels well except for nasal congestion and postnasal discharge associated with a probable viral upper respiratory tract infection from which he is recovering. He reports that when he was in his 20s and 30s, he belonged to a heavy-metal band. His medical history is significant for hyperlipidemia. There is no recent head trauma, fever or chills, headache, stiff neck, or ear drainage.

On physical examination, the external auditory canal and tympanic membranes are normal. The remainder of the physical and neurologic examination are unremarkable. On Weber testing, the patient reports hearing louder sound in the right ear.

Which of the following is the most appropriate next step in management?

(A) Reassurance
(B) Nasal decongestant and oral antibiotics
(C) Audiometry if not resolved in 1 week
(D) CT of the head
(E) Prednisone and emergent otorhinolaryngologic referral

Item 99

A 70-year-old woman is evaluated in the emergency department for severe headache, left eye pain, nausea, and vomiting that began several hours earlier in the evening. She reports that on the way to the hospital, the streetlights seemed to have fuzzy halos. She has a history of diabetes and hypertension. She has never needed prescription corrective lenses.

On physical examination, she is in marked distress. Her left eye is firmer to palpation than the right. The pupil is moderately dilated (5 mm) and unreactive, and there is diffuse ocular erythema, especially at the limbus. Visual acuity is reduced in the left eye.

Which of the following is the most likely diagnosis?

(A) Acute anterior uveitis
(B) Hyperacute bacterial conjunctivitis
(C) Acute angle-closure glaucoma
(D) Vitreous hemorrhage

Item 100

A 73-year-old man is evaluated for long-standing bilateral lower-extremity edema and a feeling of leg heaviness. Treatment with diuretics has not reduced the swelling. Medical history includes gastroesophageal reflux disease, emphysema, and hypertension treated with ranitidine, albuterol, furosemide, and lisinopril.

On examination, the pulse rate is 76/min, respiration rate is 12/min, and blood pressure is 144/84 mm Hg. There is no jugular venous distention. On cardiopulmonary examination, his heart rhythm is normal, and he has no murmurs or gallops and only a few scattered bibasilar crackles on auscultation. The lower legs are diffusely hyperpigmented, and there is pitting edema above the indurated tissue and over the feet, with no warmth, ulcerations, drainage, or toe involvement. Examination of the right lower extremity is **shown.**

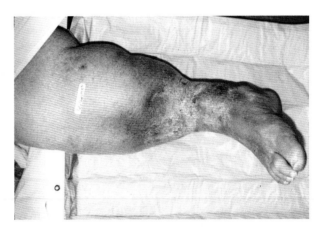

Laboratory studies include a blood urea nitrogen level of 22 mg/dL (7.86 mmol/L), serum creatinine level of 1.4 mg/dL (123.79 μmol/L), and a serum thyroid-stimulating hormone level of 8.4 mU/mL (8.4 μU/L).

Which of the following is the most likely diagnosis?

(A) Lipedema
(B) Lymphedema
(C) Lipodermatosclerosis
(D) Pretibial myxedema

Item 101

A 29-year-old woman is evaluated during a follow-up visit for recurrent bouts of depression she has experienced for approximately 7 years and for which she has taken antidepressant therapy. Her depression has been well controlled with sertraline, and she denies feeling depressed or experiencing anhedonia on this visit. She has been considering going back to graduate school but finds she is too embarrassed to do so because she has always found it difficult to go out in public and avidly avoids being the center of attention. She also reports having nightmares in which she attends class in her underwear or trips and falls in front of the whole class. The patient does not use alcohol but reports that her father was an alcoholic.

The physical examination is unremarkable. Laboratory studies, including complete blood count, liver chemistry and renal function tests, serum electrolyte and thyroid-stimulating hormone levels, and urinalysis, are normal.

In addition to cognitive behavioral therapy, which of the following is the most appropriate treatment option for this patient?

(A) Add clonazepam
(B) Increase sertraline
(C) Taper sertraline over next 2 weeks
(D) Substitute paroxetine for sertraline

Item 102

A 35-year-old farmer is evaluated for an extremely itchy rash on his face, arms, and legs. While wearing a mask, he was raking and burning brush along his driveway and was briefly engulfed in smoke. Several days later, he noticed itching and irritation developing in areas that had not been covered by the mask or his clothing. Medical history is unremarkable. The skin findings are remarkable for multiple lines of vesicles in a linear distribution surrounded by erythema and edema on the calves, forearms, and hands. The rest of the physical examination, including vital signs, is normal.

What is the first-line treatment for this condition?

(A) Topical, high-potency corticosteroids
(B) Topical pimecrolimus
(C) Avoiding contact with vesicles
(D) Oral corticosteroids for 5 days
(E) Oral corticosteroids for 14 days

Item 103

A 55-year-old man is evaluated for consideration of gastric bypass surgery. The patient has been overweight all his life. He has tried a balanced calorie-restricted diet over the past 6 months and has increased his exercise to include walking for 20 minutes three times weekly. Although he was initially successful in losing weight, he has not been able to maintain the weight loss. He works as a high school teacher and believes that his weight has interfered with his success in being asked to take leadership positions in his field. He does not smoke, and he drinks alcohol occasionally in a social context. His medical history is significant for hyperlipidemia and hypertension, both controlled with medications.

On physical examination, the pulse rate is 65/min, and the blood pressure is 142/88 mm Hg. The BMI is 40.

Laboratory studies:

Plasma glucose (fasting)	106 mg/dL (5.88 mmol/L)
Serum low-density lipoprotein cholesterol	120 mg/dL (3.1 mmol/L)
Serum total cholesterol	204 mg/dL (5.28 mmol/L)
Serum creatinine	1.2 mg/dL (106.1 µmol/L)

A chest radiograph shows borderline cardiomegaly, and the electrocardiogram is normal.

Which of the following is supported by the best evidence for sustained weight loss in this patient?

(A) Sibutramine
(B) Orlistat
(C) A low-carbohydrate diet
(D) A restricted-fat diet
(E) Gastric bypass surgery

Item 104

A 64-year-old man is evaluated for worsening urinary symptoms, including difficulty starting his stream, decreased urinary stream, and dribbling, for the past few days. He has a history of mild lower urinary tract symptoms self-treated with saw palmetto. One week ago, he developed a viral upper respiratory tract infection with nasal congestion, sneezing, and cough, for which he has been taking over-the-counter oral diphenhydramine.

On examination, the temperature is normal, and the blood pressure is 137/78 mm Hg. His bladder is not distended, and his prostate is smooth, nontender, and moderately enlarged. Laboratory studies indicate a blood urea nitrogen level of 19 mg/dL (6.78 mmol/L) and a serum creatinine of 0.9 mg/dL (79.58 µmol/L). Two to three erythrocytes and one to two leukocytes per high-power field with occasional bacteria are detected.

Which of the following is the most appropriate management of this patient's disorder?

(A) Stop oral antihistamines
(B) Perform transurethral resection of the prostate
(C) Prescribe finasteride
(D) Prescribe terazosin
(E) Continue saw palmetto therapy

Item 105

A 63-year-old man is evaluated for a symptomatic deep venous thrombosis in his right femoral vein following a total knee replacement. He was initially treated with low-molecular-weight heparin and is now receiving a therapeutic dose of warfarin 1 week after diagnosis. He has a history of hypertension, type 2 diabetes mellitus, and mild emphysema. His medications include lisinopril, metformin, and an albuterol oral inhaler.

On physical examination, the temperature is normal, pulse rate is 76/min, and blood pressure is 132/68 mm Hg. His lungs are clear to auscultation, and the heart examination is normal. The circumference of the right calf is 44 cm (17 in) and of the left calf is 38 cm (15 in). There is pitting edema, but no erythema or warmth.

Which of the following is the most appropriate next step in preventing the postphlebitic syndrome in this patient?

(A) Diuretics
(B) Elastic compression stockings
(C) Intermittent pneumatic compression
(D) Prolonged oral anticoagulation

Item 106

A 77-year-old man who wears glasses is evaluated for symptoms of increasing visual glare when he is out at night, but he reports no problems with bright sunlight, reading, or watching television. He no longer drives because he lives in a downtown condominium and prefers to walk and use public transportation. His history is negative for diabetes, corticosteroids, and cigarette smoking. His corrected visual acuity is 20/25 in each eye. Direct ophthalmoscopy reveals bilateral red reflexes with central opacities, but the optic disks and retinal vessels are normal.

Which of the following is the most appropriate management for this patient's visual symptoms?

(A) Cataract extraction
(B) Vitamin E supplementation
(C) β-Carotene supplementation
(D) Monitoring of visual status
(E) Topical ophthalmic prostaglandin

Item 107

A 37-year-old woman is evaluated for a 2-week history of sinus congestion. She initially thought she had a cold and felt better after taking an over-the-counter combination of oral pseudoephedrine and diphenhydramine; however, her symptoms returned, and she began having low-grade fevers and increased nasal secretions. She has no drug allergies.

On physical examination, the temperature is 37.4 °C (99.4 °F). There is right maxillary tenderness, erythematous turbinates, and yellowish-green nasal secretions.

Which of the following is the most appropriate management for this patient's disorder?

(A) Oral amoxicillin
(B) Oral nonsedating antihistamine
(C) Sinus radiography
(D) Sinus CT
(E) Oral amoxicillin–clavulanate

Item 108

A 42-year-old woman is evaluated during a routine examination. She has been married and monogamous for 21 years. Her history includes celiac sprue, which was diagnosed at age 25 years and for which she maintains a gluten-free diet that limits her symptoms. She also has mild rosacea and frequent urinary tract infections. Her mother was recently diagnosed with hypothyroidism, but the patient reports no fatigue or hot or cold intolerance, and she has had no changes in weight, hair, skin, and nails. The patient exercises regularly. She reports no polyuria or polydipsia.

On physical examination, the patient is fair-skinned. BMI is 18.9, and weight has been stable. The pulse rate is 68/min, and blood pressure is 102/66 mm Hg. The remainder of the physical examination is unremarkable.

Which of the following is the most appropriate management for this patient?

(A) Thyroid-stimulating hormone measurement
(B) Bone-density test
(C) Screening for *Chlamydia trachomatis* infection
(D) Diabetes screening
(E) Colon cancer screening

Item 109

A 52-year-old woman with atrial fibrillation and heart failure requests a flu shot. She takes warfarin for atrial fibrillation. She reports a milk allergy.

Which of the following is the most appropriate management of this patient?

(A) Inactivated influenza vaccine
(B) Live influenza vaccine
(C) No influenza vaccine
(D) Neuraminidase inhibitor therapy

Item 110

A 68-year-old man is evaluated in the emergency department with a 5-day history of shortness of breath. He describes being jarred in an elevator 5 days earlier and sustaining a large bruise on his right flank. That evening, he had trouble sleeping from the pain, but finally managed to rest while sitting in a recliner. Over the past 5 days he has had progressive shortness of breath; originally it was related to exertion, but it now occurs at rest. He continues to sleep in the recliner for comfort. He does not smoke.

On physical examination, an ecchymosis is evident on his right flank. He is mildly dyspneic with conversation. BMI is 25.7. Temperature is 38.3 °C (100.9 °F), pulse rate is 112/min, respiration rate is 26/min, and blood pressure is 142/72 mm Hg bilaterally. Pulse oximetry is 93% on room air. The trachea is midline, and jugular venous pressure is 6 cm. Lungs are dull to percussion, and there are decreased breath sounds on the right side of the chest. Cardiovascular point of maximal impulse is at the fifth intercostal space, midclavicular line. He has tachycardia.

No rubs, murmurs, or gallops are heard, and there is no evidence of edema.

The electrocardiogram shows sinus tachycardia without acute ST- or T-wave changes.

Which of the following is the most likely diagnosis?

(A) Pneumonia
(B) Pulmonary embolism
(C) Hemothorax
(D) Pleural effusion
(E) Chylothorax

Item 111

A 46-year-old man is evaluated for a 2- to 3-week history of neck pain, as well as pain, tingling, and intermittent numbness of his right mid-forearm into the middle of his palm. He states that the symptoms are not positional. He reports no weakness, recent trauma, fevers, or headache.

On physical examination, triceps reflex in his right arm is less than that in his left. Neck flexion toward his chest and toward the right side aggravates the symptoms in his right arm. Proprioception, light touch, and motor strength are normal bilaterally, although the examination is limited because of pain. There is no spasticity in the arm or other long-track signs.

Which of the following is the most appropriate management of this patient?

(A) Prednisone therapy
(B) NSAID therapy
(C) MRI of the cervical spine
(D) CT myelography
(E) Electromyography/nerve conduction studies

Item 112

A 24-year-old woman with Down's syndrome is evaluated for hair loss. Hair comes out in patches when she washes or brushes it. She feels well and has had no recent stressors or changes in her routine. She takes no medication. She is not fatigued and has had no recent change in weight.

On examination, she has a well-demarcated bald patch in the occipital area. The area shows a small oval patch of smooth skin with no scale or redness. Wood's light examination is negative.

Which of the following is the most likely diagnosis?

(A) Telogen effluvium
(B) Trichotillomania
(C) Tinea capitis
(D) Alopecia areata

Item 113

A 35-year-old woman is evaluated for a 3-year history of chronic pain with intercourse and severe debilitating lower abdominal cramps. She has been divorced for 6 years and recently became sexually active with a new partner. She has urinary frequency and feels a fullness in her lower abdomen; she reports no vaginal discharge. She has no history of sexually transmitted disease, and she had tubal ligation 8 years ago. Bowel movements are normal. She currently takes no medications, smokes 1 pack of cigarettes daily, and does not drink alcohol or use illicit drugs. She denies depression or anhedonia.

On examination, she is anxious and at times tearful. Pulse rate is 106/min, and blood pressure is 132/86 mm Hg. Her abdomen is soft, with tenderness to palpation in the lower quadrants. External genitalia and cervix are normal. She has no cervical motion tenderness, but she has pain on bilateral deep pelvic palpation. Rectal tone is increased, and stool is guaiac negative. Complete blood count and urinalysis are normal. An antidepressant is prescribed.

Screening for which of the following would be most appropriate for this patient?

(A) Attention deficit disorder
(B) Posttraumatic stress disorder
(C) Conversion disorder
(D) Malingering
(E) Hypochondriasis

Item 114

A 64-year-old man with end-stage metastatic prostate cancer is experiencing worsening skeletal pain throughout his back and bilateral lower extremities. He has already experienced disease progression with anti-hormonal therapy, has refused further chemotherapy, and has received the maximal dose of radiation to the spine and metastatic lesions. He had been controlling his pain with regular NSAID use but now requires short-acting narcotics almost every 4 to 6 hours. He is requesting a long-acting medication for his pain control, and his current health insurance does not include a pharmacy benefit.

The remainder of the medical history is noncontributory.

On physical examination, no focal neurologic findings are noted. Results of renal function and liver chemistry tests are normal.

Which of the following is the most cost-effective choice for long-acting analgesic medication in this patient?

(A) Long-acting morphine
(B) Long-acting oxycodone
(C) Transdermal fentanyl
(D) Duloxetine

Item 115

A 52-year-old man telephones his physician to report a 4-week history of episodic left-sided chest pain lasting 3 to 5 minutes, often occurring at rest, and resolving spontaneously. He is unsure whether the episodes are related to meals. He has not had any shortness of breath, orthopnea, exertional dyspnea, nausea or vomiting, or skin changes. His history is significant for hyperlipidemia, childhood asthma, and adopting a sedentary lifestyle for the past several years until 3 months ago when he began exercising. The patient is experiencing significant stress related to his job; he is also in the midst of a divorce. The physician recalls that the patient's most recent physical examination, including blood pressure, was normal, and that he was healthy.

During the course of the phone interview, the patient is asked to determine whether he feels any pain while pressing on his chest over the lateral aspects of the sternum. The patient reports that this maneuver does vaguely reproduce his pain.

Which of the following is the most appropriate management strategy at this time?

(A) Immediate evaluation in the emergency department
(B) NSAIDs and avoidance of strenuous activity
(C) Benzodiazepines
(D) High-dose proton pump inhibitor

Item 116

A 55-year-old woman is evaluated during a routine visit and seeks medication to help her lose weight. The patient had begun to put on weight after menopause at age 49 years. She has tried multiple diets but has failed to maintain the weight loss she initially achieves with each diet. She does not smoke or drink alcohol. Her medical history is significant for hypertension, for which she takes three medications.

On physical examination, the pulse rate is 65/min, and the blood pressure is 142/90 mm Hg. The BMI is 33. The remainder of the physical examination is normal.

Which of the following medications is the most appropriate treatment for this patient?

(A) Sibutramine
(B) Phentermine
(C) Mirtazapine
(D) Orlistat

Item 117

A 42-year-old man is evaluated for a nonpruritic, nonpainful spreading rash he has noticed over the past several weeks. The patient has been outdoors more often over the past few weeks as the weather has warmed, and his skin is beginning to tan. He has used over-the-counter corticosteroid cream without success. His medical history is significant for hyperlipidemia controlled with simvastatin.

The findings of the skin examination are **shown**. Laboratory examination indicates a serum total cholesterol level of 190 mg/dL (4.91 mmol/L) and serum low-density lipoprotein cholesterol level of 110 mg/dL (2.84 mmol/L). Findings of direct microscopic examination of scale with 10% potassium hydroxide show large, blunt hyphae and thick-walled budding spores in a "spaghetti and meatballs" pattern. Liver chemistry tests are normal.

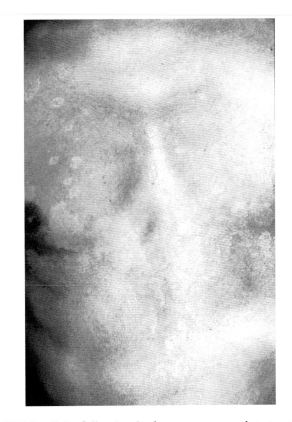

Which of the following is the most appropriate treatment for this patient?

(A) Oral terbinafine
(B) Oral itraconazole
(C) Topical triamcinolone
(D) Topical ketoconazole
(E) Oral griseofulvin

Item 118

A 37-year-old man is evaluated for frontal headaches, nasal congestion, and mucopurulent nasal drainage that have persisted intermittently for several years. He also has fatigue, a nighttime cough, and decreased sense of smell. Over the past 4 months, he has received three successive courses of antibiotics for worsening symptoms—initially with week-long courses of trimethoprim–sulfamethoxazole and doxycycline. Most recently, he completed a 3-week course of amoxicillin–clavulanate in combination with a nasal steroid inhaler, nasal saline irrigation, and an oral decongestant. This treatment regimen provided only partial relief. He has no history of allergic rhinitis, eczema, or drug allergy.

On physical examination, he is afebrile. The turbinates are edematous, with yellowish mucus between the right middle turbinate and lateral nasal wall. The septum is deviated to the right but with no nasal polyps. Percussion of his right maxillary sinus elicits mild tenderness.

Which of the following is the most appropriate management for this patient's condition?

(A) Allergy testing
(B) Nasal swab cultures

(C) Sinus MRI

(D) Sinus CT

(E) Sinus radiography

Item 119

During a little league softball game, one of the players is accidentally struck in the mouth with a bat, avulsing a permanent front tooth. A physician is in attendance, who notes that the injured player is in pain, but other than a swollen lip, appears to have no other injuries and has not lost consciousness. The player initially spit the tooth on the ground but now has his avulsed tooth in his hand.

Which of the following is the best method for transporting this patient's tooth to the dentist?

(A) Replaced into the socket

(B) In saline solution

(C) In milk solution

(D) On ice

Item 120

A 37-year-old man is evaluated during a routine visit and reports feeling depressed. He meets the criteria for major depression and generalized anxiety disorder. The medical history is otherwise noncontributory.

The physical examination, including vital signs, is normal. Laboratory studies are unremarkable.

Which of the following is the most appropriate treatment option for this patient?

(A) Paroxetine

(B) Bupropion

(C) Clonazepam

(D) Risperidone

Item 121

A 53-year-old man is evaluated for chronic nasal congestion, rhinorrhea, postnasal drainage, and sneezing. He does not have itchy or watery eyes. His medical history includes hypertension. Skin testing showed that he is allergic to grass and weeds. He hired someone to mow his lawn and used chlorpheniramine for his allergy, but he stopped the medication because it made him drowsy.

On physical examination, he is afebrile, with patent nares, pale turbinates, and clear, watery secretions. He has no nasal polyps, septal deviation, or conjunctival erythema.

Which of the following is the most appropriate long-term management of this patient's disorder?

(A) Leukotriene inhibitor

(B) Nasal decongestant

(C) Nasal corticosteroid

(D) Nonsedating oral antihistamine

(E) Oral decongestant

Item 122

A 54-year-old woman undergoes urgent preoperative evaluation before resection of a partially obstructing mass in the descending colon. She has lost 9 kg (20 lb) over the past 6 months. Her history includes moderately severe chronic obstructive pulmonary disease (COPD) but no known coronary artery disease. She smokes 1 pack of cigarettes daily. Her only medication is a combined ipratropium–albuterol oral inhaler.

On physical examination, she appears ill. The blood pressure is normal. Weight is 48.9 kg (108 lb). Oxygen saturation is 88% on room air. On cardiopulmonary examination, the lungs are clear, with distant breath sounds and a prolonged expiratory phase, and the heart has a regular rhythm without murmur or gallop. On abdominal examination, high-pitched bowel sounds are heard, and a 6-cm mass, tender to palpation, is detected in the left lower quadrant of the abdomen. Laboratory tests are normal except for a hemoglobin of 10.0 g/dL (100 g/L) and a serum albumin level of 2.9 g/dL (29 g/L). The chest radiograph shows only changes consistent with COPD, and the electrocardiogram is normal.

In addition to routine use of scheduled bronchodilator treatments and supplemental oxygen, which of the following strategies is most appropriate in preventing postoperative pneumonia in this patient?

(A) Intravenous hyperalimentation

(B) Prophylactic corticosteroids

(C) Prophylactic antibiotics

(D) Incentive spirometry

(E) Enteral hyperalimentation

Item 123

A 68-year-old man is evaluated for left hip and knee pain. His history includes a recent diagnosis of renal cell carcinoma for which he underwent left nephrectomy. The pain has been present for a few weeks and is worsening. It occurs with activity and occasionally at night, waking him from sleep. In the past, similar pains responded to rest, heat, acetaminophen, and NSAIDs, but these are not effective for the current symptoms. He completed chemotherapy 4 months ago but has recently been depressed and less active. He also has hypertension controlled with hydrochlorothiazide.

On examination, BMI is 29.2. Temperature is 37.1 °C (98.8 °F), pulse rate is 102/min, and blood pressure is 136/74 mm Hg. He has no pain on palpation of the hip but has limited range of motion with external rotation, flexion, and abduction. Palpation and range of motion at the knee are normal.

Which of the following diagnostic tests is most appropriate?

(A) Positron emission tomography

(B) CT–guided arthrocentesis

(C) Bone scan

(D) Synovial fluid analysis

Item 124

A 67-year-old woman is evaluated because she is worried that her memory is not what it used to be. She has trouble remembering where she places her keys and purse and sometimes has difficulty remembering where she parked her car on shopping trips. She is otherwise well and is fully independent in performing her activities of daily living. She denies depression or anhedonia and plays a round of golf each week. Her medical history includes hypertension and hypothyroidism well controlled with hydrochlorothiazide, lisinopril, and levothyroxine. She takes no herbal supplements, and her only other medications are low-dose enteric-coated aspirin, calcium, and vitamin D.

On physical examination, her Mini–Mental State Examination score is 28/30. The remainder of her examination is unremarkable.

Her most recent laboratory studies of 4 months ago, including complete blood count, mean corpuscular volume, liver chemistry tests, and serum creatinine, electrolyte, blood urea nitrogen, calcium, and thyroid-stimulating hormone levels, were normal.

Which of the following is the most appropriate management option for this patient?

(A) Donepezil
(B) Depression screening
(C) MRI of the head
(D) Rapid plasma reagin, serum folate, and B_{12} measurement

Item 125

A 30-year-old woman is evaluated for a 3-day history of vaginal discharge, itching, and irritation. During the past 12 months, she has had five similar episodes and has treated her symptoms successfully with an over-the-counter vaginal yeast cream. Three months ago, a fasting plasma glucose measurement was normal. She is monogamous and has had one male partner for the past 6 months. Vaginal examination during an office visit reveals inflammation of the external genitalia and a nonodorous vaginal discharge adherent to the vaginal walls. Upon microscopic examination of the vaginal discharge with potassium hydroxide slide preparation, pseudohyphae and budding filaments are noted. A pregnancy test is negative. She would like to discuss what she can do to prevent recurrences.

Which of the following is the most appropriate next step in management?

(A) Ingest lactobacillus cultures daily
(B) Begin weekly douching
(C) Avoid simple sugars
(D) Treat partner with antifungal cream
(E) Begin weekly oral fluconazole

Item 126

A 60-year-old man is evaluated for a 1-month history of bilateral lower-extremity pain. He describes the pain as an ache in both calves and upper legs that worsens after exercise and at night, but he denies predictable occurrence while active. His medical history includes hypercholesterolemia, hypertension, and osteoarthritis for which he takes fluvastatin, atenolol, and aspirin. His family history is negative for coronary artery disease.

On physical examination, blood pressure is 140/85 mm Hg. Dorsalis pedis pulses and sensation to light touch bilaterally are normal. The remainder of the examination is unremarkable.

Laboratory studies:

Serum creatinine kinase	Normal
Serum total cholesterol	215 mg/dL (5.56 mmol/L)
Serum triglycerides	300 mg/dL (3.39 mmol/L)
Serum high-density lipoprotein cholesterol	35 mg/dL (0.91 mmol/L)
Serum low-density lipoprotein cholesterol	120 mg/dL (3.1 mmol/L)

Which of the following is the most appropriate next step in the management of this patient?

(A) Cholestyramine
(B) Fibric acid derivative
(C) Further lifestyle changes
(D) Pentoxifylline
(E) Substitution of another statin for fluvastatin

Item 127

A 43-year-old man is evaluated for a 1-year history of upper epigastric discomfort that occurs once every other month and lasts for 2 to 3 weeks without progression in severity. He describes the discomfort as a gnawing, mild pain that waxes and wanes and is associated with mild nausea and, occasionally, bloating. His history is negative for changes in stool patterns, NSAID use, weight loss, or tobacco use. He drinks alcohol occasionally and has no risk factors for alcohol misuse.

The physical examination is unremarkable, including rectal examination, complete blood count, and fecal occult blood testing.

Which of the following is the most cost-effective initial step in the management of this patient?

(A) *Helicobacter pylori* infection testing and treatment
(B) Upper endoscopy
(C) Empiric *H. pylori* eradication therapy
(D) Double-contrast barium meal
(E) Proton-pump inhibitor

Item 128

A 30-year-old man was evaluated for a 4-day history of acute unilateral eye pain with a foreign-body sensation in the eye. He reported no antecedent trauma, and the pain was worse in the morning on awakening. The medical history was noncontributory.

On physical examination, there was conjunctival erythema of the affected eye, with no evidence of a foreign body. Results of fluorescein staining indicated a corneal ulcer. The patient was prescribed pain medication and was counseled to call the next day if there was no resolution or worsening of symptoms. The patient calls the next day, stating that his pain has gotten progressively worse and there is a mucopurulent discharge from his eye.

Which of the following possible patient factors is likely to be helpful in establishing a diagnosis?

(A) History of diabetes mellitus
(B) Contact lens use
(C) Swimming
(D) History of chronic allergic conjunctivitis
(E) History of systemic lupus erythematosus

Item 129

A 54-year-old woman is evaluated for a 5-day history of sore throat, nonproductive cough, and low-grade fever. She has not had any contact with persons who are ill. She takes no prescription medications and has no drug allergies. The remainder of the medical history is noncontributory.

On physical examination, the patient is not in any acute distress, and the temperature is 37.3 °C (99.2 °F). Pulmonary examination is normal. The oropharynx is erythematous without exudates. She has no cervical lymphadenopathy.

Which of the following is the most appropriate management of this patient?

(A) Oral amoxicillin–clavulanate
(B) Oral penicillin
(C) Rapid streptococcal detection test
(D) Throat culture
(E) Symptomatic treatment

Item 130

A 43-year-old woman is evaluated during an initial visit. She has brought with her a written list of health problems, including headaches, muscle pain and weakness, abdominal pain, diarrhea, sinusitis, and frequent urinary tract infections. She also reports problems with sexual intimacy. For the past 4 years, her health problems have interfered with her ability to work. Previous treatments for headache have included venlafaxine, verapamil, propranolol, and gabapentin. For each of these, she reports no relief or an intolerance to the medication. Previous evaluation by a neurologist, gastroenterologist, and rheumatologist yielded no diagnosis of her medical problems. Previous laboratory studies, including complete blood count; erythrocyte sedimentation rate; serum B_{12}/folate, electrolyte, creatinine, blood urea nitrogen, and thyroid-stimulating hormone levels; liver chemistry tests; serum lipid panel; serum rheumatoid factor and antinuclear antibody assays; heterophile antibody testing; and urinalysis, were normal. Results of MRI of the head, colonoscopy, and CT of the abdomen were negative. She has not had any tick exposures or bites

nor any memory of experiencing an expanding red rash. The patient describes health problems in response to each portion of the general review of systems. When she is asked if she feels depressed, she becomes visibly angry.

The physical examination, including vital signs, is normal.

Which of the following is the most appropriate management option for this patient?

(A) Repeated MRI of the head
(B) Cognitive behavioral therapy
(C) Enzyme-linked immunosorbent assay for *Borrelia burgdorferi*
(D) Lumbar puncture and cerebral fluid analysis
(E) Switch from nortriptyline to venlafaxine

Item 131

A 63-year-old man is evaluated for urinary incontinence characterized by leaking, dribbling urine, occurring throughout the day and requiring him to wear pads. His symptoms of incontinence began after he underwent radical prostatectomy 3 years ago for prostate cancer, and they have persisted since then. Treatment with tolterodine has not been helpful. He works as a businessman and travels frequently and states that his symptoms are beginning to interfere with performance of his daily activities. His medical history also includes depression, for which takes sertraline.

On physical examination, there are no palpable prostatic or rectal masses. The remainder of the physical examination is normal. The serum prostate-specific antigen level is undetectable.

Which of the following is the most appropriate next step in treatment?

(A) Discontinue sertraline
(B) Begin oxybutynin
(C) Institute behavioral therapy
(D) Perform bulbourethral sling procedure

Item 132

A 22-year-old woman is evaluated for acne on her face that has worsened over the past few weeks and includes inflammatory and small nodular lesions. The patient has a history of moderate-to-severe acne outbreaks occurring since she was age 14 years. Her parents and siblings also had serious acne. She has been taking topical retinoid and antibiotic preparations with no improvement. She is otherwise healthy. She takes combined oral contraceptives for birth control and has regular menses.

On physical examination, she has several papulonodular lesions on the face. The lesions are tender, and some have pustules.

Which of the following is the most appropriate next step in the management of this patient?

(A) Change to a barrier method of contraception
(B) Prescribe oral tetracycline

(C) Prescribe oral isotretinoin

(D) Prescribe a course of oral corticosteroids

Item 133

A 42-year-old woman is evaluated for a lump in her left breast she noticed several weeks ago. She thought the mass would resolve after her menstrual period, but it has persisted. She is otherwise healthy. She began menarche at age 10 years, had her first child at age 31 years, and did not breast-feed. She is sexually active and takes oral estrogen-progestin contraceptives. Results of mammography performed when she was ages 40 and 41 years were negative. Her mother was diagnosed with breast cancer at age 68 years.

On physical examination, a dominant 1 cm × 2-cm mass is palpated in the upper outer quadrant of the left breast. Examination of the right breast demonstrates glandular tissue similar to that of the left breast but no dominant mass. There is no axillary lymphadenopathy. Bilateral diagnostic mammography is performed, the results of which are interpreted as negative, with a Breast Imaging Reporting and Data System (BIRADS)-1 reading.

Which of the following is the most appropriate next step in the management of this patient?

(A) Repeated bilateral diagnostic mammography in 6 months

(B) Repeated clinical breast examination in 4 to 6 weeks, after a menstrual cycle

(C) Recommendation to avoid caffeine and repeated clinical breast examination in 3 months

(D) Fine-needle aspiration of the mass

(E) MRI of the left breast

Item 134

A 22-year-old woman is evaluated during a routine examination. She has no medical problems except for feeling tired all the time, which she attributes to working part-time while attending classes full-time and her many social activities. She denies depression, anhedonia, or constipation, and, although she has not gained weight, she has not lost any weight despite being on a diet for years. She has occasional heartburn, particularly after alcohol consumption, which she successfully self-treats two to three times per week with calcium carbonate, 500 mg. She admits to occasional binge drinking, once or twice yearly, but her CAGE score is 0/4. She smokes because it helps her to control her weight.

On physical examination, she is slightly overweight, with a BMI of 27. Her heart rate is 68/min and her blood pressure is 188/62 mm Hg. The oropharynx is remarkable for an excoriation at the back of the throat and mild bilateral parotid gland swelling. The remainder of the physical examination is normal. Complete blood count and serum thyroid-stimulating hormone level are unremarkable. Serum electrolytes are notable for mildly decreased serum potassium, slightly elevated serum bicarbonate, and mildly decreased serum chloride levels. The serum creatinine/blood urea nitrogen levels, liver chemistry tests, and urinalysis are unremarkable.

Which of the following is the most likely diagnosis?

(A) Bulimia nervosa

(B) Anorexia nervosa

(C) Primary aldosteronism

(D) Surreptitious diuretic ingestion

(E) Renal tubular acidosis

Item 135

A 50-year-old man undergoes a routine evaluation. He has type 2 diabetes mellitus, diagnosed 5 years ago. He reports measuring his plasma glucose level in the morning and sporadically throughout the day and has noted no foot or eye problems. Medical history is also significant for hypertension, hyperlipidemia, and coronary artery disease treated with stenting 3 years ago. He reports experiencing rare episodes of chest pain. Medications include metformin, 1000 mg twice daily; aspirin, 81 mg daily; lovastatin, 80 mg daily; lisinopril, 20 mg daily; and atenolol, 25 mg daily.

Physical examination findings, including blood pressure of 120/80 mm Hg, are unremarkable.

Laboratory studies:

Hemoglobin A_{1C}	6.9%
Serum creatinine	Normal
Serum potassium	Normal
Serum total cholesterol	185 mg/dL (4.78 mmol/L)
Serum triglycerides	150 mg/dL (1.69 mmol/L)
Serum high-density lipoprotein cholesterol	45 mg/dL (1.16 mmol/L)
Serum low-density lipoprotein cholesterol	110 mg/dL (2.84 mmol/L)

Which of the following is the most appropriate next step in the management of this patient?

(A) Increase lovastatin dose

(B) Continue periodic monitoring of serum cholesterol level

(C) Substitute atorvastatin for lovastatin

(D) Add gemfibrozil

Item 136

A 25-year-old woman is evaluated for a 3-day history of malodorous vaginal discharge. She denies any itching or irritation. She has been sexually active with the same partner for 6 months, using condoms to avoid pregnancy. Her medical history is unremarkable.

On physical examination, external genitalia are normal. Internal vaginal examination reveals a homogenous, white, malodorous discharge that does not adhere to the vaginal walls, without the presence of vaginal erythema. Bimanual examination reveals no cervical motion tenderness. Mixing the vaginal discharge with a normal saline preparation reveals the presence of clue cells.

Which of the following is the most likely diagnosis?

(A) Candidal vaginitis
(B) *Trichomonas vaginalis*
(C) Physiologic discharge
(D) Bacterial vaginosis

Item 137

A 78-year-old black woman is evaluated because she is concerned that she is losing her memory; she is accompanied by her daughter. The daughter confirms that the patient is forgetful and does not recall conversations that have occurred in recent days. The patient lives alone and receives some assistance with tasks such as shopping and cleaning. She appears cheerful, has no problems with eating or sleeping, and enjoys visiting with friends and watching television. Her medical history includes hypertension controlled with medications.

On physical examination, the patient is well-groomed and friendly. She is oriented to person, place, and time. The pulse rate is 70/min, and the blood pressure is 132/80 mm Hg. No focal neurologic deficits are noted. Laboratory studies, including complete blood count, serum chemistries, and serum thyroid-stimulating hormone level, are normal. A noncontrast-enhanced CT scan shows findings of an old lacunar stroke.

Which of the following is the most appropriate next step in the assessment of this patient's cognitive impairment?

(A) Katz Index of Activities of Daily Living
(B) Barthel Index
(C) Mini–Mental State Examination
(D) Geriatric Depression Scale

Item 138

A 20-year-old male college student is having trouble sleeping because of an itchy rash on his hands and inner aspect of his arm. His pruritus has been recurring for several years, becoming more severe in the winter despite his use of a daily moisturizer. His history is remarkable for seasonal allergies, and the only medication he uses is a nasal corticosteroid in the fall.

The physical examination, including vital signs, is normal, exception for the skin examination, **shown**.

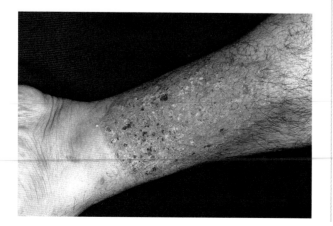

Which of the following is the most appropriate treatment for this patient's condition?

(A) Topical corticosteroids
(B) Topical tacrolimus
(C) Oral antibiotics
(D) Topical antifungals
(E) Oral corticosteroids

Item 139

A 50-year-old woman is evaluated for a 2-month history of hot flushes and night sweats. She has irregular menstrual periods that are light and not bothersome. She has read about hormone replacement therapy, wants to avoid a prescription medication, and wonders whether a nonprescription treatment is available for her hot flushes. Her medical history is noncontributory.

Physical examination, including vital signs, is normal.

Which of the following is the most appropriate recommendation for this patient?

(A) Topical progesterone cream
(B) Dong quai
(C) Black cohosh
(D) Vitamin E

Item 140

A 72-year-old man is evaluated for decreased central vision, poor night vision, and floaters. The patient has a 20-year history of type 2 diabetes mellitus controlled with oral medications, a 20-pack-year smoking history, and hypertension. The patient has not had an eye examination in over 5 years but was told at that time that he had some early changes in his eyes due to diabetes.

On physical examination, the blood pressure is 135/89 mm Hg. The ophthalmoscopic examination shows microaneurysms, cotton-wool spots, dilated retinal vessels, and new formation of retinal vessels.

Neurologic evaluation is remarkable for decreased sensation in the lower extremities. Laboratory studies include a hemoglobin A_{1C} of 7.9% and a fasting plasma glucose level of 160 mg/dL (8.88 mmol/L).

Which of the following is the most appropriate next step in the treatment of this patient's vision?

(A) Daily aspirin
(B) Enalapril
(C) Laser photocoagulation
(D) Vitrectomy
(E) Insulin

Item 141

A 19-year-old woman is evaluated in the University Health clinic for sudden-onset blindness. School has been in session for 2 weeks, and she admits that this is the first time she has been away from home, and she misses her family. During class before taking a quiz, she began to have vision problems, consisting of a loss of color vision for approximately 5 minutes in which "everything was in black and white," followed by complete vision loss. She has been having mild headaches for the past 6 weeks, located in the frontal area, and not associated with prodromes or other neurologic symptoms. Her medical history is otherwise noncontributory, and her family history includes a grandmother with multiple sclerosis.

On physical examination, the vital signs are normal. The pupils are equally round and reactive to light, and the optic discs are without evidence of papilledema or retinopathy. The remainder of her physical examination, including neurologic evaluation, is normal.

Which of the following is the most likely diagnosis?

(A) Optic neuritis
(B) Temporal arteritis
(C) Conversion disorder
(D) Macular edema
(E) Compression of optic chiasm

Item 142

An 18-year-old woman is evaluated for acne. She has had intermittent outbreaks of acne over the past 5 years. She is currently a college student who experiences stress associated with her studies. Because of her busy schedule, she often eats fast food and snacks on chocolate bars. She has tried over-the-counter topical salicylic acid and antibiotic medications to treat her acne without benefit. She is sexually active and uses barrier contraception.

On physical examination, she has comedonal acne with open (blackheads) and closed (whiteheads) comedones on her face. There are no nodular lesions.

Which of the following is the most appropriate management strategy for this patient's acne?

(A) Avoidance of fast foods and chocolate
(B) Topical retinoid medications
(C) Oral corticosteroids
(D) Oral tetracycline

Item 143

A 27-year-old woman is evaluated for abdominal pain and discomfort occurring intermittently over the past 2 years. She describes the pain as crampy, occurring diffusely in the lower quadrant. She experiences some relief with defecation. The abdominal pain is usually associated with 3 to 5 days of loose, watery stools. Between episodes, she feels fine and has normal, formed stools. She has not had fecal urgency, hematochezia, weight loss, fever, arthralgia, or rashes. Her medical history includes depression occurring after the death of her father when she was aged 22 years, for which she received 6 months of antidepressant therapy with good response. She is not currently depressed. Her family history is negative for colon cancer and inflammatory bowel disease.

On physical examination, she is well developed and appears well nourished. Vital signs, including temperature and blood pressure, are normal. The remainder of her examination is unremarkable. Laboratory studies obtained within the past 6 months, including complete blood count, renal function and liver chemistry tests, and serum thyroid-stimulating hormone, electrolyte, and calcium levels, were normal.

Which of the following treatment options is most appropriate for this patient?

(A) Nortriptyline
(B) Sertraline
(C) Loperamide
(D) Alosetron
(E) Psyllium

Item 144

A 35-year-old woman is evaluated for a red right eye that is also tearing; her symptoms have developed over the past 24 hours. Her vision is not altered, and she denies eye pain, trauma to the eye, changes in visual acuity, or pruritus.

On physical examination, the right conjunctiva is diffusely red, and the eye is tearing with clear discharge. The left eye appears normal. The vision is 20/20 in both eyes.

Which of the following is the most appropriate next step in the management of this patient?

(A) Topical antibiotics
(B) No further treatment
(C) Topical antihistamines
(D) Urgent referral to an ophthalmologist
(E) Topical corticosteroids

Item 145

A 62-year-old woman is evaluated after total knee replacement surgery complicated by postoperative pneumonia. She is now beginning to ambulate. While she was bedridden, a sequential compression device (SCD) was used for deep venous thrombosis prophylaxis. The patient is overweight.

Now that she is ambulating, which of the following is the best approach to ongoing prophylaxis during hospitalization?

(A) Standard support hose, in bed and ambulating
(B) SCD while in bed
(C) Enoxaparin, 30 mg subcutaneously, twice daily
(D) Unfractionated heparin, 5000 U subcutaneously, three times daily
(E) Warfarin with a target INR of 1.5–2.0

Answers, Critiques, and Bibliographies

Item 1   Answer: D

The patient has acute sciatica with likely L5-S1 nerve-root involvement. Nonsurgical treatment is appropriate initial management because she has no evidence of cord compression or cauda equina syndrome. Controlled trials demonstrate that NSAIDs provide effective short-term symptomatic relief for patients with acute low back pain with or without sciatica. Narcotic analgesics should be reserved for patients with severe pain and prescribed for only a limited time. Spinal manipulation, physical therapy, and muscle relaxants also demonstrate modest benefit in patients with acute back pain. Surgical intervention should be considered only if symptoms persist for more than 6 weeks or she develops progressive neurologic deficits. Two or 3 days of bed rest may be appropriate for patients with severe pain and disability. Available evidence shows no difference in pain relief or functional status between bed rest and symptom-limited activity for patients with sciatica, although activity is more beneficial for patients without sciatica. Prolonged bed rest (7 days) can lead to cardiovascular deconditioning, bone demineralization, and increased subsequent absenteeism from work. MRI of the lumbar spine early in the course of low back pain is not helpful because the false-positive rate is high. Patients undergoing early MRI are more likely to undergo surgery—and incur higher care costs—than patients evaluated with only radiography, but clinical outcomes are similar for both groups. However, routine plain films are appropriate in patients older than 50 years because they are at increased risk for malignancy and osteoporotic fractures. Back exercises are not helpful for treating acute low back pain but may help patients with chronic low back pain return to normal activities.

KEY POINTS

- **Surgical intervention of patients with low back pain should be considered only if symptoms persist for more than 6 weeks or if progressive neurologic deficits develop.**
- **Controlled trials demonstrate that NSAIDs provide effective short-term symptom relief for patients with acute low back pain with or without sciatica.**

Bibliography

1. **Jarvik JG, Deyo RA**. Diagnostic evaluation of low back pain with emphasis on imaging. Ann Intern Med. 2002;137:586-97. [PMID: 12353946]
2. **Jarvik JG, Hollingworth W, Martin B, Emerson SS, Gray DT, Overman S, et al**. Rapid magnetic resonance imaging vs radiographs for patients with low back pain: a randomized controlled trial. JAMA. 2003;289:2810-8. [PMID: 12783911]

Item 2   Answer: D

This patient has a typical presentation of benign positional vertigo (BPV). The spinning sensation he describes is classic for vertigo, and BPV is the most common specific cause of vertigo. The occurrence of symptoms upon awakening and going to bed suggests that change of head position, particularly lying down, turning over in bed, and arising, is the usual trigger for brief spells of vertigo. Although BPV can occur in any age group, it becomes increasingly common with increasing age. Two types of nonpharmacologic treatments—habituation exercises and the canalolith repositioning (Epley's) maneuver—have proved beneficial for patients with BPV in small clinical trials. Habituation exercises can be done at home and consist of the patient lying down with the head in a position that reproduces vertigo and repeating this maneuver 10 to 15 times several times per day. Canalolith repositioning is a set of head positioning maneuvers performed in the office setting.

Diagnostic testing is usually not indicated in the initial management of the dizzy patient and is not helpful in evaluating BPV. CT of the head is primarily warranted in dizzy patients with focal neurologic symptoms or signs. Electronystagmography (ENG) is most commonly performed by an otolaryngologist or other specialist expert in interpreting this test. Although the operating characteristics and clinical utility of ENG as a diagnostic test are not optimally characterized, this test is often reserved for patients with persistent, unexplained dizziness, especially when the clinician is attempting to ascertain the presence and location (central vs. peripheral) of a vestibular cause not evident by history and physical examination. Meclizine is frequently overprescribed for dizziness and is best reserved for patients with acute, disabling attacks of vertigo, such as those associated with labyrinthitis or Meniere's disease. The patient has well-controlled hypertension with no evidence of orthostatic hypotension or electrolyte abnormalities; therefore, there is no reason to suspect that the use or dose of hydrochlorothiazide is related to the patient's dizziness. Moreover, dizziness due to antihypertensive medication is typically presyncopal in nature rather than vertiginous.

KEY POINTS

- **The change of head position, particularly lying down, turning over in bed, and arising, is the usual trigger for brief spells of vertigo.**
- **Two types of nonpharmacologic treatments—habituation exercises and the canalolith repositioning (Epley's) maneuver—have proved beneficial for patients with BPV in small clinical trials.**

Bibliography

1. **Parnes LS, Agrawal SK, Atlas J**. Diagnosis and management of benign paroxysmal positional vertigo (BPPV). CMAJ. 2003;169:681-93. [PMID: 14517129]

Item 3   Answer: A

Epistaxis occurs commonly, and the source is usually anterior; 80% of cases occur in Kiesselbach's plexus, where the circulation areas of branches of three arteries converge in the septum. Most (80%) epistaxis is idiopathic or due to trauma, hyperemia with allergic or viral rhinitis, intranasal drug use, foreign body, or antiplatelet or anticoagulant drugs. The source of the nosebleed should be assumed to be anterior in patients with epistaxis in whom no bleeding site is obvious and fluid resuscitation and airway management are not needed. Pressure is usually successful in stopping bleeding but should be followed by anterior packing if bleeding recurs.

Posterior nosebleeds are uncommon and should be suspected if bleeding continues despite anterior packing. Packing for posterior bleeding is a more complicated procedure, and these patients usually receive referral to an otorhinolaryngologist. Topical oxymetazoline is often recommended and used in patients with epistaxis, but there are no data supporting its efficacy. Silver nitrate cautery should not be attempted if a bleeding vessel is not visualized. The role of hypertension and controlling blood pressure is unclear in patients with epistaxis. Increased blood pressure may result from distress and anxiety rather than be the cause of the nosebleed. Nasal tumors or aneurysms are rare causes of epistaxis. Indications for emergent or urgent referral include suspicion of posterior bleeding, need for electrocautery, uncontrolled bleeding with packing, and recurrent bleeding within 1 to 2 days requiring possible arterial ligation or embolization. Hospitalization should be considered for patients who are frail, likely to be noncompliant to prompt follow-up within 3 days for removal of packing and prevention of pressure necrosis, and those with posterior packing.

KEY POINTS

- **Epistaxis occurs commonly and the source is usually anterior.**
- **Most cases of epistaxis occur in Kiesselbach's plexus, are idiopathic, or are due to trauma, hyperemia with allergic or viral rhinitis, intranasal drug use, foreign body, or antiplatelet or anticoagulant drugs.**
- **The source of the nosebleed should be assumed to be anterior in patients with epistaxis in whom no bleeding site is obvious and fluid resuscitation and airway management are not needed.**

Bibliography

1. **Kucik CJ, Clenney T**. Management of epistaxis. Am Fam Physician. 2005;71:305-11. [PMID: 15686301]

Item 4   Answer: D

This patient has trigeminal neuralgia. Although there is little evidence on efficacious therapies for this disorder, in a meta-analysis of three placebo-controlled studies, carbamazepine was associated with a number needed to treat of 2.5 (95% CI, 2.0 to 3.4) for improvement of pain (typically a 50% reduction in pain), without any higher incidence of major adverse events compared with placebo. No other anticonvulsant agent has been adequately studied in randomized, placebo-controlled trials for treatment of this disorder.

Narcotic analgesia is only modestly effective at treating neuropathic pain and should be reserved only for patients whose pain is recalcitrant to non-narcotic treatments.

Although gabapentin is increasingly being used for patients with neuropathic pain, there is no clinical trial evidence for its efficacy in treating trigeminal neuralgia. In addition, compared with carbamazepine, gabapentin has not been found to be superior in treating other neuropathic syndromes, is considerably more expensive, and requires more frequent dosing.

Tricyclic antidepressants are efficacious in treating several neuropathic pain syndromes, although these agents have not been studied in patients with trigeminal neuralgia.

Cannabinoids are the natural constituents of marijuana (cannabis) and consist of delta-9-tetrahydrocannabinol (THC), cannabinol, and cannabidiol. Cannabinoids are currently being studied as treatment for chronic pain but have not yet been proved efficacious in patients with neuropathic pain syndromes.

KEY POINT

- **Carbamazepine improves pain in patients with trigeminal neuralgia without any higher incidence of major adverse events compared with placebo.**

Bibliography

1. **Wiffen P, Collins S, McQuay H, Carroll D, Jadad A, Moore A**. Anticonvulsant drugs for acute and chronic pain. Cochrane Database Syst Rev. 2005:CD001133. [PMID: 16034857]

Item 5   Answer: A

This patient takes nortriptyline, which can cause symptoms of urge incontinence through its anticholinergic effects. Therefore, discontinuation of nortriptyline is indicated, and another class of antidepressant should be initiated.

Several classes of drugs are associated with an increase in symptoms of urinary incontinence. In most cases, discontinuation of the causative drug will lead to an improvement in the symptoms of incontinence. Drugs that block cholinergic receptors in the bladder can lead to a disorder of bladder emptying. α- and β-adrenergic agonists can lead to disorders of bladder filling and urinary storage and manifest with symptoms of frequency, urgency, nocturia, nocturnal enuresis, or incontinence. Medications in this category include α-adrenergic blockers such as prazosin, which is used for its antihypertensive effect. β-Blockers are not associated with bladder filling and urinary storage disorders. Calcium channel blockers may be associated with urinary retention. However, the use of a calcium channel blocker in this patient did not coincide with the onset of her urinary incontinence symptoms. Discontinuation of an offending agent is preferable before initiating a new incontinence therapy that may cause side effects. Although estrogen hormone therapy has been used in the past to treat urge incontinence, recent randomized clinical trials from the Women's Health Initiative have found that estrogen therapy worsens symptoms of incontinence. Other drugs that can act on cholinergic receptors to cause symptoms of incontinence include antihistamines, antipsychotic agents, and tricyclic antidepressants. Anticholinergic agents used to treat urge incontinence due to detrusor instability (oxybutynin and tolterodine) can also cause disorders of bladder filling and urinary storage and manifest with symptoms of urgency, nocturia, nocturnal enuresis, and incontinence.

KEY POINT

- **Nortriptyline can cause symptoms of urge incontinence through its anticholinergic effects.**

Bibliography

1. **Thomas DR**. Pharmacologic management of urinary incontinence. Clin Geriatr Med. 2004;20:511-23, vii-viii. [PMID: 15341812]
2. **Hendrix SL, Cochrane BB, Nygaard IE, Handa VL, Barnabei VM, Iglesia C, et al**. Effects of estrogen with and without progestin on urinary incontinence. JAMA. 2005;293:935-48. [PMID: 15728164]

Item 6   Answer: C

Based on current guidelines, the best screening intervention for this patient is a Pap smear with screening for chlamydial infection. The Centers for Disease Control and Prevention recommend annual screening for sexually active women aged 25 years and younger and for other women at increased risk for *Chlamydia trachomatis* infection (women with new or multiple sex partners, history or current symptoms of sexually transmitted disease, or history of unprotected intercourse). Age younger than 25 years is the strongest predictor of chlamydial infection in both men and women. Untreated chlamydial infection can lead to pelvic inflammatory disease (PID) and subsequent infertility. Randomized controlled trials have shown that routine screening for *C. trachomatis* prevents PID. In Sweden, screening has been associated with decreases in both gonorrheal and chlamydial infection rates and with a dramatic decline in PID.

Endocervical and urethral swab specimens for culture were the gold standard for diagnosis, but new amplified DNA assays (polymerase chain reaction [PCR], ligase chain reaction, and strand displacement assay) using first-void urine specimens have better test characteristics (PCR sensitivity, 82% to 100%; specificity, 98% to 100%).

Patients with high cumulative levels of sun exposure and those with prior skin cancers should be encouraged to wear sunscreen and protective clothing, although the benefit of such counseling is unknown. However, this patient demonstrates no evidence of excessive sun exposure and does not have a history of skin cancer; therefore she does not require encouragement about proper sunscreen use.

A multivitamin with folic acid supplement is recommended for pregnant women to prevent neural tube birth defects; it is unnecessary in this patient since she is not pregnant and has adequate birth control. Obtaining a fasting blood glucose level is not recommended for routine screening in adults without risk factors for cardiovascular disease or type 2 diabetes.

KEY POINT

- **Annual chlamydial screening for sexually active women aged 25 years and younger and for other women at increased risk for *Chlamydia trachomatis* infection is recommended.**

Bibliography

1. **Nelson HD, Helfand M**. Screening for chlamydial infection. Am J Prev Med. 2001;20:95-107. [PMID: 11306238]

Item 7   Answer: D

Bupropion is the best treatment option for this patient because it has the least proclivity toward sexual dysfunction and does not cause weight gain. Anorgasmia is a common side effect of selective serotonin reuptake inhibitors (SSRIs), including citalopram, and there is no good evidence suggesting one SSRI has fewer sexual side effects than another SSRI. Although mirtazapine is associated with fewer sexual side effects than are SSRIs, it stimulates the appetite, resulting in weight gain; therefore, although mirtazapine might be a good treatment choice in a thin patient with anorexia, it is not appropriate in this case. Venlafaxine causes a slight increase in blood pressure and should be used cautiously in patients with less than ideally controlled blood pressure.

KEY POINTS

- **Bupropion has the least proclivity toward sexual dysfunction and does not cause weight gain.**
- **Anorgasmia is a common side effect of selective serotonin reuptake inhibitors (SSRIs), including citalopram, and there is no good evidence suggesting one SSRI has fewer sexual side effects than another SSRI.**

Bibliography

1. **Fergusson D, Doucette S, Glass KC, Shapiro S, Healy D, Hebert P, et al**. Association between suicide attempts and selective serotonin reuptake inhibitors: systematic review of randomised controlled trials. BMJ. 2005;330:396. [PMID: 15718539]

2. **Kroenke K, West SL, Swindle R, Gilsenan A, Eckert GJ, Dolor R, et al**. Similar effectiveness of paroxetine, fluoxetine, and sertraline in primary care: a randomized trial. JAMA. 2001;286:2947-55. [PMID: 11743835]

Item 8   Answer: E

Contact dermatitis is an inflammatory response of the skin to an allergen or irritant. It can appear as an acute eczematous dermatitis with erythematous papules and vesicles and, occasionally, bullae. The patient in this case has an acute presentation with a limited area of involvement and manifested by swelling and itching of the entire upper lid, including the inner canthus. Eyelids are particularly sensitive to allergens in nail polish, shampoos, hair sprays, and other aerosolized products. Chronic dermatitis is characterized by plaques of lichenification, consisting of deepening of the skin lines in a parallel or rhomboidal pattern, with satellite, small firm rounded or flat-topped papules, and signs of excoriation and hyperpigmentation. It generally causes discomfort and itch, and, if subacute, can appear as well-demarcated plaques of mild erythema with dry scales of superficial desquamation, sometimes associated with papules. Contact dermatitis affects twice as many women as men and can have unusual distributions. It is sometimes difficult to identify the underlying cause, but nickel, potassium dichromate, and paraphenylenediamine are the most common antigens. When it involves the eyelid, contact dermatitis may be confused with seborrheic blepharitis because of the scaling and flaking. Seborrheic blepharitis is a chronic condition that usually causes pain with blinking and burning eye irritation with watering. Frequently, scale is visible around the lashes, and sometimes there is crusting at the medial canthus. Occasionally, patients have decreased vision or photophobia. In its chronic course, intermittent exacerbations are typical, and it is frequently associated with seborrheic dermatitis involving the scalp, nasal folds, and eyebrows. The patient in this case has a much more limited area of involvement that does not include her lower eyelashes or chronic scaling.

Rosacea is a chronic skin disorder that most often affects the nose, cheeks, and forehead. Its classic patchy, flushed discoloration mimics sunburn. Rosacea can involve the eyelids, and many patients have irritated eyes with a bloodshot appearance. It typically appears between ages 30 and 50 years, and may emerge slowly and expand to more surface area of the face. Flushing is common, but itch is not a predominant symptom. Examination of this patient does not disclose a specific erythroderma of the face, only isolated swelling and irritation of the eyelids.

Dermatomyositis does not itch and is usually accompanied by proximal muscle weakness, although skin findings can precede muscular weakness. The typical eyelid finding in dermatomyositis is a heliotrope or violaceous discoloration around the eyes (raccoon-like). The heliotrope rash is generally not itchy and is associated with a more circumferential periorbital edema. It rarely involves scale.

Lichen simplex is known as the "scratch that itches." It is a form of chronic dermatitis, in which inflammation causes the skin to become scaly, producing the sensation of itch. Chronic itching and scratching cause further changes in the skin, and the thickening epidermal layers and leather-like texture result in a persistent scratch-itch cycle. It is frequently exacerbated by stress and is more common in women. The typical skin examination in lichen simplex demonstrates changes at the area chronically irritated by the scratching, unlike the findings in this patient.

KEY POINT

- **Chronic dermatitis is characterized by plaques of lichenification, consisting of deepening of the skin lines in a parallel or rhomboidal pattern, with satellite, small firm rounded or flat-topped papules, and signs of excoriation and hyperpigmentation.**

Bibliography

1. **Rietschel RL**. Clues to an accurate diagnosis of contact dermatitis. Dermatol Ther. 2004;17:224-30. [PMID: 15186368]

Item 9   Answer: D

The patient has risk factors for postoperative delirium (increasing age, cognitive impairment, and benzodiazepine use), which is characterized by acute, fluctuating mental status changes, with difficulty in focusing or maintaining attention, and disorganized thinking. The appropriate next step in management is to complete a full evaluation, including metabolic profile, chest radiography, electrocardiography, and review of medications, to determine the cause(s) of delirium. Potential causes of postoperative delirium include hyponatremia, severe hyperglycemia, marked decline in hemoglobin, hypoxemia, infection, unstable coronary syndrome, pneumonia, and opiate medications. Once the initial evaluation is completed, haloperidol or newer antipsychotics can be prescribed for sedation, and empiric antibiotics and CT or MRI of the head can be performed if indicated. A recent trial showed that newer antipsychotic agents were not superior to haloperidol in management of delirium, nor have they been shown to be more effective or have fewer adverse effects than haloperidol in these patients. Empiric sedation alone may obscure the signs of ongoing delirium.

A quiet, supportive environment with orientation cues, nutrition, and hydration is indicated in this setting; restraints should be avoided because they may increase the patient's anxiety and fear and worsen agitation. Because this patient's clinical scenario is not suggestive of infection, central nervous system malignancy, subarachnoid hemorrhage, demyelinating diseases, or the Guillain-Barré syndrome, performing lumbar puncture is not indicated.

KEY POINT

- In addition to a physical examination, most patients with postoperative delirium should be evaluated with electrocardiography, chest radiography, and metabolic panel.

Bibliography

1. **Amador LF, Goodwin JS**. Postoperative delirium in the older patient. J Am Coll Surg. 2005;200:767-73. [PMID: 15848371]
2. **Csernansky JG, Mahmoud R, Brenner R**; Risperidone-USA-79 Study Group. A comparison of risperidone and haloperidol for the prevention of relapse in patients with schizophrenia. N Engl J Med. 2002 Jan 3;346(1):16-22. Erratum in: N Engl J Med 2002 May 2;346(18):1424. [PMID: 11777998]

Item 10 Answer: D

Persistent rhinitis symptoms in the setting of nasal decongestant spray overuse suggests rhinitis medicamentosa. Repeated use of nasal decongestants causes a decreased sensitivity to their vasoconstrictor effect and a rebound phenomenon with increased nasal congestion and discharge. Management involves immediately withdrawing the vasoconstrictor and initiating treatment with a nasal corticosteroid spray. Allergic rhinitis is unlikely in this patient given his lack of allergy symptoms, such as sneezing and nasal itching, and because the symptoms are occurring when the patient's allergens are not in season. The absence of purulent drainage, fever, and sinus pain and the presence of pale turbinates argue against a diagnosis of bacterial sinusitis. Although nonallergic or vasomotor rhinitis can possibly be a complication of allergic rhinitis, environmental changes, such as air pollution, temperature or humidity changes, or nonspecific irritants, such as spicy foods, strong odors, perfume, exhaust fumes, cigarette smoke, and solvents, usually precipitate vasomotor symptoms. Most viral upper respiratory infections resolve within 1 week; long-term symptoms usually indicate a secondary bacterial infection.

KEY POINT

- Persistent rhinitis symptoms in the setting of nasal decongestant spray overuse suggests rhinitis medicamentosa.

Bibliography

1. **Long A, McFadden C, DeVine D, Chew P, Kupelnick B, Lau J**. Management of allergic and nonallergic rhinitis. Evid Rep Technol Assess (Summ). 2002:1-6. [PMID: 12173440]

Item 11 Answer: C

This patient may have an abnormality of her endometrial lining not detected by transvaginal ultrasonography. Possibilities include endometrial polyps, endometrial hyperplasia, or endometrial cancer. In premenopausal patients,

ultrasonography is a fairly reliable test for determining the presence of fibroids, but it may miss polyps and endometrial abnormalities. A more thorough assessment of the endometrial lining is recommended, making an endometrial biopsy an appropriate next step. If an endometrial biopsy is nondiagnostic, further testing may be indicated, including a hysteroscopy, to ensure that this patient does not have endometrial cancer.

Uterine artery embolization is appropriate for irregular bleeding from uterine fibroids, but not for undiagnosed bleeding. Placement of a progesterone intrauterine device will reduce the incidence of bleeding, but it is appropriate only if the endometrium has been thoroughly assessed and no problem has been discovered. Because this patient's transvaginal ultrasonography was negative, the test is likely missing the source of her problem. Additional transvaginal ultrasonography is unlikely to be helpful.

KEY POINT

- Endometrial biopsy is the gold standard evaluation for diagnosis of abnormal uterine bleeding.

Bibliography

1. **Farquhar C, Ekeroma A, Furness S, Arroll B**. A systematic review of transvaginal ultrasonography, sonohysterography and hysteroscopy for the investigation of abnormal uterine bleeding in premenopausal women. Acta Obstet Gynecol Scand. 2003;82:493-504. [PMID: 12780419]

Item 12 Answer: B

This patient has a furuncle, and he is at risk for methicillin-resistant *Staphylococcus aureus* (MRSA) infection because of the history of similar lesions in members of his wrestling team. If at all possible, the most appropriate first step in this case would be to obtain a culture of the fluid to evaluate for MRSA, and this can best be accomplished with incision and drainage. Doxycycline is an appropriate empiric treatment for MRSA and can be administered while culture results are pending. Outbreaks of MRSA have occurred in several populations, including competitive athletes such as football players, rugby players, and wrestlers, likely owing to hygiene issues. Other populations at risk for this infection include military personnel, children, prisoners, homeless persons, men who have sex with men, and injection drug users. Community-acquired MRSA should be considered in populations at risk for this infection and in patients who do not respond well to empiric β-lactam therapy. Although furuncles and cutaneous skin abscesses constitute the most common presentation of community-acquired MRSA, cellulitis can also occur. In athletes playing on artificial turf, abscesses at the site of skin abrasions caused by turf contact are common.

Levofloxacin and other quinolones, in addition to first-generation cephalosporins such as cephalexin, do not effectively treat patients with MRSA. Other empiric antibiotic therapy for use in patients with suspected MRSA includes trimethoprim–sulfamethoxazole, minocycline, and clindamycin. In patients in whom MRSA or β-hemolytic streptococci are suspected, β-lactam, in addition to one of the above antibiotics, is recommended.

KEY POINT

- Community-acquired methicillin-resistant *Staphylococcus aureus* should be considered in populations at risk for this infection and in patients who do not respond well to empiric β-lactam therapy.

Bibliography

1. Kazakova SV, Hageman JC, Morrison M, Sanza LT, Como-Sabetti K, Jernigan JA, et al. A clone of methicillin-resistant *Staphylococcus aureus* among professional football players. N Engl J Med. 2005;352(5):468-75. [PMID: 15689585]
2. Kowalski TJ, Berbari EF, Osmon DR. Epidemiology, treatment, and prevention of community-acquired methicillin-resistant *Staphylococcus aureus* infections. Mayo Clin Proc. 2005;80(9):1201-7; quiz 1208. [PMID: 16178500]

Item 13   Answer: B

Patients with uncontrolled asthma or the presence of wheezes have an increased risk for pulmonary complications; therefore, this patient requires improved asthma control before undergoing surgery to avoid such complications. Wheezing confers an increased risk for worsening postoperative bronchospasm and laryngospasm on intubation. Hip and gynecologic surgery do not increase the risk for postoperative pulmonary complications compared with emergency, thoracic, abdominal aortic, other vascular, or neck surgery and neurosurgery. Contrary to traditional belief, obesity does not increase the risk for pulmonary complications. The risk for pulmonary complications in the setting of OSA has not been well studied; current evidence suggests some increased airway risk in the immediate postoperative period, so there is no need to delay the hip replacement to evaluate the patient for surgical correction of OSA. Preoperative spirometry is helpful in the diagnosis of obstructive pulmonary disease, but it does not predict the risk for pulmonary complications better than clinical evaluation alone and would therefore not change the management of this patient.

KEY POINT

- Patients with uncontrolled asthma or the presence of wheezes have an increased risk for postoperative pulmonary complications.

Bibliography

1. Smetana GW, Lawrence VA, Cornell JE. Preoperative pulmonary risk stratification for noncardiothoracic surgery: systematic review for the American College of Physicians. Ann Intern Med. 2006;144:581-95. [PMID: 16618956]
2. Qaseem A, Snow V, Fitterman N, Hornbake ER, Lawrence VA, Smetana GW, et al. Risk assessment for and strategies to reduce perioperative pulmonary complications for patients undergoing noncardiothoracic surgery: a guideline from the American College of Physicians. Ann Intern Med. 2006;144:575-80. [PMID: 16618955]

Item 14   Answer: B

The most likely cause of this patient's current problem is the daily use of butalbital-aspirin-caffeine. Migraines or tension headache can "transform" into chronic daily headaches if analgesic use becomes too frequent. Although there are no data on how frequently analgesic preparations may be safely taken, most experts recommend taking them no more than three times per week. Nearly any analgesic, including acetaminophen, NSAIDs, butalbital-aspirin-caffeine, isometheptene-dichloralphenazone acetaminophen, and the triptans, can lead to chronic daily headache.

Cerebral artery aneurysm is unlikely in this patient because she has a history of migraine headache and her headaches have been chronic, not acute in onset. In addition, patients with cerebral artery aneurysm describe their pain as "the worst headache in their life," whereas this patient's pain and symptoms are consistent with her severe, chronic, and sometimes debilitating headaches. Status migrainosus and medication seeking are not likely in this patient based on her clinical scenario.

KEY POINT

- Migraines or tension headache can "transform" into chronic daily headaches if analgesic use becomes too frequent.

Bibliography

1. Snow V, Weiss K, Wall EM, Mottur-Pilson C. Pharmacologic management of acute attacks of migraine and prevention of migraine headache. Ann Intern Med. 2002;137:840-9. [PMID: 12435222]

Item 15   Answer: C

Plantar fasciitis is the most common cause of heel pain; the gradual onset of symptoms, morning pain, and inferior heel tenderness are characteristic findings. Obesity, prolonged standing, and running (repetitive microtrauma) are risk factors for this condition. Conservative treatments for plantar fasciitis include rest, icing, exercises, NSAIDs, orthotics, and cushioned soles, although rigorous evidence for these interventions is lacking. Corticosteroid injections produce short-term symptomatic relief in patients with plantar fasciitis, but the evidence for extracorporeal shock-wave therapy is inconclusive. Case series suggest that surgical procedures could be considered for patients with refractory symptoms persisting for at least 6 months.

Diffuse or focal posterior heel pain, tenderness, and swelling at the insertion site of the Achilles tendon on the calcaneus are characteristic of Achilles tendonitis. Compressing the calcaneus (squeeze test) typically elicits pain in calcaneal stress fractures. A Tinel's test (tapping the posterior tibial nerve with a finger or reflex hammer over the medial aspect of the heel just below and behind the medial malleolus) or dorsiflexion and eversion of the foot can reproduce the burning, tingling heel discomfort of tarsal tunnel syndrome. The pain from this entrapment neuropathy, which can radiate towards the toes and up the leg, is often most bothersome at night, although it can also be aggravated by prolonged standing or walking on hard surfaces.

KEY POINTS

- Plantar fasciitis is the most common cause of heel pain; the gradual onset of symptoms, morning pain, and inferior heel tenderness are characteristic findings.
- Conservative treatment for plantar fasciitis includes rest, ice application, exercises, NSAIDs, orthotics, and cushioned soles.

Bibliography

1. **Buchbinder R**. Clinical practice. Plantar fasciitis. N Engl J Med. 2004;350:2159-66. [PMID: 15152061]
2. **Crawford F, Thomson C**. Interventions for treating plantar heel pain. Cochrane Database Syst Rev. 2003:CD000416. [PMID: 12917892]

Item 16   Answer: A

Dry eyes have multiple causes and can be recalcitrant to moisture-replacement therapy. Keratoconjunctivitis sicca (KCS) is a common cause of dry eyes, which result from a reduction in the aqueous component of tears. Although this infection may be caused by Sjogrens syndrome, the symptoms of KCS may precede the presence of confirmatory evidence for this syndrome, such as a positive antinuclear antibody or anti-SSA antibody assay or indications of other systemic involvement.

Cevimeline is a cholinergic agent with muscarinic agonist activity prominently affecting the M1 and M3 receptors prevalent in exocrine glands and is a useful secretagogue therapy for the treatment of dry eyes recalcitrant to moisture-replacement therapy. Pilocarpine is another such cholinergic secretagogue, but its use is not practical because of its side effect profile, particularly excessive sweating.

Guaifenesin is a mucolytic agent that theoretically may improve nasopharyngeal congestion and lacrimal drainage, although this agent has not been studied for this indication. However, this mechanism of action would only be relevant if there were an excessive tearing problem resulting from poor lacrimal drainage and not dry eyes. Cyclosporine, corticosteroids, and topical NSAIDs are used for treating keratoconjunctivitis when there is an inflammatory component and are very expensive.

KEY POINTS

- Dry eyes, commonly caused by keratoconjunctivitis sicca, can often become recalcitrant to standard treatment with ocular moisture therapy.
- Cevimeline is a useful secretagogue therapy for the treatment of dry eyes unresponsive to moisture-replacement therapy.

Bibliography

1. **Ono M, Takamura E, Shinozaki K, Tsumura T, Hamano T, Yagi Y, et al**. Therapeutic effect of cevimeline on dry eye in patients with Sjögren's syndrome: a randomized, double-blind clinical study. Am J Ophthalmol. 2004;138:6-17. [PMID: 15234277]

Item 17   Answer: B

This patient has classic symptoms of insomnia, including awakening at night and symptoms interfering with daytime functioning. Food and Drug Administration (FDA)-approved medications for insomnia consist primarily of traditional benzodiazepines or nonbenzodiazepine-benzodiazepine-receptor agonists. The latter category of agents has greater selectivity for the γ-amino butyric acid A receptor and an improved safety and tolerability profile compared with traditional benzodiazepines. An appropriate hypnotic agent for this patient is the nonbenzodiazepine-benzodiazepine-receptor agonist zolpidem. This category of hypnotic medication confers less risk for a withdrawal reaction, addiction, carryover sedation, or reduced coordination and psychomotor skills compared with benzodiazepines.

Kava and certain other herbal medications, although often recommended for insomnia, have a poor evidence base. Selective serotonin reuptake inhibitors (SSRIs) can be effective in treating underlying mood disorders. However, these drugs do not have a hypnotic effect and may cause insomnia as an adverse reaction. If an SSRI is prescribed as primary treatment for a mood disorder, then another medication should be given to treat insomnia in conjunction with the SSRI. Diphenhydramine has been used as an off-label treatment for insomnia because of its sedating effects; however, anticholinergic side effects, including constipation, urinary retention, confusion, and delirium, may occur with the use of this drug. In addition, residual fatigue in the morning may occur with the use of diphenhydramine because of its long half-life. Patients may also become tolerant to the sedating effects of diphenhydramine. Triazolam is a short-acting benzodiazepine with an elimination half-life of 1.5 to 5.5 hours and is FDA approved for the short-term treatment of insomnia. However, the very short half-life of triazolam may limit its effectiveness in working throughout the night. Because this patient falls asleep without difficulty but awakens several times during the night, she is not a good candidate for triazolam. One selective benzodiazepine receptor agonist, eszopiclone, has recently been approved for long-term use based on clinical trials with 6-month follow-up. A recent meta-analysis found that melatonin was effective in reducing sleep-onset latency, increasing sleep efficiency, and increasing total sleep duration. Ramelton, a nonbenzodiazepine hypnotic, has received FDA approval for insomnia, but its clinical role has not been fully determined.

KEY POINT

- Food and Drug Administration-approved medications for insomnia consist primarily of traditional benzodiazepines or nonbenzodiazepine-benzodiazepine-receptor agonists.

Bibliography

1. **Silber MH**. Clinical practice. Chronic insomnia. N Engl J Med. 2005;353:803-10. [PMID: 16120860]

2. **Brzezinski A, Vangel MG, Wurtman RJ, Norrie G, Zhdanova I, Ben-Shushan A, et al.** Effects of exogenous melatonin on sleep: a meta-analysis. Sleep Med Rev. 2005;9:41-50. [PMID: 15649737]

Item 18   Answer: D

This patient may have onychomycosis of several toenails. Culturing to confirm an infection is recommended first, because thickened and dystrophic nails can be caused by other conditions, such as psoriasis. It is best to culture the nail bed debris from the most proximal part of the infection. Treatment of onychomycosis is recommended for patients with peripheral vascular disease, diabetes, or other conditions that increase risk of morbidity. Onychomycosis may also require treatment when it is a risk factor for recurrent cellulitis. A case–control study indicated that patients evaluated for cellulitis of the leg were more likely to have onychomycosis and tinea infections of the feet than other problems.

Besides terbinafine, additional approved oral treatments for onychomycosis include griseofulvin and itraconazole. Both drugs can be given in a pulse-dosing regimen. Mycologic cure rates vary as follows: terbinafine, 76% to 78%; pulse itraconazole over approximately 1 year, 63% to 75%; continuous itraconazole, 59% to 63%; and griseofulvin, 55% to 60%. Clinical cure rates (defined by nail appearance) are usually lower than mycologic cure rates because nails may not always return to their normal appearance after treatment.

Ciclopirox is a topical lacquer that is also approved for treatment of onychomycosis. The cure rate is low, at about 14%, and recurrence after discontinuation of treatment is common. However, topical treatment is recommended as initial therapy when superficial invasion of the nailbed is noted without nail thickening. Although nail debridement helps relieve pressure that footwear exerts on toes, this intervention does not address the patient's concern about the appearance of her toenails.

> **KEY POINT**
>
> - It is best to confirm the presence of an infection with a culture of debris under the nail in patients with suspected onychomycosis to rule out other conditions.

Bibliography

1. **Roberts DT, Taylor WD, Boyle J**. Guidelines for treatment of onychomycosis. Br J Dermatol. 2003;148:402-10. [PMID: 12653730]

2. **Roujeau JC, Sigurgeirsson B, Korting HC, Kerl H, Paul C**. Chronic dermatomycoses of the foot as risk factors for acute bacterial cellulitis of the leg: a case-control study. Dermatology. 2004;209:301-7. [PMID: 15539893]

Item 19   Answer: A

A common reason for social isolation in the elderly is functional decrease in vision and/or hearing. Hearing and vision assessments are simple to conduct in the office and are helpful prior to performing assessments requiring the patient to respond to oral or written questions or prompts. Elderly patients who take more than four prescription medications are at increased risk for falls and may need to receive fewer medications, but reducing medications at this time is unlikely to address her current symptoms. Depression is a possible explanation for her increasing social isolation, but a score of less than 2 on the Five-Item Geriatric Depression Screen is considered a negative depression screening result and does not necessitate initiation of antidepressant therapy. Neuropsychologic testing may be indicated, but a clinical cognitive assessment could first be conducted in the office with a tool such as the Folstein Mini–Mental State Examination.

> **KEY POINT**
>
> - A common reason for social isolation in the elderly is functional decrease in vision and/or hearing.

Bibliography

1. **Ensberg M, Gerstenlauer C**. Incremental geriatric assessment. Prim Care. 2005;32:619-43. [PMID: 16140119]

Item 20   Answer: D

This patient has evidence of metabolic syndrome, an insulin-resistant state with a threefold increased risk for coronary artery disease (CAD). He needs aggressive lifestyle-modification counseling to reverse progression of disease.

The metabolic syndrome is a constellation of predisposing conditions that increase an individual's risk for diabetes and cardiovascular disease. Diagnosis requires any three of the following: increased waist circumference, elevated serum triglyceride level, decreased serum high-density lipoprotein (HDL) level, elevated blood pressure, and elevated fasting plasma glucose level. The parameters are 1) waist circumference ≥102 cm (40 in) in men, ≥88 cm (35 in) in women; 2) triglyceride level ≥150 mg/dL (1.69 mmol/L), or on drug treatment to decrease triglyceride level; 3) HDL level <40 mg/dL (1.03 mmol/L) in men, <50 mg/dL (1.29 mmol/L) in women, or on drug treatment to increase HDL level; 4) blood pressure ≥130 mm Hg systolic or ≥85 mm Hg diastolic, or on antihypertensive drug treatment because of history of hypertension; and 5) fasting plasma glucose level ≥100 mg/dL (5.55 mmol/L), or on drug treatment to decrease glucose level. The primary goals of management for persons with metabolic syndrome are to reduce the risk for clinical atherosclerosis and to prevent type 2 diabetes mellitus. The cornerstone of management is intensive lifestyle changes to reduce modifiable risk factors (obesity, physical inactivity, and atherogenic diet).

Electron-beam CT correlates with some markers of CAD, including C-reactive protein, but there is insufficient evidence on its prognostic value for clinical coronary events to recommend it as a screening test for CAD.

Red wine may increase HDL levels but has no effect on insulin resistance. It would also add calories to this patient's diet and has the potential for addiction or abuse. Antihypertensive therapy is not warranted when based on a single value obtained in a clinical setting. The Framingham Risk Index is the most accepted and validated predictor of 5- and 10-year risk for CAD. In this patient, the index corresponds to a 5% probability of a CAD event in 5 years and a 10% probability within 10 years. Given this level of risk and the patient's lack of symptoms, an exercise treadmill test is not indicated at this time. Although abnormalities on exercise stress testing may identify persons with CAD, the prevalence of significant CAD is low in asymptomatic adults, rendering the predictive value of a positive test low (that is, false-positive results are more common than true positive results), and abnormalities on exercise testing do not accurately predict major coronary events in asymptomatic persons.

KEY POINT

- Patients with the metabolic syndrome must have any three of increased waist circumference, elevated serum triglyceride level, decreased serum high-density lipoprotein level, elevated blood pressure, and elevated fasting plasma glucose level.

Bibliography

1. **Grundy SM, Cleeman JI, Daniels SR, Donato KA, Eckel RH, Franklin BA, et al**. Diagnosis and management of the metabolic syndrome: an American Heart Association/National Heart, Lung, and Blood Institute Scientific Statement. Circulation. 2005;112:2735-52. [PMID: 16157765]
2. **Thompson GR, Partridge J**. Coronary calcification score: the coronary-risk impact factor. Lancet. 2004;363:557-9. [PMID: 14976978]

Item 21   Answer: C

Abdominal CT is superior to MRI or ultrasonography for imaging most conditions involving the bowel. It is also better than MRI for evaluating urolithiasis, although the latter is an unlikely diagnosis in this patient. CT is less costly than MRI and requires less patient cooperation. It has some limitations in visualizing common bile duct stones and the female pelvic organs, but this patient is a male, and biliary obstruction is not suspected based on his clinical presentation.

MRI of the abdomen is effective in viewing parenchymal lesions, especially in the liver. However, there is nothing in this patient's history or physical examination findings suggestive of hepatobiliary disease, and MRI is more costly than CT. Magnetic resonance cholangiopancreatography is a noninvasive option to endoscopic retrograde resonance cholangiopancreatography for evaluating biliary or pancreatic abnormalities and would typically be reserved for patients in whom clinical evaluation, laboratory tests, or initial imaging studies suggested a biliary or pancreatic lesion.

CT colonography has principally been studied as an alternative to colonoscopy for colorectal cancer screening rather than for the diagnostic evaluation of chronic abdominal pain. Its sensitivity and specificity is slightly inferior to that of colonoscopy and would not be warranted in this patient whose colonoscopy results were normal. Ultrasonography is a rapid, inexpensive option, particularly useful in establishing a diagnosis of gallbladder disease, including common bile duct stones, but the presence of gallbladder disease is unlikely in this patient based on his clinical scenario. Ultrasonography is also more operator dependent than other imaging techniques and may have poor resolution in the setting of obesity.

KEY POINTS

- Abdominal CT is superior to MRI or ultrasonography for imaging most conditions involving the bowel, is less costly than MRI, and requires less patient cooperation.
- CT has limitations in evaluating the female pelvic organs or visualizing common bile duct stones.

Bibliography

1. **Romagnuolo J, Bardou M, Rahme E, Joseph L, Reinhold C, Barkun AN**. Magnetic resonance cholangiopancreatography: a meta-analysis of test performance in suspected biliary disease. Ann Intern Med. 2003;139:547-57. [PMID: 14530225]
2. **Mulhall BP, Veerappan GR, Jackson JL**. Meta-analysis: computed tomographic colonography. Ann Intern Med. 2005;142:635-50. [PMID: 15838071]

Item 22   Answer: D

The patient has moderate lower urinary tract symptoms based on his AUA symptom index score of 13 (mild = 0 to 7, moderate = 8 to 19, severe = 20 to 35). However, these symptoms are nonspecific, and urinalysis would identify the presence of bacteria, leukocytes, glucose, and erythrocytes. Abnormal findings on urinalysis would guide further diagnostic evaluation and treatment. Serum creatinine should also be measured routinely in this patient. Drug treatment, with an α-adrenergic antagonist or 5-α-reductase-inhibitor, is an appropriate option for men with normal urinalysis and renal function who are bothered by their urinary symptoms.

An intravenous pyelogram would be appropriate for evaluating gross or microscopic hematuria but is not considered a first-line diagnostic test for evaluating lower urinary tract symptoms. Postvoid residual measurements have poor reproducibility, and there is no level of residual urine that would preclude conservative therapy. Prostate-specific antigen (PSA) measurement is recommended for select patients—those with at least a 10-year life expectancy and for whom knowledge of prostate cancer would change management—after an informed discussion of risks and benefits. In the absence of a suspicious rectal examination, PSA testing would be inappropriate given this patient's age and comorbidities. Results from urine flow-rate studies are not well correlated with lower urinary tract symptoms, and a decreased urinary flow could arise from obstructive uropathy or poor bladder contractility. Although urinary flow rates are often used to measure treatment success, these studies are considered optional tests for evaluating lower urinary tract symptoms.

KEY POINT

- **Patients with nonspecific urinary tract symptoms should undergo urinalysis and serum creatinine measurement.**

Bibliography

1. AUA Practice Guidelines Committee. AUA Guideline on management of benign prostatic hyperplasia (2003). Chapter 1: diagnosis and treatment recommendations. [PMID: 12853821]

Item 23   Answer: B

The patient's examination findings, consisting of widespread superficial tenderness, pain on axial loading of the skull, and inconsistent straight-leg-raising tests (should be positive both when the patient is sitting and supine), suggest a nonorganic component to his back pain. These findings (Waddell's signs) are considered nonorganic because they do not correspond to anatomic distributions or make physiologic sense. The examination findings and the pending disability claim also suggest that the patient is at high risk for persistent symptoms. Psychologic evaluation is appropriate because Waddell's signs have been correlated with hypochondriasis and hysteria, and the patient may benefit from antidepressants or cognitive behavioral therapy. There is no convincing evidence that epidural corticosteroids benefit patients with chronic low back pain resulting from herniated discs or spinal stenosis; no controlled trials have evaluated patients without neurologic deficits. A meta-analysis found no convincing evidence that the antispasmodic cyclobenzaprine is more effective than placebo for treating chronic low back pain. However, cyclobenzaprine does provide modest treatment benefits for patients with acute low back pain, although adverse effects are common. The patient does not have any red flags warranting plain radiography, such as trauma, age older than 50 years, history of malignancy, fever, immunosuppression, substance abuse, or neurologic deficits. An MRI is not indicated because there are no red flags necessitating early imaging and no reason for considering back surgery in this patient.

KEY POINT

- **Psychologic evaluation is appropriate in patients with Waddell's signs, which are correlated with hypochondriasis and hysteria.**

Bibliography

1. Deyo RA, Weinstein JN. Low back pain. N Engl J Med. 2001;344:363-70. [PMID: 11172169]

2. Waddell G, McCulloch JA, Kummel E, Venner RM. Nonorganic physical signs in low-back pain. Spine. 1980;5:117-25. [PMID: 6446157]

Item 24   Answer: D

This patient has posttraumatic stress disorder (PTSD). In conjunction with cognitive behavioral therapy (CBT) and some element of gradual re-exposure (often by using war movies and other video materials) or re-exploration of the traumatic event, both sertraline and paroxetine are appropriate for use in patients with PTSD, are Food and Drug Administration approved for this indication, and are particularly useful for patients with comorbid mood or anxiety disorders. The atypical antipsychotic and anticonvulsant drugs have not been studied in patients with PTSD and would therefore not be appropriate for use in this patient.

There is strong support for the efficacy of CBT across a range of trauma groups, including victims of assault, terrorism, motor vehicle accidents, combat, and childhood abuse and refugees. Exposure therapy has proven to be a reliably effective and safe intervention; however, relatively few randomized-controlled trials of CBT for PTSD have been conducted, and those that have are typically based on small samples.

KEY POINT

- **Sertraline and paroxetine have Food and Drug Administration approval for treating posttraumatic stress disorder but should generally be used with psychotherapy and are useful in patients with comorbid mood or anxiety disorders.**

Bibliography

1. McDonagh A, Friedman M, McHugo G, Ford J, Sengupta A, Mueser K, et al. Randomized trial of cognitive-behavioral therapy for chronic posttraumatic stress disorder in adult female survivors of childhood sexual abuse. J Consult Clin Psychol. 2005;73:515-24. [PMID: 15982149]

2. Ehlers A, Clark DM, Hackmann A, McManus F, Fennell M, Herbert C, et al. A randomized controlled trial of cognitive therapy, a self-help booklet, and repeated assessments as early interventions for posttraumatic stress disorder. Arch Gen Psychiatry. 2003;60:1024-32. [PMID: 14557148]

Item 25   Answer: B

True syncope is an abrupt, transient loss of consciousness due to global cerebral hypoperfusion without focal neurologic deficit and with spontaneous recovery. This patient experienced situational syncope, in which syncope is associated with a particular situation. It includes syncope associated with vagal stimulation, such as straining at micturition, defecation, cough, and, occasionally, swallowing, especially very cold liquids. Vertebrobasilar transient ischemic attacks (TIAs) may cause transient loss of consciousness but usually involve focal neurologic deficits, such as hemianopsia or ataxia; carotid TIAs involve focal neurologic deficits without loss of consciousness. Carotid sinus syncope, also vagally mediated, is caused by pressure on the carotid sinus due to turning the head, a tight collar, shaving, a tumor, or vascular dissection. Prodromal aura, secondary incontinence, slowness in regaining full consciousness (>5 minutes), and postictal disorientation are characteristic of generalized seizure, although syncope may be associated with brief prodromal nausea or sweating.

KEY POINT

- Situational syncope is associated with a particular situation and includes syncope associated with vagal stimulation, such as straining at micturition, defecation, cough, and, occasionally, swallowing, especially very cold liquids.

Bibliography

1. Benditt DG, van Dijk JG, Sutton R, Wieling W, Lin JC, Sakaguchi S, et al. Syncope. Curr Probl Cardiol. 2004;29:152-229. [PMID: 15107784]

2. Brignole M, Alboni P, Benditt DG, Bergfeldt L, Blanc JJ, Thomsen PE, et al. Guidelines on management (diagnosis and treatment) of syncope-update 2004. Executive Summary. Eur Heart J. 2004;25:2054-72. [PMID: 15541843]

Item 26 Answer: C

The most appropriate treatment of microbial otitis externa consists of physical evacuation of the ear canal, antibiotic treatment, and efforts to decrease inflammation to allow sufficient drainage of the ear. Topical acetic acid has an antibiotic effect through the acidification of the canal. Corticosteroids are effective at decreasing inflammatory swelling of the canal, which then allows optimal drainage.

Cerumenolytics (for example, triethanolamine polypeptide oleate) are effective at maintaining patency of the ear canal and thereby facilitating drainage, but they are insufficient at decreasing inflammation and local cellulitis in the ear canal.

Polymyxin/neomycin, oral antibiotics, and acetic acid (which has a topical antibiotic effect) used by themselves are effective antimicrobials, but they are ineffective in patients with insufficient ear canal drainage due to lack of patency.

Acetic acid alone (without the use of concomitant corticosteroid drops) is associated with a lower cure rate at 2 weeks (57% versus 80%), and a twofold higher risk for recurrence compared with the combination of acetic acid or polymyxin/neomycin with concomitant corticosteroid drops, confirming the premise that a combined strategy of an antimicrobial agent with canal patency intervention is necessary in patients with otitis externa.

KEY POINT

- The most appropriate treatment of microbial otitis externa consists of the combination of physical evacuation of the ear canal, topical antibiotic treatment, and efforts to decrease inflammation to allow sufficient drainage of the ear canal.

Bibliography

1. van Balen FA, Smit WM, Zuithoff NP, Verheij TJ. Clinical efficacy of three common treatments in acute otitis externa in primary care: randomised controlled trial. BMJ. 2003;327:1201-5. [PMID: 14630756]

Item 27 Answer: D

Acute joint pain and fever should raise suspicions for septic arthritis. It is an urgent problem; the longer it goes unrecognized, the higher the potential for permanent damage to the joint and risk for developing a chronic infection. Instrumentation of the genitourinary tract and recurrent genitourinary infections are risk factors for development of septic arthritis and vertebral osteomyelitis. Other potential contributors are diabetes mellitus, contiguous decubitus ulcers, and certain hardware or prosthetic joints. Radiographic evidence is usually delayed 7 to 10 days in the acute setting but should not delay diagnosis. Joint aspiration with culture is essential and may be combined with blood cultures. Gram stain alone has limited sensitivity when compared with culture. Positive results from the aspirate or blood cultures dictate antibiotic selection. Analysis of synovial fluid from joint aspiration helps to differentiate from among hemarthrosis, gout, or pseudogout as alternative diagnoses. This patient's condition should be treated as a medical emergency because of the potential for bone destruction.

Acute infection with *Borrelia burgdorferi* (Lyme disease) does not cause arthritis or arthralgias. It is characterized by fever, headache, and fatigue with the characteristic erythema migrans skin lesion. When left untreated, intermittent arthritis syndrome with severe joint pain and swelling occur after several months. Infection with *B. burgdorferi* most frequently involves the large joints, particularly the knees. This patient's history does not suggest exposure to Lyme disease, because he has no known tick bite or extended exposure from outdoor activities such as camping, hiking, or landscaping.

Gonococcal arthritis is a sexually acquired infection presenting with a complex of symptoms, including polyarthralgias (at times migratory), tenosynovitis, arthritis, and skin rash, usually on extensor surfaces. It generally affects those at risk for other sexually transmitted diseases. This patient does not have other symptoms and is not at high risk for this infection. For patients at high risk, demonstrated mucosal infection with *N. gonorrhoeae* may confirm the diagnosis, because synovial fluid and blood culture results are usually negative.

Although rheumatologic disorders such as systemic lupus erythematosus and rheumatoid arthritis may present with hip pain, the constellation of a recent genitourinary procedure and acute pain and fever is more supportive of septic arthritis. Fever may complicate diagnosis of autoimmune processes by confusing them with infection, but in a patient with recent instrumentation of his genitourinary tract, infection must be ruled out first. Systemic lupus erythematosus is nine times more common in women than in men, and usually strikes between ages 15 and 45 years, although it may present in older adults. Rheumatoid arthritis has a similar predilection for women over men (3:1). The incidence increases with age, with onset most likely during the fourth and fifth decades; in 80% of patients, the disease develops between ages 35 and 50 years. Rheumatoid arthritis generally presents insidiously with fatigue, anorexia, generalized weakness, and vague musculoskeletal symptoms until synovitis becomes apparent. Small joints are first affected, usually symmetrically. In about 10% of patients, rheumatoid arthritis develops more acutely with fever, lymphadenopathy, and splenomegaly.

Bone scan is sensitive for defining osteoblastic activity in the bone but is not specific and will not differentiate between septic arthritis and other destructive bone processes.

KEY POINT

- **Acute joint pain and fever should raise suspicions for septic arthritis.**

Bibliography

1. **Berendt T, Byren I**. Bone and joint infection. Clin Med. 2004;4:510-8. [PMID: 15656476]

Item 28   Answer: C

The clinical history and ophthalmoscopic findings in this patient suggest dry age-related macular degeneration (AMD). AMD is the leading cause of legal blindness among people aged 65 years or older in the United States. It is a degenerative disorder of the retinal pigment epithelium and neurosensory retina. This patient has several risk factors for this disease, including female sex, white race, older age, and cigarette-smoking history. Patients with this disorder typically have unilateral symptoms of gradual or sudden central vision loss. The diagnosis is established by findings of ophthalmoscopic examination. Patients with dry AMD (nonneovascular) have soft drusen, pigmentary abnormalities, and geographic atrophy (well-defined areas of retinal pigment epithelium loss) as noted in this patient's ophthalmoscopic examination. Risk factors associated with cataracts are the same as those associated with AMD. Patients with cataracts typically have cloudy or blurry vision, a perception that colors are faded, difficulty with night vision, and frequent changes in eyeglass prescriptions. However, on physical examination, an opacity of the lens is observed in patients with cataracts rather than the retinal findings observed in this patient.

Proliferative diabetic retinopathy is characterized by microaneurysms, cotton wool spots, dilated retinal vessels, and new formation of retinal vessels, findings not present in this patient. Wet (neovascular) AMD is characterized by an exudative process consisting of choroidal neovascularization that is not present in this patient. Patients with open-angle glaucoma have elevated intraocular pressure and optic disc cupping, symptoms not noted in this case.

KEY POINTS

- **Age-related macular degeneration is the leading cause of legal blindness among people aged 65 years or older in the United States.**
- **Patients with this disorder typically have unilateral symptoms of gradual or sudden central vision loss.**

Bibliography

1. **Gottlieb JL**. Age-related macular degeneration. JAMA. 2002;288:2233-6. [PMID: 12425683]
2. **Solomon R, Donnenfeld ED**. Recent advances and future frontiers in treating age-related cataracts. JAMA. 2003;290:248-51. [PMID: 12851280]

Item 29   Answer: A

Because this patient is experiencing significant symptoms of hot flushing and is interested in rapid and effective treatment, she can benefit from short-term hormone replacement therapy after a discussion of its risks and benefits. Using hormone replacement therapy to improve menopause-related vasomotor symptoms is clearly documented in studies that confirm a reduction of 6 to 22 hot flushes per week. Estrogen can be given orally or via a transdermal patch with progestin in women with an intact uterus to reduce the risk for endometrial cancer. Low-dose therapy that can reduce hot flushes includes conjugated equine estrogen (0.3 mg), estradiol (0.5 mg), and transdermal estradiol (2.5 µg).

Although the antidepressants venlafaxine, paroxetine, and fluoxetine have been shown to be helpful, duloxetine has not been studied for treatment of hot flushes. Cognitive behavioral therapy may be helpful to this patient for other reasons, but no evidence supports its use to resolve hot flushes. The botanical agent red clover has been commercially promoted as treatment for reducing hot flushes, but studies do not support its effectiveness.

There is no clear benefit of one estrogen product over another. Atypical vaginal bleeding and breast tenderness are the most common adverse effects of hormone replacement. Contraindications to estrogen use include undiagnosed vaginal bleeding, breast cancer, other estrogen-sensitive cancers, current or previous history of venous or arterial thrombosis, or liver dysfunction or disease. With long-term use, the Women's Health Initiative Studies indicate estrogen therapy is associated with an increased risk for breast cancer, coronary artery disease, stroke, venous thromboembolism, dementia and cognitive decline, and urinary incontinence. Quality-of-life measures are not clinically improved by hormone use.

The Food and Drug Administration recommends using the smallest effective dose of hormone replacement therapy for the shortest duration possible to treat menopausal symptoms only. No hormonal treatment is recommended for prevention of chronic conditions, although estrogen effectively prevents osteoporosis. A trial of discontinuing or decreasing this patient's estrogen dosage should be attempted as soon as she is willing to make this attempt. In women who have been taking estrogen replacement for a long time, gradual reduction is recommended by lowering the daily dose, the days per week estrogen is taken, or a combination or these approaches. Women who discontinue hormone therapy that they began taking for vasomotor symptoms will experience a recurrence of these symptoms after discontinuing the therapy.

KEY POINTS

- **Using hormone replacement therapy to improve menopause-related vasomotor symptoms is clearly documented in studies.**
- **The Food and Drug Administration recommends using the smallest effective dose of hormone replacement therapy for the shortest duration possible to treat menopausal symptoms only.**

Bibliography
1. **Grady D**. Postmenopausal hormones—-therapy for symptoms only. N Engl J Med. 2003;348:1835-7. [PMID: 12642636]
2. Treatment of menopause-associated vasomotor symptoms: position statement of The North American Menopause Society. Menopause. 2004;11:11-33. [PMID: 14716179]

Item 30   Answer: A

Simple topical treatments containing salicylic acid appear to be effective and safe for treating common warts. This patient's wart is responding to the treatment, indicating that it should continue. Six to 12 weeks of therapy may be necessary to completely eradicate the wart. Reassurance that the treatment is working is indicated.

No clear evidence has shown cryotherapy more effective than topical salicylic acid therapy. This patient has a periungual wart, which can be quite resistant to therapy, especially if it is under a fingernail. Periungual cryotherapy should be used with extreme caution because of possible complications, including matrix destruction and nail distortion. Other treatments that have not been approved by the Food and Drug Administration may be considered for resistant and recurrent warts, including topical imiquimod and mumps or intralesional injection of *Candida* antigens. In small open-label studies, these treatments have resulted in 70% to 80% cure rates. These treatments would not be appropriate for this patient at this time because salicylic acid therapy is reducing the size and pain of the common wart.

KEY POINT

- **Simple topical treatment containing salicylic acid is an effective and safe initial therapy for common warts.**

Bibliography
1. **Gibbs S, Harvey I, Sterlin JC, Stark R**. Local treatments for cutaneous warts. Cochrane Database Syst Rev. 2003:CD001781. [PMID: 12917913]
2. **Micali G, Dall'Oglio F, Nasca MR, Tedeschi A**. Management of cutaneous warts: an evidence-based approach. Am J Clin Dermatol. 2004;5:311-7. [PMID: 15554732]

Item 31   Answer: C

Endometriosis is a common cause of pelvic pain that cycles with menses. Diagnostic clues include a change in menstrual discomfort after a history of pain-free menses, lower back pain, and tenderness in cul-de-sac or uterosacral ligaments. Transvaginal ultrasonography is 100% sensitive and specific for endometriosis in the ovary; it is much less useful in identifying disease in other sites. MRI can be helpful for identifying retroperitoneal disease, and new cytokine assays are being studied as diagnostic tools. Laparoscopy with biopsy of endometrial tissue on serosal surfaces used to be the gold standard for definitive diagnosis, but it has considerable limitations: its utility depends on the experience of the surgeon, the disease may not be grossly apparent, and it is inconvenient, expensive, and invasive, with some risk of complications.

Laparotomy is not indicated unless the cause of abdominal pain is less certain than in the scenario described.

Colonoscopy is indicated for symptoms involving the lower gastrointestinal tract, such as diarrhea, tenesmus, or blood in the stool. Cystoscopy is sometimes used to evaluate endometriosis and help determine whether the disease involves the bladder or ureter. However, patients usually report dysuria or hematuria when the genitourinary tract is involved.

Hysterosalpingography is indicated in the evaluation of infertility and recurrent miscarriage to rule out mechanical obstruction within the fallopian tube. Any obstruction seen on this study would not be diagnostic and would require further testing to confirm the leading diagnosis of endometriosis in this patient.

KEY POINTS

- **Diagnostic clues for endometriosis include a change in menstrual discomfort after a history of pain-free menses, lower back pain, and tenderness in cul-de-sac or uterosacral ligaments.**
- **Transvaginal ultrasonography is 100% sensitive and specific for endometriosis in the ovary; it is much less useful in identifying disease in other sites.**

Bibliography
1. **Valle RF**. Endometriosis: current concepts and therapy. Int J Gynaecol Obstet. 2002;78:107-19. [PMID: 12175711]

Item 32   Answer: A

Basal cell carcinoma is the most common malignancy in humans. Early basal cell cancers are small, nodular lesions usually of flesh or pearly color, with areas of translucency and surface telangiectasia. They usually occur on sun-exposed skin and, with time, invade locally both out and down into surrounding tissue. Often, patients describe a nonhealing sore that bleeds easily even with minimal trauma. Early identification with prompt treatment prevents the disfiguring effect of local tissue destruction from expanding tumors.

The characteristics of this patient's lesion do not coincide with those of squamous cell carcinoma (SCC). SCC is characterized by hyperkeratotic, ulcerated, and fast-growing lesions and is associated with a 2% to 6% incidence of metastasis. Higher-risk SCC lesions grow noticeable within 1 to 3 months, show deeper tissue invasion, have ill-defined borders, and are less differentiated on biopsy than lower-risk lesions.

Keratoacanthoma originates in the pilosebaceous glands and typically grows rapidly over a few weeks; it appears on sun-exposed areas. It is generally a solitary reddish-colored, dome-shaped papule with a smooth shiny surface and a central ulceration or keratin plug (horn). Keratoacanthoma spontaneously resolves over 4 to 6 months.

Sebaceous hyperplasia occurs in about 1% of healthy adults. One or more lesions may be present, typically on the nose, cheeks, or forehead. The lesions are soft, discrete, and yellowish, with a smooth or slightly rough surface. Sebaceous hyperplasia is completely benign and does not require treatment.

KEY POINT

- Early basal cell cancers are small, nodular lesions usually of flesh or pearly color, with areas of translucency and surface telangiectasia, frequently occurring on sun-exposed skin.

Bibliography

1. **Rubin AI, Chen EH, Ratner D**. Basal-cell carcinoma. N Engl J Med. 2005;353:2262-9. [PMID: 16306523]

Item 33   Answer: A

Given her history of multiple pregnancies and deliveries and only recent perimenopausal status, available evidence indicates it is reasonable to perform a complete blood count to rule out anemia in this patient before she undergoes major abdominal surgery. This healthy patient has had no bleeding difficulties associated with prior surgery, childbirth, or tooth extraction or history of epistaxis or alcohol abuse; therefore, preoperative screening for coagulopathy is not indicated. The INR, PT, PTT nor bleeding test is indicated in this patient. The bleeding test, a test of platelet function, is notoriously imprecise and does not correlate with bleeding problems or add information to results of other hematologic tests.

KEY POINTS

- **Healthy patients with no history of bleeding difficulties, epistaxis, or alcohol abuse do not require coagulopathy screening before major abdominal surgery.**
- **Performing a routine complete blood count is reasonable in women who are premenopausal or only recently perimenopausal to rule out anemia before major abdominal surgery.**

Bibliography

1. **Smetana GW, Macpherson DS**. The case against routine preoperative laboratory testing. Med Clin North Am. 2003;87:7-40. [PMID: 12575882]

Item 34   Answer: A

This patient has mild, or subclinical, hypothyroidism. Patients with mild or moderate hypothyroidism can safely undergo surgery. Because levothyroxine's half-life is 5 to 9 days, mildly hypothyroid and euthyroid patients who are fasting can go without replacement therapy for several days. For patients with severe hypothyroidism, elective surgery should be delayed until thyroid hormone is partly or fully replaced. Severely hypothyroid patients who need urgent or emergent surgery should have an endocrinologic consultation and intravenous levothyroxine, triiodothyronine, and corticosteroids as needed for possible adrenal insufficiency.

Patients with mild hyperthyroidism need not delay elective surgery. In moderate or severe hyperthyroidism, elective surgery should be delayed and β-blockers should be administered until a normal thyroid level is achieved. Patients with moderate or severe disease who need urgent or emergent surgery should have an endocrinologic consultation and β-blockers, thyroid antagonists (for example propylthiouracil), and corticosteroids as needed for possible hypoadrenalism.

KEY POINT

- **Patients with mild or moderate hypothyroidism can safely have surgery.**

Bibliography

1. **Schiff RL, Welsh GA**. Perioperative evaluation and management of the patient with endocrine dysfunction. Med Clin North Am. 2003;87:175-92. [PMID: 12575889]
2. **Stathatos N, Wartofsky L**. Perioperative management of patients with hypothyroidism. Endocrinol Metab Clin North Am. 2003;32:503-18. [PMID: 12800543]

Item 35   Answer: D

The patient's history is suspicious for a meniscal tear. The most appropriate treatment at this time is knee-strengthening exercises without weights. Patients with meniscal tears may complain of a clicking or locking of the knee secondary to loose cartilage in the knee but often have pain only on walking, particularly going up or down stairs. Pain on the joint line is sensitive (76%) for meniscal tears, and findings of the McMurray test are specific for this condition (97%).

She has no history of trauma or wrenching of the knee, more characteristic of ligamentous injury. Ligamental tears tend to produce immediate swelling, whereas meniscal tears cause less swelling that is more delayed in onset.

In the hands of experienced clinicians, the physical examination of patients with suspected meniscal injuries is as effective in yielding a diagnosis as is MRI. Therefore, it is not necessary to obtain an MRI in a patient considering her classic findings for meniscal tear on physical examination and history. Arthrocentesis, in the presence of significant swelling, can be therapeutic because it removes some of the fluid; however, this patient's effusion is minimal, and the history and physical examination do not suggest an infectious or crystalline cause. Although knee-strengthening exercises are appropriate in this case, stair-stepper exercises would be inappropriate this soon in rehabilitation. Most authorities recommend surgical repair only if pain and disability persist for 2 to 4 weeks.

KEY POINT

- Patients with meniscal tears may have a clicking or locking of the knee, secondary to loose cartilage in the knee, but often have pain only on walking, particularly going up or down stairs.

Bibliography

1. Jackson JL, O'Malley PG, Kroenke K. Evaluation of acute knee pain in primary care. Ann Intern Med. 2003;139:575-88. [PMID: 14530229]

Item 36 Answer: B

This patient has anorexia nervosa and should be immediately hospitalized. Criteria for hospitalization of these patients include severe malnutrition or dehydration, electrolyte disturbances, cardiac arrhythmias, physiologic instability, failure of outpatient treatment, acute food refusal, uncontrollable bingeing and purging, acute medical complication of malnutrition, suicidal ideation, and the presence of comorbid problems interfering with treatment. This patient requires hospitalization because she is orthostatic, severely malnourished, and has hypokalemia and hypophosphatemia. She is at high risk for the refeeding syndrome and could become profoundly hypophosphatemic because malnourished patients have depleted intracellular phosphate stores; this condition can worsen as patients switch from fat to carbohydrate metabolism.

Although patients with anorexia nervosa commonly have psychiatric comorbidities, pharmacologic antidepressants, such as citalopram, are not indicated as monotherapy. In patients who can be managed on an outpatient basis, referral to a psychiatrist that specializes in eating disorders or management by a multidisciplinary team, including a nutritionist, mental health worker, and internist, are both acceptable treatment options; however, the results of this

patient's physical examination and laboratory studies indicate the need for in-hospital care. Although there have been a few case reports suggesting olanzapine to be effective in patients with anorexia nervosa, its widespread use cannot be recommended until better clinical trials have established its efficacy.

KEY POINT

- Criteria for hospitalization of patients with anorexia nervosa include severe malnutrition or dehydration, electrolyte disturbances, cardiac arrhythmias, physiologic instability, failure of outpatient treatment, acute food refusal, uncontrollable bingeing and purging, acute medical complication of malnutrition, suicidal ideation, and the presence of comorbid problems interfering with treatment.

Bibliography

1. Golden NH, Katzman DK, Kreipe RE, Stevens SL, Sawyer SM, Rees J, et al. Eating disorders in adolescents: position paper of the Society for Adolescent Medicine. J Adolesc Health. 2003;33:496-503. [PMID: 14642712]

2. Pike KM, Walsh BT, Vitousek K, Wilson GT, Bauer J. Cognitive behavior therapy in the posthospitalization treatment of anorexia nervosa. Am J Psychiatry. 2003;160:2046-9. [PMID: 14594754]

3. Kaye WH, Bulik CM, Thornton L, Barbarich N, Masters K. Comorbidity of anxiety disorders with anorexia and bulimia nervosa. Am J Psychiatry. 2004;161:2215-21. [PMID: 15569892]

Item 37 Answer: E

The patient described in this scenario is asymptomatic and needs to be told the benefits and harms of prostate-specific antigen (PSA) testing before any other diagnostic tests are performed. Screening for prostate cancer continues to be controversial owing to the poor sensitivity and specificity of serum PSA testing. With a cutoff of 4 ng/mL (4 µg/L), a single PSA assay has a sensitivity of 70% to 80% and a specificity of 60% to 70%. In asymptomatic patients, it has a positive predictive value of 30%, meaning that fewer than one in three men with an elevated PSA level actually has prostate cancer. Levels can be normal in the presence of prostate cancer or elevated without cancer present. There are age and racial differences in normal values, although use of these values is not recommended for clinical use. The U.S. Preventive Services Task Force cites the level of evidence for screening with PSA as insufficient for determining whether the benefits outweigh the harms because of mixed and inconclusive evidence that early detection improves health outcomes. Screening is associated with frequent false-positive results, unnecessary anxiety, biopsies, and complications associated with treatment of some cancers that may never have affected the patient's health.

Digital rectal examination is unreliable, because physicians have relatively low inter-rater agreement on findings. The combination of PSA and digital rectal examination provides an overall rate of cancer detection higher than either test alone. However, this strategy should be preceded by adequate discussion with the patient about its benefits and harms. Several tools have been developed to assist providers in this discussion (http://www.aafp.org/).

Transrectal ultrasonography with biopsy is an invasive test used in the workup of an established problem, such as a palpable nodule or a rising PSA level. Given its low sensitivity and low positive predictive value, it is a poor screening test and not feasible in most practices. Transrectal ultrasonography is not indicated in this patient.

KEY POINT

- In patients with no symptoms of prostate disease, prostate-specific antigen (PSA) testing has a positive predictive value of 30%; PSA levels can be normal in the presence of prostate cancer or elevated without cancer present.

Bibliography

1. **Donovan JL, Martin RM, Neal DE, Hamdy FC**. Prostate cancer: screening approaches. Br J Hosp Med (Lond). 2005;66:623-6. [PMID: 16308948]

Item 38   Answer: B

This patient's symptoms suggest acute bacterial epididymitis. In sexually active young adults, it is frequently caused by sexually transmitted pathogens, including *Chlamydia trachomatis* or *Neisseria gonorrhoeae*. It can also be caused by enteric pathogens in men who engage in receptive anal intercourse. In men 35 years or older, nonsexually transmitted epididymitis is associated with urinary tract infections, recent genitourinary instrumentation or surgery, indwelling catheters, or anatomic abnormalities of the urinary tract. Urine culture is usually positive in epididymitis, but urethral culture for gonococcus and urine DNA amplification test for gonorrhea and chlamydia can provide valuable additional information.

Treatment of acute bacterial epididymitis includes bed rest and scrotal elevation with oral antibiotics. The Centers for Disease Control and Prevention recommend ceftriaxone and doxycycline in combination for treatment of epididymitis most likely caused by gonococcal or chlamydial infection. Fluoroquinolone monotherapy (ofloxacin or levofloxacin) is recommended in patients in whom enteric organisms are more likely, in those who are allergic to cephalosporins and tetracyclines, and in those older than 35 years.

Doxycycline alone is effective against *C. trachomatis* but does not adequately treat *N. gonorrhoeae*. Amoxicillin has no activity against either of these pathogens. Trimethoprim—sulfamethoxazole has adequate gram-negative coverage but is not effective against the pathogens most likely causing this patient's symptoms.

Any health care episode possibly related to sexually transmitted disease is an opportunity to educate patients about safe sex practices and to screen for other sexually transmitted infections, specifically HIV infection and syphilis. Discussion should include risks of unprotected sex and potential infections. When patients have confirmed or suspect infection with *N. gonorrhoeae* or *C. trachomatis*, they should be instructed to refer their sexual partners for evaluation and treatment and to avoid sexual intercourse until they and their sexual partners are cured (or therapy is completed with no further symptoms).

KEY POINTS

- In sexually active young adults, bacterial epididymitis is frequently caused by sexually transmitted pathogens or enteric pathogens in men who engage in receptive anal intercourse.
- Treatment of acute bacterial epididymitis includes bed rest and scrotal elevation with oral antibiotics.

Bibliography

1. **Hagley M**. Epididymo-orchitis and epididymitis: a review of causes and management of unusual forms. Int J STD AIDS. 2003;14:372-7; quiz 378. [PMID: 12816663]

Item 39   Answer: A

This patient has symptoms of urge incontinence. The mechanism primarily involves detrusor muscle overactivity and is mediated by acetylcholine. Anticholinergic agents are the mainstay of treatment. Side effects limiting the use of anticholinergic medications include dry mouth as experienced by this patient. Tolterodine was found to confer a lower risk for dry mouth than oxybutynin in a Cochrane Systematic Review and therefore is an appropriate alternative therapy. Tolterodine also crosses the blood-brain barrier in only negligible amounts and is associated with a lower incidence of central nervous system side effects than oxybutynin. Doxepin is a tricyclic antidepressant and is used as an off-label medication for urge incontinence. Its mechanism of action is thought to involve an anticholinergic effect; however, this drug is not Food and Drug Administration approved for urge incontinence. Midodrine is an α-adrenergic agonist used as an off-label treatment for stress, but not urge, incontinence. This agent is also associated with elevated blood pressure and is not indicated in patients with hypertension. Duloxetine is a selective serotonin and norepinephrine reuptake inhibitor and has been found to be effective in the treatment of stress, but not urge, incontinence.

KEY POINT

- Tolterodine crosses the blood-brain barrier in only negligible amounts and is associated with a lower incidence of central nervous system side effects than oxybutynin.

Bibliography

1. **Thomas DR**. Pharmacologic management of urinary incontinence. Clin Geriatr Med. 2004;20:511-23, vii-viii. [PMID: 15341812]
2. **Hay-Smith J, Herbison P, Ellis G, Morris A**. Which anticholinergic drug for overactive bladder symptoms in adults. Cochrane Database Syst Rev. 2005:CD005429. [PMID: 16034974]

Item 40   Answer: A

Breast pain, which can be cyclical or noncyclical, is a commonly occurring symptom. The risk of breast cancer among patients with breast pain as an only symptom is 0.8 to 2%. However, localized breast pain followed by the detection of a lump is the presenting symptom in up to 18% of patients with breast cancer. A clinical breast examination is indicated and a mammography should be considered in all patients older than 35 years with breast pain. If the clinical breast examination and mammogram are negative, then reassurance and monitoring of symptoms are appropriate. Cyclical breast pain resolves spontaneously within 3 months in 20% to 30% of women. Clinical trials have not found vitamin E or evening primrose oil to be effective treatments for breast pain. Clinical trials of a methylxanthine-restricted diet (avoidance of coffee, tea, chocolate, and cola beverages) resulted in no better symptom relief than placebo in clinical studies. Danazol is a Food and Drug Administration–approved medication for breast pain. This drug has been found to reduce cyclical mastalgia compared with placebo after 12 months but is associated with adverse effects, including weight gain, deepening of the voice, menorrhagia, and muscle cramps. Danazol is contraindicated in women with a history of thromboembolic disease and is teratogenic. Given these complications, a trial of reassurance versus danazol therapy is the appropriate first option. Among women who are treated for cyclical breast pain, up to 60% develop recurrent symptoms within 2 years. Breast ultrasonography is not indicated as part of the workup unless a discrete mass were to be palpated.

The American College of Radiology has established the Breast Imaging Reporting and Data System (BIRADS) in which mammograms are rated in 6 categories: 0 (needs additional imaging); 1 (negative); 2 (benign finding); 3 (probably benign finding); 4 (suspicious abnormality); and 5 (highly suggestive of malignancy).

KEY POINTS

- A clinical breast examination is indicated and a mammography should be considered in all patients older than 35 years with breast pain.
- Cyclical breast pain resolves spontaneously within 3 months in 20% to 30% of women.

Bibliography

1. Smith RL, Pruthi S, Fitzpatrick LA. Evaluation and management of breast pain. Mayo Clin Proc. 2004;79:353-72. [PMID: 15008609]
2. Bundred N. Breast pain. Clin Evid. 2002:1840-8. [PMID: 12603972]

Item 41   Answer: A

This patient has chronic fatigue, which is defined as disabling fatigue lasting for longer than 6 months. Of these patients, only a small minority (one in seven) meet the criteria for chronic fatigue syndrome (CFS), which include physical and mental fatigue exacerbated by physical and mental effort in the absence of a known physical or mental disorder, as in this patient. After discussion with this patient of the probable diagnosis and prognosis of CFS, a therapeutic program consisting of cognitive behavioral therapy (CBT) and graded exercise should be implemented.

A systematic review of interventions for CFS showed that only CBT and graded exercise were beneficial in improving, but not curing, symptoms. Therefore, a rehabilitative outpatient program based on appropriately managed increases in activity, as graded exercise therapy or CBT, are the therapies of choice for this patient. The aim of therapy in patients with CFS is to maximize functioning and quality of life while minimizing the risk of iatrogenic harm. In a recent randomized controlled trial of CBT among adolescents, patients in the therapy group reported a significantly greater decrease in fatigue severity and functional impairment and a significant increase in attendance at school. They also reported a significant reduction in several accompanying symptoms. Self-reported improvement was largest in the therapy group.

Randomized controlled trial evidence has shown that fluoxetine, galantamine, and combination hydrocortisone and fludrocortisone do not improve CFS symptoms.

There is recent clinical trial evidence that methylphenidate improves the symptoms of patients with CFS with frequent concentration disturbance, although it has not been compared directly with CBT.

KEY POINT

- Only two interventions, cognitive behavioral therapy and graded exercise, were found to be beneficial in improving, but not curing, symptoms of chronic fatigue syndrome.

Bibliography

1. Whiting P, Bagnall AM, Sowden AJ, Cornell JE, Mulrow CD, Ramírez G. Interventions for the treatment and management of chronic fatigue syndrome: a systematic review. JAMA. 2001;286:1360-8. [PMID: 11560542]
2. Stulemeijer M, de Jong LW, Fiselier TJ, Hoogveld SW, Bleijenberg G. Cognitive behaviour therapy for adolescents with chronic fatigue syndrome: randomised controlled trial. BMJ. 2005;330:14. [PMID: 15585538]
3. Blockmans D, Persoons P, Van Houdenhove B, Bobbaers H. Does methylphenidate reduce the symptoms of chronic fatigue syndrome? Am J Med. 2006;119:167.e23-30. [PMID: 16443425]

Item 42   Answer: A

Management of patients taking chronic warfarin varies according to the planned surgery and reason for anticoagulation. This patient is low risk for thromboembolism due to atrial fibrillation with short-term discontinuation of warfarin. Patients undergoing dermatologic, cataract, and dental surgery can usually continue taking warfarin; bleeding risks may actually be higher for patients who continue taking antiplatelet medications. Reducing the warfarin dose to produce a lower target INR is usually not necessary, nor is stopping the warfarin before dermatologic, cataract, or dental surgery. Changing to bridging heparin with therapeutic low-molecular-weight or unfractionated heparin is indicated only in patients at high risk for thromboembolism while not taking warfarin.

KEY POINT

- Temporary use of heparin to maintain therapeutic anticoagulation is needed only in patients at high risk for thromboembolism.

Bibliography

1. Geerts WH, Pineo GF, Heit JA, Bergqvist D, Lassen MR, Colwell CW, et al. Prevention of venous thromboembolism: the Seventh ACCP Conference on Antithrombotic and Thrombolytic Therapy. Chest. 2004;126:338S-400S. [PMID: 15383478]

Item 43   Answer: D

A landmark trial of 1548 critically ill surgical patients compared outcomes associated with conventional and tight blood glucose control. Conventional glucose control with insulin infusion as needed to maintain blood glucose levels <215 mg/dL (11.93 mmol/L) was compared with tight glucose control with insulin infusion to achieve levels of 80–110 mg/dL (6.11 mmol/L). The group randomly assigned to tight control had significantly lower hospital and 1-year mortality, sepsis, acute renal failure, and critical-illness polyneuropathy, and fewer days of intensive care and ventilatory support. Benefit was greatest for patients requiring more than 5 days of intensive care for sepsis and multiorgan failure. Tight control with insulin infusion to maintain blood glucose levels <110 mg/dL (6.11 mmol/L) is optimal for critically ill surgical patients.

KEY POINT

- Critically ill surgical patients who received insulin infusion to maintain blood glucose <110 mg/dL had significantly lower hospital and 1-year mortality, sepsis, acute renal failure, and critical-illness polyneuropathy, and fewer days of intensive care and ventilatory support compared with those who received conventional glucose control with an insulin infusion to maintain glucose at <215 mg/dL.

Bibliography

1. van den Berghe G, Wouters P, Weekers F, Verwaest C, Bruyninckx F, Schetz M, et al. Intensive insulin therapy in the critically ill patients. N Engl J Med. 2001;345:1359-67. [PMID: 11794168]

Item 44   Answer: D

This patient has the classic signs and symptoms of migraine headaches. In addition, she has cutaneous allodynia, the perception of pain produced by innocuous stimulation of normal skin. The best treatment option for this patient is metoclopramide. Several antiemetic agents have been shown effective in aborting acute migraine headaches.

Triptans are effective abortive therapy for most migraines, but they have been reported to be much less effective than antiemetics once allodynia occurs during a migraine attack. Although 97% of migraines improve or resolve with the use of triptans, only 15% of patients with allodynia respond to these agents. Because allodynia takes 1 to 4 hours after headache onset to develop, triptans are effective if initiated before allodynia begins. While clearly superior to placebo, and probably as effective as meperidine, meta-analyses suggest that antiemetics and triptans as well as dihydroergotamines combined with an antiemetic are all superior to ketorolac in acute migraine treatment. Ketorolac is a nonspecific pain medication, although it has been evaluated in numerous clinical trials of patients with migraines with mixed results.

KEY POINTS

- Cutaneous allodynia is the perception of pain produced by innocuous stimulation of normal skin.
- Triptans are effective abortive therapy for most migraines, but are much less effective in the setting of allodynia during a migraine attack.

Bibliography

1. Snow V, Weiss K, Wall EM, Mottur-Pilson C. Pharmacologic management of acute attacks of migraine and prevention of migraine headache. Ann Intern Med. 2002;137:840-9. [PMID: 12435222]

2. Moja PL, Cusi C, Sterzi RR, Canepari C. Selective serotonin re-uptake inhibitors (SSRIs) for preventing migraine and tension-type headaches. Cochrane Database Syst Rev. 2005:CD002919. [PMID: 16034880]

3. Colman I, Brown MD, Innes GD, Grafstein E, Roberts TE, Rowe BH. Parenteral dihydroergotamine for acute migraine headache: a systematic review of the literature. Ann Emerg Med. 2005;45:393-401. [PMID: 15795718]

Item 45   Answer: A

This patient has varicose veins, a common manifestation of chronic venous disease that often presents with symptoms of leg heaviness, aching, fatigue, and swelling. Uncommon complications that require aggressive treatment include bleeding, superficial thrombophlebitis, and ulceration. For a symptomatic patient without complications, appropriate initial management includes elastic compression stockings (unless there is arterial insufficiency) with leg elevation, avoidance of prolonged standing, and weight loss (if appropriate). Furosemide is not effective in treating varicose veins, and the patient has only minimal edema. Patients with more severe chronic venous insufficiency should undergo cautious institution of diuresis because edema fluid is hard to mobilize, and aggressive diuresis can lead to intravascular volume depletion. Laser therapy is effective for telangiectasias and reticular veins but is not indicated for varicose veins. Patients who do not respond to 3 to 6 months of conservative treatment or who are very bothered by the cosmetic appearance of the varicose veins should be considered for surgery, such as vein stripping or ligation, or sclerotherapy. Duplex ultrasonography is often performed to accurately locate incompetent venous sites, although there is no evidence that preoperative imaging improves surgical outcomes. A meta-analysis suggested that surgery has poorer short-term, but better long-term, outcomes than sclerotherapy, although there is insufficient evidence to preferentially recommend either treatment.

> ### KEY POINT
>
> - **For a symptomatic patient with varicose veins without complications, appropriate initial management includes elastic compression stockings (unless there is arterial insufficiency) with leg elevation, avoidance of prolonged standing, and weight loss as appropriate.**

Bibliography

1. **Rigby KA, Palfreyman SJ, Beverley C, Michaels JA**. Surgery versus sclerotherapy for the treatment of varicose veins. Cochrane Database Syst Rev. 2004:CD004980. [PMID: 15495134]

Item 46   Answer: D

Ankle sprains are classified according to clinical signs and functional loss. This patient has a grade II (moderate) ankle sprain from an incomplete ligament tear. Patients with grade II sprains have moderate pain, swelling, tenderness, and ecchymosis; mild or moderate joint instability; slightly limited range of motion; and pain with weight bearing. Conservative treatment with a compression bandage, as well as rest, ice, and elevation, is the most appropriate management choice for this patient. A grade I sprain occurs when the ligament is stretched, symptoms are mild, and there is no joint instability, loss of function, or problems with ambulating. A grade III sprain indicates a complete ligament tear; these patients have severe symptoms, joint instability, loss of function, and are unable to bear weight. MRI may be reasonable if symptoms persist for several months to rule out another pathologic process but is not indicated in the acute setting. Based on the Ottawa ankle rules as **shown**, radiography of the ankle is not indicated in

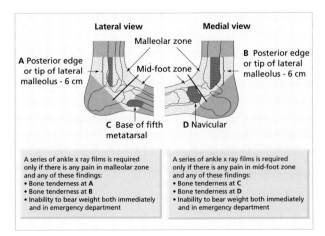

this patient because she is able to bear weight and does not have bony tenderness over the lateral malleolus or fifth metatarsal bone. Patients with moderate ankle sprains usually are not treated with cast immobilization, which can delay return to normal activities compared with functional therapy. There is insufficient evidence from randomized trials to determine the effectiveness of surgical interventions even for grade III sprains. Given the risks for complications and costs associated with surgery, conservative treatment is generally the best option for a grade II sprain.

> ### KEY POINTS
>
> - **Based on the Ottawa ankle rules, radiography of the ankle is not indicated in patients with ankle injury who can bear weight and have no bony tenderness over the lateral malleolus or fifth metatarsal bone.**
> - **Patients with moderate ankle sprains usually are not treated with cast immobilization, which can delay return to normal activities compared with functional therapy.**

Bibliography

1. **Bachmann LM, Kolb E, Koller MT, Steurer J, ter Riet G**. Accuracy of Ottawa ankle rules to exclude fractures of the ankle and mid-foot: systematic review. BMJ. 2003;326:417. [PMID: 12595378]
2. **Kerkhoffs GM, Handoll HH, de Bie R, Rowe BH, Struijs PA**. Surgical versus conservative treatment for acute injuries of the lateral ligament complex of the ankle in adults. Cochrane Database Syst Rev. 2002:CD000380. [PMID: 12137612]

Item 47   Answer: E

Heart failure is as significant a cardiac risk factor as is ischemic disease. The recently validated Revised Cardiac Risk Index assigns one point each for the following six variables: high-risk surgery, history of ischemic heart disease, history of congestive heart failure, history of cerebrovascular disease, diabetes treated with insulin, and serum creatinine level >2.0 mg/dL (176.84 µmol/L). According to their score, patients fall into one of four risk strata: 0, 1, 2 or ≥3 points. This patient has excellent exertional capacity (able to achieve and sustain >4 metabolic equivalents [METS]), but his Revised Cardiac Risk Index score is 3 as indicated by the presence of ischemic heart disease and ischemic cardiomyopathy in the setting of a high-risk procedure. Nonetheless, patients with compensated, asymptomatic heart failure can generally proceed to surgery if the level of other risk factors is acceptable. In those with stable, infrequent angina and compensated heart failure, no further preoperative testing of left ventricular function with echocardiography or nuclear imaging and stress testing is indicated. The role of plasma B-type natriuretic peptide measurement in preoperative risk assessment is currently undefined.

> ### KEY POINT
>
> - **Patients with compensated, asymptomatic heart failure can generally proceed to surgery if the level of other risk factors is acceptable.**

Bibliography

1. **Hernandez AF, Newby LK, O'Connor CM**. Preoperative evaluation for major noncardiac surgery: focusing on heart failure. Arch Intern Med. 2004;164:1729-36. [PMID: 15364665]

Item 48   Answer: C

This patient has symptoms of a viral upper respiratory infection (URI), for which there are a myriad of treatments available, although relatively few have been proven effective at improving symptoms or modifying the course of the illness. Effective therapies with good evidence for patients with viral URIs include pseudoephedrine, ipratropium nasal inhaler, cromolyn sodium nasal inhaler, and humidified air; however, their efficacy is based largely on their effect of reducing nasal congestion severity and not the course of the illness itself. Pseudoephedrine is safe for use in patients with hypertension whose blood pressure is adequately controlled, because the increase in blood pressure and heart rate caused by this agent, on average, is only slightly higher than that of placebo.

Therapies with insufficient evidence to support their use in patients with viral URI symptoms include vitamin C, zinc, antihistamines, and antitussives. There is sufficient randomized trial evidence indicating that echinacea is not effective for viral URI symptoms or illness duration. New antiviral agents targeting the rhinovirus genus are being actively studied.

KEY POINTS

- **Effective therapies for reducing the severity of nasal congestion in patients with viral upper respiratory infections include pseudoephedrine, ipratropium nasal inhaler, cromolyn sodium nasal inhaler, and humidified air.**
- **Pseudoephedrine is safe in patients with well-controlled hypertension.**

Bibliography

1. **Bye CE, Cooper J, Empey DW, Fowle AS, Hughes DT, Letley E, et al**. Effects of pseudoephedrine and triprolidine, alone and in combination, on symptoms of the common cold. Br Med J. 1980;281:189-90. [PMID: 6996784]
2. **Eccles R, Jawad MS, Jawad SS, Angello JT, Druce HM**. Efficacy and safety of single and multiple doses of pseudoephedrine in the treatment of nasal congestion associated with common cold. Am J Rhinol. 2005;19:25-31. [PMID: 15794071]
3. **Salerno SM, Jackson JL, Berbano EP**. Effect of oral pseudoephedrine on blood pressure and heart rate: a meta-analysis. Arch Intern Med. 2005;165:1686-94. [PMID: 16087815]

Item 49   Answer: B

The clinical presentation and physical findings in this case are suggestive of psoriasis. When the plaques of psoriasis are localized and involve less than 5% of the total body area, treatment with a topical agent is appropriate. In this case, high-potency corticosteroids should be used for approximately 2 weeks. Topical corticosteroid therapy can then be rotated with other topical therapies, including topical vitamin D analogs, retinoids, anthralin, or tar preparations. Topical coal tar can be used as a corticosteroid-sparing drug in resistant cases and is very effective when combined with ultraviolet B phototherapy. However, the rate of patient acceptability of coal tar therapy is low because of its unpleasant odor and staining, and some evidence from animal studies suggests an increased risk for skin and uroepithelial cancer associated with this treatment. Topical tacrolimus (a nonsteroidal agent with topical anti-inflammatory activity) is helpful for treatment of psoriasis on the face and intertriginous areas but is of limited benefit on chronic plaques in other areas. Phototherapy is effective in the treatment of plaque or guttate psoriasis; it is generally used when large areas of the body are involved and topical therapy is not practical or in cases in which the patient has been resistant to topical therapy. Methotrexate is an established systemic treatment for psoriasis but is not indicated in this patient with involvement of less than 5% of total body area and who has not yet undergone a trial of high-potency topical corticosteroid therapy. Methotrexate has antiproliferative effects and can cause bone marrow toxicity, stomatitis, gastrointestinal intolerance, fever, and alopecia. Methotrexate is associated with chronic hepatotoxicity and requires monitoring of liver function, although a baseline liver biopsy is no longer indicated in patients who take this drug. Methotrexate is a teratogen and cannot be prescribed to women who are pregnant or considering conception. Other systemic medications that are Food and Drug Administration approved for treating psoriasis are the immunosuppressive agents fumarates or cyclosporine or the new immune response modifier biologic agents, including alefacept, efalizumab, and adalimumab.

KEY POINT

- **When the plaques of psoriasis are localized and involve less than 5% of the total body area, treatment with a topical agent is appropriate.**

Bibliography

1. **Saporito FC, Menter MA**. Methotrexate and psoriasis in the era of new biologic agents. J Am Acad Dermatol. 2004;50:301-9. [PMID: 14726893]
2. PIER: Physicians' Information and Education Resource [online database]. Philadelphia: American College of Physicians; 2006. Updated June 29, 2006. Available at http://online.statref.com/Document/Document.aspx?DocId=2505&FxId=50&Scroll=1&Index=0&SessionId=67AF72RVWVGLXLYO.

Item 50   Answer: D

Several recent studies have shown that early treatment with a statin is associated with decreased mortality and morbidity in patients with acute coronary syndrome, manifested as unstable angina in this case. Treatment should be initiated while the patient is in the hospital, if possible. In one recent study, investigators compared standard treatment (pravastatin, 40 mg daily) with intensive treatment (atorvastatin, 80 mg daily) in patients with acute coronary syndrome. Serum low-density lipoprotein cholesterol levels decreased to 95 mg/dL (2.46 mmol/L) in the standard-treatment group and to 62 mg/dL (1.6 mmol/L) in the intensive-treatment group. After an average of 24 months, fewer deaths and vascular problems (myocardial infarction, unstable angina requiring hospitalization, revascularization, and stroke) occurred in the intensive-treatment group (22.4%) than in the standard-treatment group (26.3%).

Although a low-cholesterol diet and an exercise program are important in reducing this patient's long-term risk for coronary artery disease, these interventions would not have the greatest impact on her outcome in the near future. Niacin would lower triglyceride levels, which is not necessary because this patient's triglyceride level is acceptable.

> **KEY POINT**
>
> - Patients with acute coronary syndromes benefit from in-hospital treatment with a statin.

Bibliography

1. Cannon CP, Braunwald E, McCabe CH, Rader DJ, Rouleau JL, Belder R, et al. Intensive versus moderate lipid lowering with statins after acute coronary syndromes. N Engl J Med. 2004;350:1495-504. [PMID: 15007110]

2. Grundy SM, Cleeman JI, Merz CN, Brewer HB Jr, Clark LT, Hunninghake DB, et al. Implications of recent clinical trials for the National Cholesterol Education Program Adult Treatment Panel III guidelines. Circulation. 2004;110:227-39. [PMID: 15249516]

Item 51   Answer: D

This patient has likely experienced improvement in her dysmenorrhea because of the contraceptive pill, but her difficulty remembering to take it as prescribed is limiting its effectiveness. Prescribing a contraceptive patch may improve her compliance because it does not require the patient to remember to take a pill every day. The patch is applied weekly for 3 concurrent weeks then left off for the fourth week when withdrawal bleeding should occur. Efficacy and adverse effects are similar to those experienced with use of the contraceptive pill, with the exception of slightly increased breast tenderness associated with the patch. Skin reactions at the application site are rare (1% to 2.4% incidence). Partial or complete detachment of the patch occurs less than 5% of the time.

Use of a condom will reduce her risk of pregnancy, but it will not help with her breakthrough bleeding, which is also likely associated with her irregular pill use. The copper intrauterine device is known to cause bleeding and cramping during periods, and it may worsen her dysmenorrhea. The progestin-only pill must be taken very regularly to be most effective. This patient's difficulty with compliance limits use of this contraceptive modality as an option. The failure rate associated with the progestin-only pill is slightly higher than that of combination oral contraceptives. The progestin-only pill is typically prescribed to lactating women because combination estrogen-progestin contraceptive pills suppress milk production. The progestin-only pill is also appropriate when combination estrogen-progestin pills are contraindicated, as would be the case in women 35 years or older with a history of smoking, hypertension, or diabetes. Combination pills are also contraindicated in women with a history of thromboembolic disease, cardiac disease, or cerebrovascular disease.

> **KEY POINT**
>
> - In patients who have difficulty complying with the daily use of oral contraceptive pills for symptomatic relief of dysmenorrhea, the contraceptive patch, with similar efficacy, may be an appropriate alternative.

Bibliography

1. Petitti DB. Clinical practice. Combination estrogen-progestin oral contraceptives. N Engl J Med. 2003;349:1443-50. [PMID: 14534338]

2. Seibert C, Barbouche E, Fagan J, Myint E, Wetterneck T, Wittemyer M. Prescribing oral contraceptives for women older than 35 years of age. Ann Intern Med. 2003;138:54-64. [PMID: 12513046]

Item 52   Answer: A

Although many practitioners and hospital guidelines prefer a broad battery of preoperative tests, the evidence-based standard is selective testing based on the patient's medical history, physical examination, and risk for surgery-specific blood loss. Multiple studies have shown that indiscriminant preoperative testing rarely identifies clinically important abnormalities, delays surgery, or predicts complications. Abnormal test results often are ignored by clinicians or prove to be false-positive results.

Electrocardiography is indicated in men older than aged 40 years, in women older than aged 50 years (based on the median age of menopause in the United States), and in patients with known coronary artery disease, diabetes mellitus, or other significant risk factors for coronary artery disease, such as hyperlipidemia, family history of coronary artery disease at a young age, and hypertension. Measurement of serum electrolytes and creatinine is indicated because of this patient's history of hypertension and diuretic therapy. Chest radiography is not indicated because the patient does not smoke, is younger than 50 years, has no respiratory symptoms, and is physically active. A complete blood count is not necessary because anticipated blood loss is minimal for the planned procedure. Coagulation studies are not warranted because the patient has no history of bleeding difficulties. Because the patient has no urinary symptoms, preoperative urinalysis is not necessary. One well-designed study has determined tests performed within 4 months do not need repeating if medications or clinical status has not changed.

Bibliography

1. Swanson DL, Vetter RS. Bites of brown recluse spiders and suspected necrotic arachnidism. N Engl J Med. 2005;352:700-7. [PMID: 15716564]

2. Vetter RS. Arachnids submitted as suspected brown recluse spiders (Araneae: Sicariidae): Loxosceles spiders are virtually restricted to their known distributions but are perceived to exist throughout the United States. J Med Entomol. 2005;42:512-21. [PMID: 16119538]

KEY POINTS

- The evidence-based standard is selective preoperative testing based on medical history, physical examination, and risk for surgery-specific blood loss.
- Multiple studies have shown that indiscriminant preoperative testing rarely identifies clinically important abnormalities, delays surgery, or predicts complications.

Bibliography

1. Smetana GW, Macpherson DS. The case against routine preoperative laboratory testing. Med Clin North Am. 2003;87:7-40. [PMID: 12575882]

2. Macpherson DS, Snow R, Lofgren RP. Preoperative screening: value of previous tests. Ann Intern Med. 1990;113:969-73. [PMID: 2240920]

Item 53   Answer: B

Brown recluse spiders are most commonly found in the south-central United States and can often be discovered in dark basements. The best treatment option for this type of bug bite is ice application, wound elevation, and avoidance of strenuous exercise in the muscles surrounding the bite. There is no antivenom available in the United States for brown recluse spider bites and no specific therapy. Although black widow spider bites are often described as being very painful, the brown recluse bite may not be felt or is felt only as a pinprick. Shortly afterwards, patients often describe a stinging sensation at the bite site. Although most U.S. brown recluse spiders have a violin pattern on the cephalothorax (the first body part to which the legs attach), some western species and younger spiders may not have this pattern.

Because the reaction to brown recluse spider bites is to the venom, antihistamines such as fexofenadine are of limited value. The efficacy of other suggested treatment modalities, such as systemic or intralesional corticosteroids, hyperbaric oxygen, and electric therapy, are not supported by good evidence. Cutting or "sucking out the poison" from a brown recluse spider bite results in more harm than good.

Most brown recluse bites heal without necrosis. Debridement should be delayed in the 10% of patients who develop necrotic lesions for 6 to 8 weeks until the eschar has formed and the surrounding tissues are healthy. Although dapsone is sometimes used to limit wound necrosis, and there is some supportive evidence for its use in animals, there are no data on its efficacy in humans with brown recluse spider bites. If dapsone is used in these patients, glucose-6-phosphate dehydrogenase levels should be checked, because deficiency in this enzyme can lead to methemoglobinemia.

KEY POINT

- The best treatment for brown recluse spider bites is ice application, wound elevation, and avoidance of strenuous exercise in the muscles surrounding the bite.

Item 54   Answer: E

Initiation of testosterone replacement therapy is temporally related to and is the most likely explanation for this patient's erythrocytosis. Higher testosterone levels stimulate erythropoiesis, and injections are more potent stimulants than transdermal preparations. The resulting increase in blood viscosity could exacerbate cardiovascular disease, particularly in the elderly. Reducing the dose or stopping the injections are appropriate measures for treating erythrocytosis. Blood counts should be monitored in men receiving testosterone-replacement therapy, initially within 1 to 2 months of initiating therapy, then every 3 to 6 months for the first year, and then annually. Although there is no convincing evidence that testosterone-replacement therapy increases the risk for prostate cancer, patients should be monitored periodically for prostate cancer with prostate-specific antigen measurement and digital rectal examination. Chronic obstructive pulmonary disease is a common secondary cause of erythrocytosis, but this patient is oxygenating well with supplemental oxygen and maintained a normal hematocrit until initiation of testosterone. Increasing supplemental oxygen is unnecessary. Obstructive sleep apnea can cause erythrocytosis, but this snoring patient did not have apneic episodes or excessive daytime somnolence, and polysomnography is therefore not warranted. Although therapeutic phlebotomy may be required in patients with erythrocytosis, it is usually reserved for those with hematocrit values >55%. An elevated leukocyte alkaline phosphatase level is a minor criterion for diagnosing polycythemia vera, a chronic myeloproliferative disorder characterized by increased hematocrit and erythrocyte mass, platelet count >400,000/μL (400 × 10^9/L), and leukocyte count >12,000/μL (12 × 10^9/μL). Patients with polycythemia vera often have hepatomegaly, splenomegaly, and/or facial cyanosis. Erythrocytosis is the only criterion for polycythemia vera met by this patient.

KEY POINTS

- Blood counts should be monitored in men receiving testosterone-replacement therapy, initially within 1 to 2 months of initiating therapy, then every 3 to 6 months for the first year, and then annually.
- Higher testosterone levels stimulate erythropoiesis, and injections are more potent stimulants than transdermal preparations.

Bibliography

1. **Rhoden EL, Morgentaler A**. Risks of testosterone-replacement therapy and recommendations for monitoring. New Engl J Med 2004; 350:482-92. [PMID: 14749457]

Item 55   Answer: D

This patient has the metabolic syndrome, indicated by the presence of elevated triglycerides, a low serum high-density lipoprotein (HDL) cholesterol level, and hypertension. He should be advised to make lifestyle changes, including diet modification, weight loss, and increased physical activity. The metabolic syndrome should be a secondary target of therapy, after low-density lipoprotein level, to reduce a patient's risk of coronary artery disease (CAD). The metabolic syndrome augments this patient's risk for CAD.

Because his serum low-density lipoprotein (LDL) cholesterol level is acceptable for his CAD risk level, a statin is not recommended. A fibric acid derivative would lower triglycerides, however this is recommended only if a patient fails to make lifestyle changes that this patient has not yet initiated. The Adult Treatment Panel of the NCEP does not specifically recommend evaluation of LDL particle size to further guide treatment, although a separate measurement of LDL size has gained popularity. Research has indicated that small, dense LDL particles may contribute to CAD, however these particles are often present when patients have other high-risk characteristics, including high triglycerides, low HDL, diabetes, and metabolic syndrome. LDL subclass measurement does not add information to typical measurements of cholesterol values.

The diagnosis of the metabolic syndrome is based on the presence of three or more risk factors. Besides the elevated triglycerides (>50 mg/dL [1.69 mmol/L]), low HDL cholesterol (HDL cholesterol <40 mg/dL [1.03 mmol/L]), and hypertension (>130/>85 mmHg or taking antihypertensive drugs) that are present in this patient, additional risk factors used to diagnose metabolic syndrome include abdominal obesity (waist circumference >102 cm [40 in] for men or >88 cm [35 in] for women) and fasting glucose >110 mg/dL (6.11 mmol/L).

KEY POINT

- **The metabolic syndrome is a secondary target of therapy, after serum low-density lipoprotein level, to reduce a patient's risk for coronary artery disease.**

Bibliography

1. National Cholesterol Education Program. Third Report of the Expert Panel on Detection, Evaluation, and Treatment of High Blood Cholesterol in Adults (Adult Treatment Panel III). [The National Heart, Lung, and Blood Institute Web site]. Available at: http://www.nhlbi.nih.gov/guidelines/cholesterol/atp3full.pdf. Accessed August 1, 2006.
2. **Sacks FM, Campos H**. Clinical review 163: Cardiovascular endocrinology: Low-density lipoprotein size and cardiovascular disease: a reappraisal. J Clin Endocrinol Metab. 2003;88:4525-32. [PMID: 14557416]

Item 56   Answer: A

Given the recent initiation of a benzodiazepine, the most likely cause of this patient's confusion is a reaction to triazolam, and the appropriate intervention would be to discontinue this medication. The elderly are at increased risk for falls, accidents, and cognitive impairment from hypnotic agents. Benzodiazepines are the class of psychotropic agents most frequently implicated in causing delirium and exacerbating pre-existing cognitive impairment in elderly patients; they are also the class of psychotropic agents most often associated with falls and hip fractures in the elderly because of their sedative properties and effects on balance.

Doses of hypnotic medications should be decreased in the elderly, but once an adverse effect such as delirium occurs, prescribing a different medication is preferable to reducing the dose. The patient's physical examination findings and laboratory studies were normal; therefore, it is not necessary to perform a full workup to evaluate for an infectious etiology or occurrence of new stroke. Diphenhydramine is used as an off-label treatment for insomnia but is also associated with delirium in the elderly and would not be an appropriate substitute medication in this clinical scenario. Cognitive behavioral therapy has established efficacy in many randomized-controlled trials in the treatment of primary insomnia. However, it is less likely to be effective in patients with significant cognitive impairment. An appropriate alternative medication for the treatment of insomnia in patients who have difficulty falling asleep is zaleplon, a short-acting nonbenzodiazepine-benzodiazepine receptor agonist hypnotic agent. This drug also has rapid clearance and has been found to reduce the time to sleep in the elderly at a dose of 5 to 10 mg without documented residual fatigue effects. Zolpidem is also a nonbenzodiazepine-benzodiazepine-receptor agonist hypnotic agent, but its half-life of 2.5 hours is longer than that of zaleplon. There is greater potential for morning residual effects and rebound insomnia after discontinuation of zolpidem compared with zaleplon.

KEY POINTS

- **Benzodiazepines are one of the most frequently implicated classes of drugs causing delirium and exacerbating pre-existing cognitive impairment in elderly patients.**
- **Benzodiazepines are the class of psychotropic agents most often associated with falls and hip fractures in the elderly.**

Bibliography

1. **Desai AK**. Use of psychopharmacologic agents in the elderly. Clin Geriatr Med. 2003;19:697-719. [PMID: 15024808]
2. **Silber MH**. Clinical practice. Chronic insomnia. N Engl J Med. 2005;353:803-10. [PMID: 16120860]

Item 57   Answer: A

The standard of weight loss against which dietary interventions are compared is counseling for exercise and a balanced low-calorie diet. Against this standard, very-low-calorie diets are more difficult to adhere to and have not been found more effective at 1 year. Low-fat and low-carbohydrate diets have limited evidence to support their long-term efficacy. Low-carbohydrate diets, in particular, have not been well evaluated in persons older than 53 years of age and/or those with comorbid conditions. There is evidence from randomized-controlled trials that participation in Weight Watchers proprietary program leads to a loss of 3.2% of initial weight at 2 years. The Weight Watchers program recommends a balanced low-calorie diet, exercise, and behavioral modification.

Obesity is defined by the World Health Organization (WHO) as patients who have a BMI of 30 or higher. This patient has class II Obesity. There are three classes of obesity; class I is associated with a BMI of 30 to 34.9, class II with a BMI of 35 to 39.9, and class III with a BMI of 40 or greater. The WHO has defined success in management of the obese patient as a 5% to 15% reduction in initial weight. This patient has several risk factors for cardiovascular disease including obesity, hypertension, and hyperlipidemia. Obesity is also a risk factor for breast cancer among postmenopausal women. Therefore, weight reduction is an important intervention with respect to risk factor modification in this patient.

KEY POINT

- **The standard of weight loss against which dietary interventions are compared is counseling for exercise and a balanced low-calorie diet.**

Bibliography

1. **Snow V, Barry P, Fitterman N, Qaseem A, Weiss K**. Pharmacologic and surgical management of obesity in primary care: a clinical practice guideline from the American College of Physicians. Ann Intern Med. 2005;142:525-31. [PMID: 15809464]

2. **Tsai AG, Wadden TA**. Systematic review: an evaluation of major commercial weight loss programs in the United States. Ann Intern Med. 2005;142:56-66. [PMID: 15630109]

Item 58   Answer: A

This patient has complex regional pain syndrome, also known as reflex sympathetic dystrophy, which is a unique chronic pain syndrome consisting of chronic pain of the extremities, often characterized by swelling, vasomotor instability, skin changes, and patchy bone demineralization. The onset of this syndrome frequently begins following an injury, surgery, or vascular event. Although general principles of pain management apply, these patients also respond to bisphosphonates, presumably through bone-associated effects on nociception.

Transcutaneous electrical stimulation, tricyclic antidepressants or selective serotonin reuptake inhibitors such as fluoxetine, and corticosteroids have all been shown to improve the severity of various chronic pain syndromes but have not been shown specifically to improve complex regional pain syndrome.

Other adjunctive treatments that have been shown to be efficacious in treating complex regional pain syndrome include gabapentin, hyperbaric oxygen therapy, spinal cord stimulation coupled with physical therapy, intrathecal baclofen in patients with associated dystonia, and transdermal or epidural clonidine.

KEY POINT

- **Patients with complex regional pain syndrome respond to bisphosphonate therapy.**

Bibliography

1. **Manicourt DH, Brasseur JP, Boutsen Y, Depreseux G, Devogelaer JP**. Role of alendronate in therapy for posttraumatic complex regional pain syndrome type I of the lower extremity. Arthritis Rheum. 2004;50:3690-7. [PMID: 15529370]

Item 59   Answer: E

True syncope is an abrupt, transient loss of consciousness caused by global cerebral hypoperfusion without focal neurologic deficit and with spontaneous recovery. Rates of 1-year cardiac mortality and sudden death are higher for patients with cardiac syncope than noncardiac or idiopathic syncope. Arrhythmia is strongly suspected in this patient because of his known coronary artery disease and bifascicular block. Long-term ($\geq$30 days) event monitoring with external or implantable continuous-loop recorders is recommended when suspicion of arrhythmia remains after inpatient telemetry and ambulatory electrocardiographic monitoring are nondiagnostic. Continuous-loop recorders require that patients activate the monitoring when symptoms occur. After activation, readings are captured for the preceding several minutes and 1 minute longer. Subcutaneously implanted recorders can now monitor for events up to 18 months. Electrophysiologic testing would be performed as a last step in diagnosis or if patients cannot self-activate a continuous-loop recorder. Increasing ambulatory electrocardiographic monitoring to 72 hours will not increase the diagnostic yield. Cardiac catheterization is not the appropriate next step in this patient given the negative results on exercise stress testing. Tilt-table testing is indicated for patients with unexplained syncope in the absence of coronary artery disease or after a cardiac cause has been excluded.

KEY POINTS

- **Arrhythmia should be strongly suspected in patients with syncope and coronary artery disease and bifascicular block.**
- **Long-term ($\geq$30 days) event monitoring with external or implantable continuous-loop recorders is recommended when suspicion of arrhythmia remains after inpatient telemetry and ambulatory electrocardiographic monitoring are nondiagnostic.**

Bibliography

1. **Grubb BP**. Clinical practice. Neurocardiogenic syncope. N Engl J Med. 2005;352:1004-10. [PMID: 15758011]

2. **Brignole M, Alboni P, Benditt DG, Bergfeldt L, Blanc JJ, Thomsen PE, et al**. Guidelines on management (diagnosis and treatment) of syncope-update 2004. Executive Summary. Eur Heart J. 2004;25:2054-72. [PMID: 15541843]

Item 60   Answer: B

Corneal abrasion associated with hard or soft contact lenses is especially susceptible to infectious keratitis. The eye is red and painful; vision loss is not usually immediately present, but it may occur as the corneal abrasion progresses or with infectious keratitis. Permanent vision loss may occur. There is an increased risk for fulminant keratitis caused by *Pseudomonas sp.*

With hypopyon (white or yellowish-white accumulation of purulence in the anterior chamber) and hyphema (blood in the anterior chamber), gravity causes inferior pooling. Both conditions are associated with acute anterior uveitis (red and painful eye with decreased visual acuity) and corneal trauma, infiltrate, or ulcer. Anterior uveitis also presents with red, painful eye, blurred vision, and vision loss, usually in young or middle-aged persons, but is not associated with contact lens use, corneal abrasion, or foreign-body sensation. There is diffuse erythema prominent at the limbus, light reflex is sluggish to unreactive, and the pupil is constricted in patients with anterior uveitis. Diagnosis of this condition usually requires slit-lamp examination, and hypopyon or hyphema may be visible at the base of the anterior chamber. Herpetic keratitis is associated with watery discharge and dendritic, or branching, pattern on fluorescein staining, and may have branching opacities. Hypopyon, infectious keratitis associated with corneal abrasion, and anterior uveitis require emergency referral to an ophthalmologist; viral keratitis should be evaluated by an ophthalmologist in 1 to 2 days.

KEY POINT

- Corneal abrasion associated with hard or soft contact lenses is especially susceptible to infectious keratitis.

Bibliography
1. **Mah-Sadorra JH, Yavuz SG, Najjar DM, Laibson PR, Rapuano CJ, Cohen EJ**. Trends in contact lens-related corneal ulcers. Cornea. 2005;24:51-8. [PMID: 15604867]
2. **Cheng KH, Leung SL, Hoekman HW, Beekhuis WH, Mulder PG, Geerards AJ, et al**. Incidence of contact-lens-associated microbial keratitis and its related morbidity. Lancet. 1999;354:181-5. [PMID: 10421298]

Item 61   Answer: B

This patient has evidence of the cauda equina syndrome, including urinary retention, saddle anesthesia, and radiculopathy, likely resulting from epidural spinal cord compression caused by metastatic prostate tumor. Suspected cauda equina syndrome is an indication for urgent evaluation and requires definitive imaging to visualize the spinal cord and epidural space. MRI is a noninvasive definitive imaging study for confirming epidural spinal cord compression. CT myelogram is also a definitive imaging study, although it requires a lumbar puncture. CT of the lumbar spine does not provide an image of the cord and epidural space as well as MRI does, and it requires longer imaging time in addition to exposing the patient to ionizing radiation. Although positron emission tomography (PET) is used to detect metastatic tumors, it has poorer anatomic resolution than MRI, and there are little data on its role in detecting spinal cord compression. Radiography of the lumbar spine can detect vertebral body collapse and lytic lesions, but it has limited sensitivity for detecting spinal cord compression. Although radionuclide bone scanning has a high sensitivity (>90%) for identifying metastases, it also cannot determine the presence of spinal cord compression.

KEY POINTS

- Cauda equina syndrome is characterized by urinary retention, saddle anesthesia, and radiculopathy.
- Cauda equina syndrome is an indication for urgent evaluation and requires definitive imaging to visualize the spinal cord and epidural space.

Bibliography
1. **Jarvik JG, Deyo RA**. Diagnostic evaluation of low back pain with emphasis on imaging. Ann Intern Med. 2002;137:586-97. [PMID: 12353946]
2. **Prasad D, Schiff D**. Malignant spinal-cord compression. Lancet Oncol. 2005;6:15-24. [PMID: 15629272]

Item 62   Answer: A

This patient has several "red flags" that should prompt immediate neuroradiologic imaging in the form of an MRI of the head, including headache onset that is acute and occurring after age 50 years and a history of malignancy. Other headache warning signs include atypical or nonreproducible symptoms, fever, rash, HIV status, pregnancy, vomiting, severe hypertension, nonresolving neurologic defects, or trauma. Encephalitis or other central nervous system infections can cause headaches, but neither her history nor physical examination suggests the presence of such an infection. Headaches can be caused by a number of medical conditions, including hyperparathyroidism, Lyme disease, hepatitis, and renal cell carcinoma, but the more urgent concern is ruling out metastatic disease in this patient through MRI of the head. A bone scan is not indicated because the patient is not displaying any symptoms suggesting bone involvement at this time, and the more immediate need is to evaluate the source of her pain through MRI. Although she has a history of migraine headaches, her current headache is different in nature from the migraines she experienced in the past, and she has been headache free for over 2 decades; therefore, triptans, which are specific agents for treating migraines, are not indicated.

- Headaches that are acute in onset, occur after age 50 years, and are associated with a history of malignancy are "red flags" prompting immediate neuroradiologic evaluation.

Bibliography

1. Taylor FR. Diagnosis and classification of headache. Prim Care. 2004;31:243-59. [PMID: 15172505]

Item 63   Answer: E

Because of her age and occupational exposure, this patient is at high risk for developing a serious varicella-zoster viral infection and should be immunized with the usual two-dose series. The varicella vaccine is recommended for all adults with no evidence of immunity to varicella-zoster virus. Special consideration is given to persons with close contact to individuals at high risk for severe disease, such as health care workers and family contacts of immuno-compromised patients. Teachers of young children and child care employees, residents and staff in institutional settings (including correctional facilities), military personnel, college students, women who may become pregnant, and international travelers are at high risk for exposure.

Patients taking less than 20 mg daily of prednisone (or the equivalent) can safely obtain vaccinations, with expectation of immunity without dissemination. Live vaccination should not be given to persons who take more than 20 mg daily of prednisone (or the equivalent), because of the risk for developing active disease. Because this patient takes 10 mg prednisone daily, the risk for development of disseminated varicella from the live attenuated vaccine is low. She may proceed with the usual vaccination series.

The live varicella vaccine causes some viral shedding in the 4 weeks after injection, so she should avoid patients who can get sick from exposure to her. Given her employment as a pediatric nurse, she should not start work for 4 weeks after the first vaccination. Also, because of a theoretical risk of Reye's syndrome, use of salicylates is discouraged in the 6 weeks after vaccination.

The live varicella vaccine has been available only since 1995, so its long-term effectiveness is still being defined. There have been breakthrough cases of the disease in vaccinated populations, notably in day-care environments. It may be that a booster will be recommended to address this issue. In addition, a vaccination for older adults who are at risk for reactivated herpes zoster (shingles) is in development.

A single dose (shortened series) is not advised for any population. Persons undergoing vaccination should get the two-dose series over 4 to 8 weeks. Persons with a family history of congenital immune disorders or with cellular immunity defects (symptomatic HIV infection) should not get the live attenuated varicella vaccine. Pregnancy is also a contraindication for this vaccine. For persons who cannot be immunized, varicella-zoster immune globulin and antiviral medications are available if they are exposed to chickenpox.

- The varicella vaccine is recommended for all adults with no evidence of immunity to varicella.

Bibliography

1. **Davis MM**. Successes and remaining challenges after 10 years of varicella vaccination in the USA. Expert Rev Vaccines. 2006;5:295-302. [PMID: 16608428]

Item 64   Answer: C

Urticaria that does not respond to usual treatment should prompt a workup for urticarial vasculitis, including erythrocyte sedimentation rate, complete blood count, and skin biopsy from the edge of the wheal. Histopathologic evidence of vascular damage, nuclear debris, or erythrocyte extravasation is diagnostic. This form of leukocytoclastic vasculitis is often limited to the skin, but, occasionally, there is organ involvement or systemic signs, such as fever, abdominal pain, or nephritis. Most cases are idiopathic, but they can also be drug-induced (ACE inhibitors, penicillin, and sulfonamide), related to rheumatic diseases such as systemic lupus erythematosus, or caused by viral disease, including hepatitis B and C infection, and infectious mononucleosis. Treatment is dictated by the underlying cause, if one is found. If not, a trial of anti-inflammatory or immunomodulating medications is indicated. Often, more than one agent must be tried before there is long-term relief.

C1 esterase inhibitor deficiency, also known as hereditary angioedema, causes cutaneous edema with tightness or tingling of the skin followed by angioedema that evolves over several hours. It is often associated with dermatographism and abdominal pain related to bowel wall edema; it may also cause life-threatening laryngeal edema. Affected women may have attacks during menses, but most episodes do not have a precipitating factor. Decreased C4 and CH50 levels are typical during attacks. Quantitative and qualitative C1 inhibitor assays are needed to confirm the diagnosis.

Skin testing is generally indicated in the evaluation of patients with suspected atopic disease, allergic rhinitis, asthma, atopic eczema, or allergic reactions to foods, venoms, or drugs. This patient does not report upper respiratory symptoms, and despite frequent episodes, he has not been able to link the attacks to a specific exposure.

Overactive and underactive thyroid syndromes can cause urticaria, but there are usually other signs and symptoms associated with these syndromes, including weight changes, bowel changes, and fatigue.

- Urticaria that does not respond to usual treatment should prompt a workup for urticarial vasculitis, including erythrocyte sedimentation rate, complete blood count, and skin biopsy from the edge of the wheal.

Bibliography

1. **Greaves MW**. Chronic urticaria. N Engl J Med. 1995;332:1767-72. [PMID: 7760895]

Item 65   Answer: D

This patient is at increased risk for venous thromboembolic disease secondary to her history of deep vein thrombosis (DVT). The levonorgestrel intrauterine device (IUD) will not increase her risk for developing embolic disease. The IUD will also sufficiently decrease the likelihood of pregnancy because only 0.1% of patients using it become pregnant during the first year. This preventive effect compares favorably with permanent sterilization, which is associated with an expected 1.85% cumulative 10-year failure rate. Although a patient may note increased menstrual bleeding and spotting during the first 3 months of using a levonorgestrel IUD, these effects usually decrease over time. Levonorgestrel will eventually help reduce the heaviness of periods. Amenorrhea can be expected in 20% to 50% of patients 1 year after insertion.

Oral and topical hormonal contraception are contraindicated in this patient because of her history of DVT. The risk for venous thromboembolism from hormonal contraception is higher in patients with thrombophilias, including plasma protein C and protein S deficiency, factor V Leiden, or the prothrombin gene mutation. However, screening for DVT is not routinely recommended before patients begin taking oral contraceptives. In the average population, the risk for venous thromboembolism increases with age and varies by type of progestin used. Desogestrel or gestodene produce a higher risk (16 to 30 excess cases per 100,000 woman-years of use, depending on age), and the remaining progestins are lower risk (6 to 12 excess cases per 100,000 woman-years of use, depending on age).

Although the diaphragm is a safe form of contraception, it will not provide the level of protection from pregnancy that the IUD provides, but it does offer protection equal to that provided by condoms.

KEY POINTS

- **In patients with a history of deep venous thrombosis (DVT), the levonorgestrel intrauterine device will not increase the risk for developing embolic disease and also sufficiently decreases the likelihood of pregnancy.**
- **Both oral and topical hormonal contraception are contraindicated in patients with a history of DVT.**

Bibliography

1. **Petitti DB**. Clinical practice. Combination estrogen-progestin oral contraceptives. N Engl J Med. 2003;349:1443-50. [PMID: 14534338]
2. **Peterson HB, Curtis KM**. Clinical practice. Long-acting methods of contraception. N Engl J Med. 2005;353:2169-75. [PMID: 16291986]

Item 66   Answer: C

This patient's diagnosis is postherpetic neuralgia from herpes zoster. Postherpetic neuralgia, causing pain after the rash heals, occurs in about 9% to 34% of patients with herpes zoster, and the incidence increases with age. Spontaneous resolution of postherpetic neuralgia is common, particularly during the first 6 months of the episode, but medical treatment may be indicated for pain that is interfering with functioning or sleep. Gabapentin, approved by the Food and Drug Administration for treatment of postherpetic neuralgia, has been shown to reduce pain and improve sleep in randomized controlled trials. Side effects of treatment include dizziness, somnolence, and peripheral edema.

Although acute treatment of herpes zoster with antiviral agents such as famciclovir can reduce the incidence of postherpetic neuralgia, the agents do not provide symptomatic relief for this condition. Prednisone is also not effective for relieving symptoms in patients with postherpetic neuralgia. Most studies evaluating other treatments for postherpetic neuralgia, including opioids, lidocaine patch, and capsaicin, are small and heterogeneous. Better-designed trials are needed.

This patient's age and history of bladder outlet obstruction from benign prostatic hyperplasia require cautious use of opioids such as oral oxycodone. Tricyclic antidepressants (off-label use) can reduce severity, duration, and prevalence of postherpetic neuralgia, especially when initiated early in the course of the illness, but side effects can limit their use.

KEY POINT

- **Gabapentin, approved by the Food and Drug Administration for treatment of postherpetic neuralgia, has been shown to reduce pain and improve sleep in randomized controlled trials.**

Bibliography

1. **Plaghki L, Adriaensen H, Morlion B, Lossignol D, Devulder J**. Systematic overview of the pharmacological management of postherpetic neuralgia. An evaluation of the clinical value of critically selected drug treatments based on efficacy and safety outcomes from randomized controlled studies. Dermatology. 2004;208:206-16. [PMID: 15118369]

Item 67   Answer: C

This patient has noncardiac chest pain; therapy with a tricyclic antidepressant would be an appropriate option in this setting.

Although not rigorously defined, a current understanding of noncardiac chest pain is chest discomfort, the character of which is inconsistent with obstructive epicardial coronary artery disease, pericardial disease, or myocardial disease, or in which standard cardiovascular testing for such diseases has sufficiently ruled out the heart as a cause for the chest pain.

Among patients with chronic noncardiac chest pain, randomized, placebo-controlled studies have demonstrated that tricyclic antidepressants, β-blockers, ACE inhibitors, L-arginine, statins, and exercise may relieve symptoms. Empiric treatment with high-dose proton pump inhibitors may be helpful in diagnosing a gastroesophageal reflux etiology, and patients with esophageal spasm may respond to sublingual nitroglycerin or calcium channel blocker therapy.

Colchicine and NSAIDs have been shown to be efficacious in the management of chest pain associated with recurrent pericarditis but have not been studied in patients with noncardiac chest pain.

Fluoxetine and tramadol have not been studied in clinical trials specifically for their efficacy in treating noncardiac chest pain; thus, there is insufficient evidence to support their use for noncardiac chest pain.

KEY POINT

- **Among patients with chronic noncardiac chest pain, randomized, placebo-controlled studies have demonstrated that tricyclic antidepressants, β-blockers, ACE inhibitors, L-arginine, statins, and exercise may relieve symptoms.**

Bibliography

1. **Bugiardini R, Bairey Merz CN**. Angina with "normal" coronary arteries: a changing philosophy. JAMA. 2005;293:477-84. [PMID: 15671433]
2. **Wang WH, Huang JQ, Zheng GF, Wong WM, Lam SK, Karlberg J, et al**. Is proton pump inhibitor testing an effective approach to diagnose gastroesophageal reflux disease in patients with noncardiac chest pain?: a meta-analysis. Arch Intern Med. 2005;165:1222-8. [PMID: 15956000]

Item 68   Answer: B

Causes of unexplained weight loss in the elderly include depression, cancer, benign gastrointestinal conditions, medication toxicities, and socioeconomic concerns. Elderly patients may be at nutritional risk because of difficulties with grocery shopping, meal preparation, or social isolation. In this case, the patient has difficulty grocery shopping. Arranging for assistance in shopping and/or meal preparation would an appropriate intervention.

The most common malignancies characterized by weight loss in the elderly are lung and gastrointestinal malignancies. Because this patient's physical examination, laboratory studies, and recent series of fecal occult blood testing and chest radiography were normal, no further workup for malignancy, including CT of the abdomen or colonoscopy, is required at this time. Depression can cause weight loss in the elderly, but this patient takes antidepressant therapy, states that her mood is good, and has a low score on the Five-Item Geriatric Depression Scale, indicating a negative depression screening result; only patients with scores of 2 or more (of a possible 5) require further evaluation for depression. Therefore, a change in antidepressant medication is not indicated. Benign gastrointestinal problems such as reflux are common causes of weight loss in the elderly, but this patient has no abdominal symptoms and takes ibuprofen only intermittently. Therefore, it is not necessary to discontinue this drug in this patient at this time.

KEY POINTS

- **Causes of unexplained weight loss in the elderly include depression, cancer, benign gastrointestinal conditions, medication toxicities, and socioeconomic concerns.**
- **The most common malignancies characterized by weight loss in the elderly are lung and gastrointestinal malignancies.**

Bibliography

1. **Ensberg M, Gerstenlauer C**. Incremental geriatric assessment. Prim Care. 2005;32:619-43. [PMID: 16140119]

Item 69   Answer: A

Vestibular rehabilitation is one of the few evidence-based treatments for chronic dizziness of various causes, including peripheral vestibular disorders, benign positional vertigo (BPV), multifactorial dizziness in the elderly, psychologic factors, and head injury. Vestibular rehabilitation can be taught to a patient by a nurse in 30 to 40 minutes and is a program of graded home-based exercises consisting of head, eye, and body movements designed to stimulate the vestibular system. This intervention can improve symptoms, postural stability, and dizziness-related challenges.

Habituation exercises can be performed at home and consist of the patient lying down with the head in a position that reproduces vertigo, with repetition of this maneuver 10 to 15 times several times per day. These exercises have limited clinical trial efficacy and have been principally tested in patients with BPV rather than other types of chronic dizziness. Although paroxetine and cognitive behavioral therapy may both benefit the somatic symptoms associated with depressive and anxiety disorders, their efficacy has not been established for dizziness in the absence of depression or anxiety. This patient has nonspecific symptoms of fatigue and trouble sleeping, but more specific symptoms of depressed mood, anhedonia, or anxiety are not present. Vestibular nerve resection is a treatment of last resort for patients with disabling Meniere's disease but is not indicated for other types of chronic dizziness. Meclizine may help some patients with acute vertiginous attacks, such as those occurring in patients with labyrinthitis and Meniere's disease, but is not indicated in patients with chronic dizziness.

KEY POINT

- **Vestibular rehabilitation is one of the few evidence-based treatments for chronic dizziness, including peripheral vestibular disorders, benign positional vertigo, multifactorial dizziness in the elderly, psychologic factors, and head injury.**

Bibliography

1. **Yardley L, Donovan-Hall M, Smith HE, Walsh BM, Mullee M, Bronstein AM**. Effectiveness of primary care-based vestibular rehabilitation for chronic dizziness. Ann Intern Med. 2004;141:598-605. [PMID: 15492339]

Item 70   Answer: C

This patient has panic disorder, for which selective serotonin reuptake inhibitors (SSRIs), such as paroxetine, are considered first-line therapy. It is recommended that the initial dose of therapy in this patient be low and titrated to moderate doses over the first month of treatment. Partial responders, those with at least a 50% improvement at 4 weeks, should receive augmentation therapy with a benzodiazepine or cognitive behavioral therapy (CBT). Nonresponders should undergo a trial of a different SSRI or a serotonin norepinephrine reuptake inhibitor. Additional augmentation with CBT, if not already initiated, or atypical neuroleptics (risperidone, 1 to 2 mg; olanzapine, 5 to 10 mg; or quetiapine, 25 to 50 mg) should be considered in patients with persistent symptoms after 6 months of therapy.

The abrupt onset of symptoms, lack of evidence of ischemia or arrhythmias during his two recent evaluations, and the lack of symptoms with strenuous exercise make a cardiac cause of his symptoms unlikely; therefore, adenosine stress testing with a thallium scan is not appropriate in this patient. Although hyperthyroidism might be responsible for some of his symptoms, symptoms of hyperthyroidism are unlikely to be so intermittent and temporally discrete as those occurring in this patient. In addition, no thyromegaly was noted on physical examination, which is present in most cases of Graves' hyperthyroidism. Pheochromocytoma can cause similar symptoms, but this patient's normal blood pressure makes this diagnosis less likely. In addition, pheochromocytoma is a rare disorder, whereas panic attacks occur commonly; therefore 24-hour urine collection for catecholamine and metanephrine measurement is not indicated. Studies to rule out pheochromocytoma should be sought, however, if the patient fails to respond to treatment. Antipsychotic medications are not first-line therapy in panic disorder but might be appropriate in patients in whom augmentation therapy has failed. Clinical trials have shown CBT to have equal efficacy with pharmacologic treatment, and the combination of CBT with pharmacologic treatment is synergistic, but CBT is not a first-line therapy for this disorder.

KEY POINT

- **First-line therapy for panic disorder consists of selective serotonin reuptake inhibitors, such as paroxetine.**

Bibliography

1. **Otto MW, Deveney C**. Cognitive-behavioral therapy and the treatment of panic disorder: efficacy and strategies. J Clin Psychiatry. 2005;66 Suppl 4:28-32. [PMID: 15842185]

Item 71   Answer: B

Although irritable bowel syndrome (IBS) occurs very commonly in patients in this age group, and many features of this patient's presentation suggest this syndrome, including the chronicity of the problem, its association with stress, and the pattern of alternating diarrhea and constipation, she also has two alarm symptoms, weight loss of greater than 4.5 kg (10 lb), and anemia; therefore, she should undergo colonoscopy.

In patients with tenesmus or hematochezia, disease is likely distal, and flexible sigmoidoscopy may be sufficient. Crohn's disease is frequently characterized by skip areas (that is, areas of normal-appearing bowel interrupted by large areas of diseased bowel) and often is associated with terminal ileitis, diagnosable with a colonoscopy; however, a small-bowel follow-through is sometimes required to find disease that does not extend to the colon. If the patient were febrile, a CT of the abdomen might be necessary to identify fistulas and abscesses, which can occur in Crohn's disease.

Fecal calprotectin is a zinc- and calcium-binding protein derived mostly from neutrophils and monocytes, and although initial studies suggest that measuring levels of this protein may be useful for distinguishing inflammatory from noninflammatory causes of chronic diarrhea, its test characteristics are not yet sufficiently defined for routine clinical use.

Rome II criteria for IBS require the presence of 3 (not-necessarily-consecutive) months of pain relieved with defecation and onset associated with change in stool frequency or consistency. In clinical practice, these criteria have a positive predictive value of 98%. Because most clinicians are unaware of these criteria, the American College of Gastroenterology recommends diagnosis of IBS based on abdominal discomfort associated with altered bowel habits. However, both of these clinical diagnostic rules should be applied only to patients who have no "alarm" symptoms suggesting a potentially serious underlying condition, such as hematochezia, weight loss greater than 4.5 kg (10 lb), family history of colon cancer, recurring fever, anemia, or chronic severe diarrhea.

KEY POINT

- **"Alarm" symptoms in patients with abdominal pain include hematochezia, weight loss >4.5 kg (10 lb), family history of colon cancer, recurring fever, anemia, or chronic severe diarrhea.**

Bibliography

1. **Carroccio A, Iacono G, Cottone M, Di Prima L, Cartabellotta F, Cavataio F, et al**. Diagnostic accuracy of fecal calprotectin assay in distinguishing organic causes of chronic diarrhea from irritable bowel syndrome: a prospective study in adults and children. Clin Chem. 2003;49:861-7. [PMID: 12765980]

2. **Pardi DS, Sandborn WJ**. Predicting relapse in patients with inflammatory bowel disease: what is the role of biomarkers? Gut. 2005;54:321-2. [PMID: 15710974]

3. **Vermeire S, Van Assche G, Rutgeerts P**. C-reactive protein as a marker for inflammatory bowel disease. Inflamm Bowel Dis. 2004;10:661-5. [PMID: 15472532]

Item 72   Answer: E

Rotator cuff tendonitis, an inflammation of the supraspinatus and/or infraspinatus tendon that can also involve the subacromial bursa, is a common overuse injury. This injury is characterized by subacromial tenderness and impingement—painful compression of the rotator cuff tendons and subacromial bursa between the humeral head and the acromion with arm elevation. Pain in patients with rotator cuff tendonitis often occurs with overhead reaching and when lying on the side. The passive painful-arc maneuver assesses the degree of impingement. The examiner places one hand on the acromion, another on the forearm, and abducts the arm while preventing the patient from shrugging. Subacromial pain at 60 to 70 degrees of abduction suggests moderate impingement, while pain at 45 degrees or less suggests severe impingement. Pain with resisted midarc abduction is a specific finding for rotator cuff tendonitis. Appropriate treatments for acute tendonitis include NSAIDs, ice, and exercises; overhead reaching and lifting should be limited in these patients.

Adhesive capsulitis (frozen shoulder) is characterized by a decreased range of shoulder motion predominantly resulting from stiffness rather than from pain or weakness. Bicipital tendonitis is also an overuse injury in which the bicipital groove may be tender, and anterior shoulder pain is elicited with resisted forearm supination or elbow flexion. Glenohumeral arthritis is often related to trauma and the gradual onset of pain and stiffness over months to years. A torn rotator cuff usually results in arm weakness, particularly with abduction and/or external rotation. A postive drop-arm test (inability to smoothly lower the affected arm from full abduction) is a very specific but relatively insensitive method for diagnosing rotator cuff tear.

KEY POINT

- **Rotator cuff tendonitis is characterized by subacromial tenderness and impingement; pain often occurs with overhead reaching and when lying on the side.**

Bibliography
1. **Koester MC, George MS, Kuhn JE**. Shoulder impingement syndrome. Am J Med. 2005;118:452-5. [PMID: 15866244]
2. **Green S, Buchbinder R, Hetrick S**. Physiotherapy interventions for shoulder pain. Cochrane Database Syst Rev. 2003:CD004258. [PMID: 12804509]

Item 73   Answer: D

This patient should be reassured that he has recurrent aphthous ulcers, not herpes simplex virus infection. Recurrent aphthous ulcers usually begin to occur in the teenaged years and recur intermittently, and their etiology is unknown.

Thalidomide has been found useful in treating severe stomatitis among patients with immunodeficiency, particularly those with HIV, but it is not indicated in this patient. Before treatment with thalidomide is initiated, clinicians are required by the manufacturer to register and ask patients to complete an informed consent, because this drug, even when transmitted by seminal fluids, can cause birth defects. Performing another HIV test is not indicated in this patient at this time. Patients with oropharyngeal candidiasis often describe a cottony sensation in the mouth, loss of taste, and, occasionally, pain induced by eating and swallowing, symptoms not present in this patient.

KEY POINT

- **Recurrent aphthous ulcers usually begin to occur in the teenaged years and recur intermittently, and their etiology is unknown.**

Bibliography
1. **Porter S, Scully C**. Aphthous ulcers (recurrent). Clin Evid. 2004:1766-73. [PMID: 15652078]

Item 74   Answer: A

This patient meets the criteria for perioperative cardioprophylaxis with a β-blocker.

The recently validated Revised Cardiac Risk Index assigns one point each for the following six variables: high-risk surgery, history of ischemic heart disease, history of heart failure, history of cerebrovascular disease, diabetes mellitus treated with insulin, and serum creatinine level >2.0 mg/dL (176.84 µmol/L). According to their score, patients fall into one of four risk strata: 0, 1, 2, or ≥3 points. This patient has excellent exertional capacity because he is able to achieve and sustain >4 metabolic equivalents (METS), but his Revised Cardiac Risk Index score of 2, determined by the presence of ischemic heart disease and coronary artery disease in the setting of a high-risk procedure, indicates that he has a high risk for postoperative cardiac complications.

If there is no contraindication, patients with coronary artery disease or significant risk factors should take perioperative β-blockers, titrated to a resting heart rate of 60/min. Patients not already taking β-blockers who meet the criteria for perioperative β-blocker therapy may also meet the criteria for long-term use of these drugs. β-Blockers should be titrated over 7 to 10 days before surgery; if this is not feasible, these drugs can be quickly titrated up preoperatively and intraoperatively. If patients do not meet criteria for long-term β-blocker therapy, this medication may be discontinued 7 to 10 days postoperatively if they are doing well and ambulating.

Neither stress testing nor echocardiography is indicated in this patient because he does not require further risk stratification before high-risk surgery, he is clinically stable without evidence of new or worsening ischemia, and it has been 5 years or less since revascularization. In a well-done randomized trial, perioperative right heart catheterization did not reduce perioperative cardiac morbidity and mortality in high-risk surgical patients.

Trials of perioperative β-antagonists have studied a range of drugs and intravenous or oral regimens; it is not clear whether the cardioprotective effects of these agents are drug-specific (atenolol, bisoprolol) or a class effect. Recent studies suggest the benefits of β-blockers are not yet fully elucidated. Although several small meta-analyses of 5 to 11 trials consistently found benefit with the perioperative use of β-blockers, a recent meta-analysis of 22 trials found no benefit in total mortality, cardiovascular mortality, or nonfatal myocardial infarction and found benefit only for a composite outcome of major perioperative cardiac complications (risk reduction 0.44; 95% CI, 0.20 to 0.97). Additionally, a large retrospective cohort study of major noncardiac surgery found β-blockers to be associated with reduced hospital mortality in patients with Revised Cardiac Index scores ≥2, no benefit in patients with a score of 1, and increased mortality in patients with a score of 0.

KEY POINT

- If there is no contraindication, patients with coronary artery disease or significant risk factors should take perioperative β-blockers, titrated to a resting heart rate of 60/min.

Bibliography

1. Eagle KA, Berger PB, Calkins H, Chaitman BR, Ewy GA, Fleischmann KE, et al. ACC/AHA guideline update for perioperative cardiovascular evaluation for noncardiac surgery—executive summary: a report of the American College of Cardiology/American Heart Association Task Force on Practice Guidelines (Committee to Update the 1996 Guidelines on Perioperative Cardiovascular Evaluation for Noncardiac Surgery). J Am Coll Cardiol. 2002;39:542-53. [PMID: 11823097]

2. Grayburn PA, Hillis LD. Cardiac events in patients undergoing noncardiac surgery: shifting the paradigm from noninvasive risk stratification to therapy. Ann Intern Med. 2003;138:506-11. [PMID: 12639086]

3. Lindenauer PK, Pekow P, Wang K, Mamidi DK, Gutierrez B, Benjamin EM. Perioperative beta-blocker therapy and mortality after major noncardiac surgery. N Engl J Med. 2005;353:349-61. [PMID: 16049209]

4. Sandham JD, Hull RD, Brant RF, Knox L, Pineo GF, Doig CJ, et al. A randomized, controlled trial of the use of pulmonary-artery catheters in high-risk surgical patients. N Engl J Med. 2003;348:5-14. [PMID: 12510037]

Item 75   Answer: A

The Canadian (Ottawa) criteria for patients with blunt trauma to the cervical spine include five factors, that, if negative, are highly sensitive for ruling out serious cervical spine injury. These factors are 1) no midline cervical tenderness on direct palpation, 2) no focal neurologic deficits, 3) normal alertness, 4) no intoxication, and 5) no painful distracting injuries. Tenderness is considered present if the patient reports pain on palpation of the posterior midline neck from the nuchal ridge to the prominence of the T1

vertebra, or if the patient experiences pain with direct palpation of any cervical spine process. Altered alertness includes a Glasgow coma scale score of 14 or lower, disorientation to person, place, time, or events, or failure to recall three objects at 5 minutes.

This patient fulfills all five criteria, and thus the negative predictive value is 99.8% for serious injury. This simple decision instrument was validated by the National Emergency X-ray Utilization Study (NEXUS), a prospective study that enrolled over 34,000 patients from 21 emergency departments in the United States. Using clinical criteria only in patients presenting with neck injury and neck pain, this instrument essentially rules out serious pathology and decreases the need for imaging. In retrospective studies to confirm these findings, the criteria were modified to include three factors related to mechanism of injury. This modification may add additional prognostic information, but it also makes the tool more complex. The simplicity of the five-factor criteria is part of its appeal.

If any one of these criteria is not present, imaging is indicated. For patients at high risk, CT is the preferred initial strategy because its sensitivity for fracture may decrease the need for further imaging.

KEY POINT

- An absence of midline cervical tenderness on direct palpation, focal neurologic deficits, intoxication, or painful distracting injuries; and normal alertness are highly sensitive for ruling out cervical spine injury.

Bibliography

1. Blackmore CC. Evidence-based imaging evaluation of the cervical spine in trauma. Neuroimaging Clin N Am. 2003;13:283-91. [PMID: 13677807]

Item 76   Answer: E

Topical ophthalmologic medications often have systemic side effects, particularly β-blockers. Fatigue, hypotension, bradycardia, and exacerbations of reactive airway disease and heart failure are recognized side effects of timolol eye drops. Neither alendronate nor glyburide are reported to cause persistent fatigue. Alendronate most often causes adverse gastrointestinal effects, and glyburide can cause hypoglycemia, particularly in elderly patients and in those with renal or hepatic insufficiency. Latanoprost, a topical ophthalmic prostaglandin, is an effective treatment for glaucoma with minimal systemic side effects. Although hypothyroidism, which would be suggestive of an insufficient levothyroxine dose, can cause fatigue, her serum thyroid-stimulating hormone level is only slightly elevated.

KEY POINT

- Fatigue, hypotension, bradycardia, and exacerbations of reactive airway disease and heart failure are recognized side effects of timolol eye drops.

Bibliography
1. **Khaw PT, Shah P, Elkington AR**. Glaucoma—2: treatment. BMJ. 2004;328:156-8. [PMID: 14726349]

Item 77   Answer: B

This patient has minor depression for which the best management approach is regular follow-up evaluation to monitor for the progression from minor to major depression. Minor depression, also known as subthreshold depression, occurs commonly, present in up to 15% of patients in primary care. Minor depression consists of the presence of either depressed mood or anhedonia (or both) with other symptoms that total more than two but less than the five total symptoms required to establish a diagnosis of major depression. Although follow-up data are sparse, the limited evidence suggests that minor depression is transient in most patients, with approximately only 10% to 15% progressing to major depression.

Although minor depression decreases functional status, several treatment trials of pharmacotherapy and psychotherapy have reported that treatment outcomes for these modalities are no better than those associated with placebo.

KEY POINTS
- Minor depression consists of the presence of either depressed mood or anhedonia (or both) with other symptoms that total more than two but less than the five total symptoms required to establish a diagnosis of major depression.
- Although minor depression decreases functional status, several treatment trials of pharmacotherapy and psychotherapy have reported that treatment outcomes for these modalities are no better than those associated with placebo.

Bibliography
1. **Kroenke K**. Minor depression: midway between major depression and euthymia [Editorial]. Ann Intern Med. 2006;144:528-30. [PMID: 16585668]
2. **Hermens ML, van Hout HP, Terluin B, van der Windt DA, Beekman AT, van Dyck R, et al**. The prognosis of minor depression in the general population: a systematic review. Gen Hosp Psychiatry. 2004;26:453-62. [PMID: 15567211]
3. **Barrett JE, Williams JW Jr, Oxman TE, Frank E, Katon W, Sullivan M, et al**. Treatment of dysthymia and minor depression in primary care: a randomized trial in patients aged 18 to 59 years. J Fam Pract. 2001;50:405-12. [PMID: 11350703]

Item 78   Answer: D

All three drugs should be temporarily discontinued perioperatively. There is increasing evidence that selective serotonin reuptake inhibitors (SSRIs) may increase the risk for bleeding because of depletion of intraplatelet serotonin stores. Estrogen and selective estrogen receptor modulators (SERMs), such as raloxifene and tamoxifen, increase the risk for thromboembolism and should be discontinued perioperatively. The length of time patients can interrupt therapy with an antineoplastic SERM should be coordinated with an oncologist. Alendronate should be discontinued until patients become ambulatory and have resumed normal eating patterns so they can safely take this drug, which requires patients to remain upright for 30 minutes after ingestion of a full glass of water.

Ginkgo and garlic can cause bleeding problems; valerian is a sedative and can be associated with a withdrawal syndrome. Stopping these drugs 1 week before surgery is based on their half-lives, potential for causing platelet dysfunction, and need to have patients undergo surgery when they are safely past valerian withdrawal; little is known of their half-lives and reversibility of effects. Naproxen is a reversible platelet inhibitor and needs to be stopped only 2 to 3 days before surgery. Anticonvulsants and non-SSRI antidepressants should be continued until surgery is performed and reinstituted as soon as possible after surgery.

KEY POINTS
- Selective serotonin reuptake inhibitors may increase the risk for surgical bleeding complications.
- Estrogen and selective estrogen receptor modulators increase the risk for thromboembolism and should be discontinued perioperatively.

Bibliography
1. **Mercado DL, Petty BG**. Perioperative medication management. Med Clin North Am. 2003;87:41-57. [PMID: 12575883]
2. **Ang-Lee MK, Moss J, Yuan CS**. Herbal medicines and perioperative care. JAMA. 2001;286:208-16. [PMID: 11448284]

Item 79   Answer: C

When hormone replacement therapy has been prescribed for vasomotor symptoms, the symptoms will recur when therapy is discontinued. The recurring symptoms are most significant on abrupt termination of hormone therapy as in this patient. She likely will benefit if her previous estrogen-progesterone combination dose is resumed and then tapered when her symptoms again become tolerable. No evidence supports a universal approach to discontinuation; however gradual reduction is recommended by lowering the daily dose, decreasing the days per week estrogen is taken, or a combination of these approaches. If intolerable hot flushes recur, this patient can maintain the lowest daily or weekly dose that controls hot flushes, then attempt further tapering in 1 to 2 months.

Regular exercise can decrease symptoms of hot flushes. However, it is not known if a limit exists on the amount of exercise that produces these benefits. Because this patient already exercises regularly, additional exercise may or may not help with her symptoms.

There is no evidence that bupropion decreases the frequency of hot flushes. Progestins alone, such as depot-medroxyprogesterone, oral medroxyprogesterone, and megestrol acetate, are off-label treatments that can help reduce hot flushes. However, the use of progestins has been linked to breast cancer in some studies. As a result, the agents are not recommended in patients with hormone-dependent tumors or those at risk for developing these tumors. In addition, using progestins alone for vasomotor symptoms has not been studied extensively. Short- and long-term benefits and harms are unknown.

KEY POINT

- When hormone replacement therapy has been prescribed for vasomotor symptoms, the symptoms will recur when therapy is discontinued.

Bibliography

1. **Grady D**. Postmenopausal hormones—-therapy for symptoms only. N Engl J Med. 2003;348:1835-7. [PMID: 12642636]
2. **Ockene JK, Barad DH, Cochrane BB, Larson JC, Gass M, Wassertheil-Smoller S, et al**. Symptom experience after discontinuing use of estrogen plus progestin. JAMA. 2005;294:183-93. [PMID: 16014592]

Item 80   Answer: D

This patient's serum thyroid-stimulating hormone level should be measured because she is experiencing symptoms consistent with hypothyroidism. Elevated cholesterol levels, which can occur in hypothyroidism, may reverse after thyroid replacement. She is at low risk for coronary artery disease (CAD) based on her risk factors. If she does not have hypothyroidism, her serum low-density lipoprotein cholesterol and triglyceride levels necessitate institution of therapeutic lifestyle changes only as a first-step approach.

A statin would be an option in this patient if diet and exercise were ineffective in reducing her cholesterol values to acceptable levels. The ATP III does not specifically recommend use of fish oil supplements. No evidence indicates that they reduce mortality or morbidity.

KEY POINT

- Hypothyroidism may be an underlying cause of elevated cholesterol levels, and thyroid replacement therapy can reverse this finding.

Bibliography

1. National Cholesterol Education Program. The Third Report of the Expert Panel on Detection, Evaluation, and Treatment of High Blood Cholesterol in Adults (ATP III) executive summary. Available at http://www.nhlbi.nih.gov/guidelines/cholesterol/atp_iii.htm. Accessed August 1, 2006.

Item 81   Answer: C

This patient has class II obesity (defined as a BMI of 35 to 39.9). Obesity is associated with an increased risk for total mortality and chronic conditions, including coronary artery disease, stroke, type 2 diabetes mellitus, heart failure, dyslipidemia, and hypertension. In trials studying the effects of diet and exercise in obese patients with impaired glucose tolerance, weight loss of approximately 5% at 1 year decreased progression to type 2 diabetes and improved control of lipid levels and hypertension. However, there is no evidence of benefits in cardiovascular mortality or overall mortality from this level of modest weight loss. Although improvement in control of cardiovascular risk factors, including hypertension, glucose intolerance, and hyperlipidemia, have been demonstrated with modest degrees of weight loss, improvement in clinical symptoms such as those caused by osteoarthritis has not been documented with modest weight loss. Social and economic benefits have been demonstrated in quality-of-life studies in patients after significant weight loss from bariatric surgery but not from modest weight loss owing to dietary interventions.

KEY POINTS

- Obesity is associated with an increased risk for total mortality and chronic conditions, including coronary artery disease, stroke, type 2 diabetes, heart failure, dyslipidemia, and hypertension.
- Weight loss of approximately 5% at 1 year decreased progression to type 2 diabetes and improved control of lipid levels and hypertension.

Bibliography

1. **Snow V, Barry P, Fitterman N, Qaseem A, Weiss K**. Pharmacologic and surgical management of obesity in primary care: a clinical practice guideline from the American College of Physicians. Ann Intern Med. 2005;142:525-31. [PMID: 15809464]

Item 82   Answer: E

Most cases of acute bronchitis are caused by viruses, with influenza, parainfluenza, coronavirus, and rhinovirus accounting for most cases, yet most patients are treated with antibiotics in practice. There has been a robust effort to reduce inappropriate antibiotic use in patients with acute bronchitis due to inappropriate overuse. With the exception of acute bronchitis in patients with underlying chronic obstructive pulmonary disease, the only bacterial infection requiring antibiotic therapy is *Bordetella pertussis* (macrolides are first-choice agents in this setting), which is typically characterized by a barking or paroxysmal cough in the setting of prolonged upper respiratory infection symptoms (>2 weeks). Antibiotics should be administered to patients with pertussis infection primarily to hasten clearance of the organism and limit transmission to susceptible contacts. Treatment of patients with pertussis infection may reduce the duration or severity of symptoms, but a benefit is unlikely when treatment is initiated after the first week of symptoms.

There is no evidence to support the use of antibiotics in patients with acute bronchitis with concomitant heart failure, diabetes mellitus, asthma, or renal failure.

Bibliography

1. **Steinman MA, Landefeld CS, Gonzales R**. Predictors of broad-spectrum antibiotic prescribing for acute respiratory tract infections in adult primary care. JAMA. 2003;289:719-25. [PMID: 12585950]

2. **Snow V, Mottur-Pilson C, Hickner JM, et al**. Principles of appropriate antibiotic use for acute sinusitis in adults. Ann Intern Med. 2001;134:495-7. [PMID: 11255527]

3. **Hewlett EL, Edwards KM**. Clinical practice. Pertussis—not just for kids. N Engl J Med. 2005;352:1215-22. [PMID: 15788498]

Item 83   Answer: D

A rehabilitative outpatient program based on appropriately managed increases in activity, as graded exercise therapy or cognitive behavioral therapy (CBT), is the nonpharmacologic therapy of choice in patients with fibromyalgia syndrome (FMS). Patient education, acupuncture, hypnosis, biofeedback, and mineral baths have also been shown to be efficacious in improving FMS symptoms.

In one randomized, controlled trial, graded exercise therapy, compared with relaxation and flexibility training, led to significantly more participants rating themselves as feeling much or very much better at 3-month follow-up (24 of 69 [35%] vs. 12 of 67 [18%], P = 0.03). Benefits were maintained or improved at 1-year follow-up when fewer participants in the exercise group no longer fulfilled the symptomatic criteria for fibromyalgia (31 of 69 vs. 44 of 67, P = 0.01). Patients in the exercise group also had greater reductions in tender point counts (4.2 vs. 2.0, P = 0.02) and in scores on the fibromyalgia impact questionnaire (4.0 vs. 0.6, P = 0.07) compared with the relaxation and flexibility training groups.

Ultrasonography, psychotherapy, and massage therapy have not been studied in clinical trials, although most patients with fibromyalgia do seek some form of complementary and alternative treatment. In one survey, the 10 most frequently used complementary alternative medicine treatments were exercise for a specific medical problem (48%), spiritual healing (prayers) (45%), massage therapy (44%), chiropractic treatments (37%), vitamin C (35%), vitamin E (31%), magnesium (29%), vitamin B complex (25%), green tea (24%), and weight-loss programs (20%).

Bibliography

1. **Goldenberg DL, Burckhardt C, Crofford L**. Management of fibromyalgia syndrome. JAMA. 2004;292:2388-95. [PMID: 15547167]

2. **Richards SC, Scott DL**. Prescribed exercise in people with fibromyalgia: parallel group randomised controlled trial. BMJ. 2002;325:185. [PMID: 12142304]

3. **Wahner-Roedler DL, Elkin PL, Vincent A, Thompson JM, Oh TH, Loehrer LL, et al**. Use of complementary and alternative medical therapies by patients referred to a fibromyalgia treatment program at a tertiary care center. Mayo Clin Proc. 2005;80:55-60. [PMID: 15667030]

Item 84   Answer: B

The leading diagnosis in this patient is primary dysmenorrhea, a common cause of lower-abdominal pain, often beginning in women in their late teens or early 20s. A key feature of dysmenorrhea is the onset of pain during the menstrual cycle. Pain is felt to be hormonally related and, typically, no anatomic abnormalities are revealed with pelvic examination and ultrasonography. NSAIDs are a generally safe and often effective initial treatment for this symptom.

Oral contraceptives may also be helpful in treating the symptoms of primary dysmenorrhea. However, in a woman who has no other indications for oral contraceptives, an empiric trial of NSAIDs may be preferable as initial treatment. Constipation associated with lower abdominal pain could also denote irritable bowel syndrome (IBS). However, the occurrence of pain principally during menstruation is not characteristic of IBS. Also, although psyllium and tegaserod are first- and second-line treatments for IBS-related constipation, their benefits for the abdominal pain of IBS are not well-established. Small trials (largely uncontrolled) suggest local anesthetic/corticosteroid injections may be beneficial in patients with abdominal wall pain. However, abdominal wall pain is characterized by very localized pain in which the most intense component can be covered by a fingertip and/or increased point tenderness with abdominal wall muscle tensing.

Bibliography

1. **Srinivasan R, Greenbaum DS**. Chronic abdominal wall pain: a frequently overlooked problem. Practical approach to diagnosis and management. Am J Gastroenterol. 2002;97:824-30. [PMID: 12003414]

Item 85   Answer: A

A comprehensive audiometric evaluation is essential in this patient with subjective tinnitus to assess for hearing loss. Hearing aids may reduce symptom bother in patients with documented conductive hearing loss by increasing ambient noise. Asymmetric high-frequency hearing loss combined with poor speech discrimination may indicate an acoustic neuroma or meningioma. MRI of the head is appropriate for evaluating asymmetric audiologic abnormalities, but neuroimaging is not recommended as an initial diagnostic test. Objective tinnitus may arise from carotid vascular anomalies, with patients reporting pulsatile sounds that may also be heard on auscultation. However, this patient's symptoms and examination are consistent with subjective tinnitus; therefore, vascular imaging with magnetic resonance angiography is not indicated. Studies have shown that tricyclic antidepressants, benzodiazepines, and cognitive behavioral therapy can improve disability and loudness of tinnitus in patients with chronic tinnitus. There is no similar evidence, however, supporting the use of selective serotonin reuptake inhibitors or newer antidepressants in this setting. Additionally, screening results for depression were negative in this patient. Tinnitus is a side effect of many medications, including NSAIDs, aminoglycosides, loop diuretics, and chemotherapeutic agents. However, aspirin—not clopidogrel—is the antiplatelet drug associated with tinnitus.

KEY POINT

- A comprehensive audiometric evaluation is appropriate in patients with subjective tinnitus to assess for hearing loss.

Bibliography

1. **Lockwood AH, Salvi RJ, Burkard RF**. Tinnitus. N Engl J Med. 2002;347:904-10. [PMID: 12239260]

Item 86   Answer: A

Intracavernous alprostadil injections are an effective and safe treatment for patients with erectile dysfunction. Peyronie's disease is a relative contraindication to this treatment approach, but this patient has no penile plaques suggestive of this disease. Patients need to be educated about the potential side effect of priapism with this treatment; erections persisting for more than 4 hours require urgent medical attention. Intraurethral alprostadil and vacuum pump devices are also effective initial treatments for patients with erectile dysfunction. Penile implants are generally considered only if medical treatment, including maximal injec-

tion therapy, is unsuccessful. Phosphodiesterase type-5 (PDE-5) inhibitors are a first-line treatment for most men with erectile dysfunction; however, nitrate therapy is a contraindication to their use. PDE-5 inhibitors should be used cautiously in patients who take α-blockers and other antihypertensive agents because combined therapy may lead to significant hypotension. Testosterone therapy is not indicated in this patient because his intact libido and normal gonadal examination suggest that hypogonadism is not causing his erectile dysfunction. Trazodone is only a marginally effective therapy that apparently works best for men with psychogenic erectile dysfunction.

KEY POINTS

- Intracavernous alprostadil injections are an effective and safe treatment for patients with erectile dysfunction.
- Phosphodiesterase type-5 inhibitors are a first-line treatment for most men with erectile dysfunction; however, nitrate therapy is a contraindication to their use.

Bibliography

1. **Beckman TJ, Abu-Lebdeh HS, Mynderse LA**. Evaluation and medical management of erectile dysfunction. Mayo Clin Proc. 2006;81:385-90. [PMID: 16529142]
2. **Morgentaler A**. A 66-year-old man with sexual dysfunction. JAMA. 2004;291:2994-3003. [PMID: 15213212]

Item 87   Answer: C

Acute shoulder pain and weakness after falling on an outstretched arm is characteristic of a rotator cuff tear. The inability to smoothly lower the affected arm from full abduction (positive drop-arm test) is a highly specific finding for a rotator cuff tear. Complete radiographic evaluation (plain films and MRI) and immediate surgical repair are recommended for younger, healthy patients with moderate or severe tears. Patients who are not surgical candidates do not need MRI; appropriate conservative management for an acute rotator cuff tear includes ice, anti-inflammatory drugs, restricted lifting, and physiotherapy. Subacromial corticosteroid injections should be considered for patients with more chronic symptoms.

Adhesive capsulitis (frozen shoulder) is characterized by a decreased range of shoulder motion predominantly resulting from stiffness, rather than from pain or weakness. Glenohumeral arthritis is often related to remote trauma and gradual onset of pain and stiffness over months to years. Rotator cuff tendonitis is a common overuse injury characterized by subacromial tenderness and impingement; arm strength is preserved in these patients. Vigorous arm lifting can lead to spontaneous rupture of a chronically inflamed biceps tendon. The characteristic physical finding is the mass of contracted muscle (Popeye sign) in the mid-upper arm. Pain and tenderness can persist in these patients for several days following rupture, but arm strength is generally well preserved.

- **Acute shoulder pain and weakness after falling on an outstretched arm is characteristic of a rotator cuff tear.**
- **The inability to smoothly lower the affected arm from full abduction (positive drop-arm test) is a highly specific finding for a rotator cuff tear.**

Bibliography

1. **Stevenson JH, Trojian T**. Evaluation of shoulder pain. J Fam Pract. 2002;51:605-11. [PMID: 12160496]

Item 88   Answer: E

This patient's ulcer has the characteristic appearance (shallow, irregular, red-based) and location (above medial malleolus) of a venous ulcer. An occlusive hydrocolloid dressing, usually composed of gelatin and pectin, can increase exudate absorption, reduce pain and odor, and help debridement and reepithelialization. Dressings are usually changed every 3 to 7 days. The patient is already receiving aspirin; randomized trials have shown faster ulcer healing with aspirin doses higher than 300 mg daily.

An antibiotic would be appropriate adjunctive therapy if the patient were to have cellulitis, however, there is no indication of infection on history or physical examination. Elastic compression stockings and intermittent pneumatic compression pumps can improve ulcer healing, particularly when used with occlusive dressings. However, this patient has evidence of occlusive arterial disease, a contraindication for using these compression modalities. Diuretics are most appropriate for patients with venous insufficiency and severe edema but should be used cautiously owing to their increased risk for intravascular volume depletion because edema fluid is poorly mobilized. Increasing diuretics would not be appropriate for this patient because his edema is minimal, his blood pressure is already low, and he is slightly azotemic.

- **An occlusive hydrocolloid dressing can increase exudate absorption, reduce pain and odor, and help debridement and reepithelialization in patients with venous ulcers.**
- **Aspirin doses higher than 300 mg daily can result in faster healing in patients with venous ulcers.**

Bibliography

1. **de Araujo T, Valencia I, Federman DG, Kirsner RS**. Managing the patient with venous ulcers. Ann Intern Med. 2003;138:326-34. [PMID: 12585831]

Item 89   Answer: B

Meniere's disease is the most common cause of recurrent, disabling attacks of vertigo. Age of onset occurs most commonly in the fourth to sixth decade of life. Episodes typically last for several hours and are accompanied by vomiting and cochlear symptoms (for example, tinnitus, ear fullness, and/or hearing loss). Episodes occur at irregular intervals over years, and patients may develop a progressive sensorineural hearing loss, initially unilateral and low-frequency in nature, but eventually bilateral in 30% to 50% of patients. Prior to identifying changes in an audiogram, the diagnosis of Meniere's disease is largely established clinically without the necessity of diagnostic testing. Treatment for acute episodes of this disorder is symptomatic and includes meclizine, benzodiazepines, antiemetics, and for frequent recurrences is prophylactic, requiring diuretics and a low-sodium diet because the presumptive pathophysiology involves increased endolymphatic fluid volume. Because spontaneous remission occurs frequently in long-term follow-up, endolymphatic shunting or other surgical treatments are reserved for a minority of patients.

Acephalgic migraine is a controversial diagnosis and a rare cause of vertigo in large series of dizzy patients. Migraine is a difficult diagnosis to establish in the absence of headache or classic visual or other prodromal features and would not be associated with abnormal audiometry results. Acoustic neuroma is a very rare tumor in which the usual symptoms are a slowly progressive unilateral hearing loss with or without tinnitus. Severe vertiginous attacks are not the usual presentation for acoustic neuromas, and MRI of the internal auditory canal and adjacent structures can identify most of these tumors. Benign positional vertigo is characterized by brief (less than 1 minute) episodes of vertigo triggered by changes of head position and not associated with vomiting or prostration. Vestibular neuritis is typically a single episode of disabling vertigo that resolves in a few days to a week and, although it may occasionally be recurrent, is rarely manifested by the chronic, episodic course or the progressive hearing loss associated with Meniere's disease. An acute episode of dizziness resembling vestibular neuritis but associated with a unilateral hearing loss typically is referred to as labyrinthitis.

- **Episodes of Meniere's disease last for several hours and involve vomiting and cochlear symptoms, and patients may develop a progressive sensorineural hearing loss.**
- **Prior to identifying changes in an audiogram, the diagnosis of Meniere's disease is largely established clinically without the necessity for diagnostic testing.**

Bibliography

1. **Baloh RW**. Clinical practice. Vestibular neuritis. N Engl J Med. 2003;348:1027-32. [PMID: 12637613]

Item 90   Answer: D

β-Blockers, oral nitrates, and most antihypertensive drugs should be continued the morning of surgery and reinstituted when patients begin eating. Abrupt discontinuation appears to increase the risk for postoperative complications. ACE inhibitors and angiotensin receptor blockers have been associated with intraoperative hypotension and should be held the morning of surgery. The anti-inflammatory and pleotrophic plaque-stabilizing effects of statins appear to reduce the risk for postoperative cardiac complications in observational studies and should be continued the morning of surgery and reinstituted when patients are eating. Oral nitrate formulations should be continued the morning of surgery. Postoperatively, intravenous nitroglycerin or transdermal formulations can be used until the patient is eating.

KEY POINTS

- β-Blockers, oral nitrates, and most antihypertensive drugs should be continued the morning of surgery and reinstituted when patients begin eating.
- The anti-inflammatory and pleotrophic plaque-stabilizing effects of statins appear to reduce the risk for postoperative cardiac complications in observational studies and should be continued the morning of surgery and reinstituted when patients begin eating.

Bibliography
1. **Mercado DL, Petty BG**. Perioperative medication management. Med Clin North Am. 2003;87:41-57. [PMID: 12575883]

Item 91   Answer: C

The U.S. Preventive Services Task Force (USPSTF) has found sufficient evidence of benefit to recommend screening for aortic abdominal aneurysm (AAA) in men aged 65 to 75 years who have ever smoked. Ultrasonography is highly sensitive and specific in detecting AAA of all sizes (sensitivity approaches 100%). Although there is good evidence on the harms of both screening and early treatment (increased surgeries with clinically significant morbidity and mortality, as well as short-term psychologic harm), overall, the net benefit seems to outweigh the harm. Almost all deaths from AAA occur in men between 65 and 80 years old, supporting the age bracket for this one-time screening test. The USPSTF does not recommend for or against screening in men who have never smoked, as the benefits and harms are too close for recommendation. The prevalence of AAA in men who have never smoked is low, so the benefit from screening in this population is small. The USPSTF recommends against routine screening for women because of evidence that it is ineffective and that associated harms outweigh any benefit. Few deaths would be prevented by screening women, because this population has a low prevalence of large AAAs. There are negligible health benefits of re-screening in persons with a prior study showing normal aortic diameter.

Carotid ultrasonography is not recommended as a screening test but as a diagnostic evaluation for persons with symptoms of cerebrovascular disease such as transient ischemic attack. There are no other good indicators for impending atherosclerosis in the cerebral circulation, because evidence suggests that bruits may be absent in high-grade stenosis. Further, medical and surgical therapies are equivalent unless the patient is at very low risk for surgical complications. This patient has no indication for a study of his carotid arteries.

Using the Framingham Risk Index, this patient is at moderate risk for developing coronary artery disease (CAD) (12% in 10 years). There is no evidence about the prognostic value of electron-beam CT as an indicator of disease. It has been correlated to other markers for CAD, including C-reactive protein, but there is insufficient evidence about its relationship to clinical coronary events. The patient's cholesterol levels do not support treatment with statin therapy.

KEY POINT

- Screening for aortic abdominal aneurysm in men aged 65 to 75 years who have ever smoked is recommended.

Bibliography
1. **Fleming C, Whitlock EP, Beil TL, Lederle FA**. Screening for abdominal aortic aneurysm: a best-evidence systematic review for the U.S. Preventive Services Task Force. Ann Intern Med. 2005;142:203-11. [PMID: 15684209]
2. Screening for abdominal aortic aneurysm: recommendation statement. Ann Intern Med. 2005;142:198-202. [PMID: 15684208]

Item 92   Answer: B

This lesion suggests a nodular melanoma. Lesions suspicious for melanoma should not be manipulated, as doing so can spread malignant cells. An excision biopsy is required. Nodular melanomas are particularly aggressive and invade deep into the skin layer early. Patients with melanoma or who are at risk for melanoma should be taught the ABCD mnemonic for suspicious lesions. Patients should seek early medical attention for lesions that have any of these characteristics: A) asymmetry (inability to draw a line down the middle to produce two mirror images, B) border that is irregular, scalloped, or poorly circumscribed, C) color (more than one in the same lesion or very dark, black, occasionally white, red, or blue), and D) diameter of 6 mm (the size of a pencil eraser) or more. Patients should also be suspicious of moles that are different from others or that change, itch, or bleed. Persons who have fair skin or a family or personal history of malignant melanoma should have a thorough skin examination yearly by a dermatologist.

Destruction of suspicious lesions could not only result in the spread of malignant cells and significantly alter the prognosis, but it also makes it impossible to diagnose or stage the lesion and thereby select the correct treatment.

Superficial shave biopsies, electrodessication, and liquid nitrogen are dangerous for this patient.

> **KEY POINT**
> - Lesions suspicious for melanoma require an excision biopsy to prevent manipulation of the lesion and the potential for the spread of malignant cells.

Bibliography
1. **Martinez JC, Otley CC**. The management of melanoma and nonmelanoma skin cancer: a review for the primary care physician. Mayo Clin Proc. 2001;76:1253-65. [PMID: 11761506]

Item 93   Answer: A

This patient is likely experiencing primary dysmenorrhea, a term that describes menstrual cramping without a pathologic cause. The mainstay treatments are oral contraceptives, which generally reduce symptoms of primary dysmenorrhea, or NSAIDs. Meclofenamate would not necessarily be the next best choice for a patient who has experienced no relief using other NSAIDs. An individual patient may respond to one NSAID when others have not been effective. However, no evidence demonstrates the superiority of one NSAID over another.

Treatment of primary dysmenorrhea with depot-medroxyprogesterone acetate (DMPA) is an off-label use that can induce hypomenorrhea or amenorrhea, resulting in decreased dysmenorrhea. However, only about 50% of patients will become completely amenorrheic during the first year of use of this agent, with the remainder continuing to experience dysmenorrhea. Other alternative therapies, including magnesium, vitamin B_6 (pyridoxine), vitamin E, and omega-3 fatty acids, have shown some benefit but have not been studied thoroughly enough to make a recommendation for use in this patient. Although tramadol may effectively reduce pain, it is not a good long-term solution.

> **KEY POINT**
> - The mainstay of treatment for primary dysmenorrhea is oral contraceptives or NSAIDs.

Bibliography
1. **Marjoribanks J, Proctor ML, Farquhar C**. Nonsteroidal anti-inflammatory drugs for primary dysmenorrhoea. Cochrane Database Syst Rev. 2003:CD001751. [PMID: 14583938]
2. **Wilson ML, Murphy PA**. Herbal and dietary therapies for primary and secondary dysmenorrhea. Cochrane Database Syst Rev. 2001:CD002124. [PMID: 11687013]

Item 94   Answer: D

Depression can be a treatable cause of insomnia, and this patient has some risks for depression, including a recent divorce and other life stressors. Screening for depression is indicated prior to treatment of primary insomnia. The diagnosis of chronic insomnia can be established clinically. It is generally defined as a complaint of insufficient or inadequate sleep when one has the opportunity to sleep. The American Psychiatric Association Diagnostic and Statistical Manual 4th Edition (DSM-IV) defines primary insomnia as difficulty initiating or maintaining sleep or nonrestorative sleep for at least 1 month. The sleep disturbance must cause clinically significant distress or impairment of functioning and not be caused by another diagnosable sleep or mental disorder.

Polysomnography is needed only in patients with insomnia who have symptoms of a sleep-related breathing disorder, narcolepsy, sleepwalking, or are employed as pilots or truck drivers. None of these criteria apply to this case. This patient has risk factors for pulmonary disorders (smoking and being overweight) and cardiac disease (smoking, being overweight, sex, and age); however, he does not have symptoms or findings indicative of chronic obstructive pulmonary disease (COPD), obstructive sleep apnea, or coronary artery disease (CAD). Therefore, further evaluation of COPD with spirometry or stress testing for CAD is not indicated. Sleep hygiene recommendations, including avoidance of strenuous exercise or alcohol within a few hours of bedtime, developing a relaxing evening routine, and avoidance of afternoon caffeine, are an appropriate first step in intervention once a diagnosis of primary insomnia is established.

> **KEY POINTS**
> - Good sleep hygiene includes avoiding strenuous exercise or alcohol close to bedtime, developing a relaxing evening routine, and avoiding afternoon caffeine.
> - Depression is a treatable underlying cause for insomnia.

Bibliography
1. **Neubauer DN**. Insomnia. Prim Care. 2005;32:375-88. [PMID: 15935191]
2. **Silber MH**. Clinical practice. Chronic insomnia. N Engl J Med. 2005;353:803-10. [PMID: 16120860]

Item 95   Answer: D

This patient should be advised to have her cholesterol levels re-measured in 5 years. The National Cholesterol Education Program (NCEP) has recommended a nine-step procedure for identifying and treating patients at risk for coronary artery disease (CAD). The first three steps are pertinent to this case. After cholesterol numbers are checked (Step 1), the presence of CAD or CAD equivalents (Step 2) should be established. The definition of CAD includes myocardial infarction, unstable angina, coronary artery procedures, or evidence of myocardial ischemia. CAD-equivalents include diabetes, symptomatic carotid artery disease, peripheral artery disease, and abdominal aortic aneurysm.

Because this patient does not have CAD or CAD-equivalents, the next step (Step 3) is to determine if she has any other risk factors, other than serum low-density lipoprotein level, for CAD. These risk factors include cigarette smoking, hypertension (blood pressure >140/90 mm Hg or taking an antihypertensive medication), low high-density lipoprotein (HDL) cholesterol levels (<40mg/dL [1.03 mmol/L]), family history of premature CAD (male first-degree relative <55 years; female first-degree relative <65 years), and age (men >45 years; women >55 years). This patient's only risk factor is her age. She is therefore at low risk for CAD. The Adult Treatment Panel of the NCEP does not recommend further treatment for her cholesterol, and her cholesterol levels should be followed regularly. A diet that is rich in plant stanols or sterols, recommended among other therapeutic lifestyle changes to lower cholesterol, is indicated for patients who have a higher risk for CAD than this patient. Treatment with either a statin or niacin is also recommended for patients at higher risk for CAD than this patient.

KEY POINT

- **Cholesterol monitoring is indicated once every 5 years in patients with only one risk factor for coronary heart disease.**

Bibliography

1. National Cholesterol Education Program. Third Report of the Expert Panel on Detection, Evaluation, and Treatment of High Blood Cholesterol in Adults (Adult Treatment Panel III) executive summary. Available at http://www.nhlbi.nih.gov/guidelines/cholesterol/atp_iii.htm. Accessed August 1, 2006.

Item 96   Answer: D

The most likely diagnosis in this patient is allergic rhinitis with associated bronchospasm; therefore, treatment with oral antihistamine and nasal corticosteroids is appropriate. In addition, inhaled β-agonists are also appropriate in this patient as they appear beneficial only in patients with wheezing or airflow limitation with end-expiratory wheezes. Antibiotics are not indicated for allergic rhinitis or viral upper respiratory infection. Although the patient has yellowish sputum, the absence of fever, chills, and progressive illness argue against current bacterial infection. Nasal decongestants may be of some symptomatic benefit, but direct treatment of the underlying allergic disorder with a nasal corticosteroid and oral antihistamine is the indicated treatment. In general, antitussives or cough suppressants are indicated only for cough that is painful, causes sleep disruption, or is debilitating in frail, elderly patients. Recent systematic reviews conclude that no antitussive is clearly superior to another for cough in adults, and elderly patients are most vulnerable to adverse effects of antitussive agents, such as confusion, nausea, and constipation.

KEY POINTS

- **Inhaled β-agonists appear beneficial only in patients with wheezing or airflow limitation with end-expiratory wheezes on examination.**
- **Antibiotics are not indicated for allergic rhinitis or viral upper respiratory infection. Although the patient has yellowish sputum, the absence of fever, chills, and progressive illness argue against current bacterial infection.**

Bibliography

1. Smucny JJ, Flynn CA, Becker LA, Glazier RH. Are beta2-agonists effective treatment for acute bronchitis or acute cough in patients without underlying pulmonary disease? A systematic review. J Fam Pract. 2001;50:945-51. [PMID: 11711010]
2. Schroeder K, Fahey T. Over-the-counter medications for acute cough in children and adults in ambulatory settings. Cochrane Database Syst Rev. 2004:CD001831. [PMID: 15495019]

Item 97   Answer: D

Because this patient meets none of the criteria for a fracture according to the Ottawa Knee Rules, the most appropriate next step in management is reassurance and symptomatic treatment.

The Ottawa rules suggest obtaining a knee film in patients who meet any of the following criteria: 1) age older than 55 years, 2) tenderness at the head of the fibula or patella, or 3) an inability to flex to 90 degrees or to bear weight both immediately and during evaluation. Because this patient does not meet these criteria, knee radiography is not necessary in this case. Although this rule is highly sensitive, patients who receive assurance and symptomatic care should be instructed to return for re-evaluation if knee pain persists.

Although this patient has some effusion of the knee, in the absence of erythema or warmth, it is unlikely that the effusion has occurred secondary to either acute gout or an infectious etiology; therefore, arthrocentesis is not required. Patients who receive assurance and symptomatic care for knee injuries should be informed that if the effusion worsens, they become febrile, or the knee becomes erythematous or warm, they should return for arthrocentesis. MRI has been found to be slightly more sensitive, but less specific, than physical examination for detecting meniscal and ligamentous injuries. Additionally, MRI frequently finds abnormalities that are of no clinical significance. Given the lack of evidence of a meniscal or ligamentous injury in the history or physical examination, any MRI findings would likely not be associated with his current problem and might instead be associated with his history as a chronic runner. However, if the patient's symptoms do not respond to symptomatic treatment, an MRI might be a future consideration. Acute treatment for a knee sprain consists of rest, ice, compression, and elevation (RICE). After application of ice when the area is thoroughly cooled, an elastic wrap should be applied to compress the injury, and anti-inflammatory medication may be used for pain relief. The patient should be advised to cease running for at least 2 weeks and to stop if pain recurs once running is continued. Crutches or a knee brace are not necessary in the absence of laxity or significant pain with stressing of the knee ligaments.

KEY POINT

- **The Ottawa rules suggest obtaining a knee film in patients who are older than age 55 years, have tenderness at the head of the fibula or patella, or have an inability to flex to 90 degrees or to bear weight both immediately and during evaluation.**

Bibliography

1. **Jackson JL, O'Malley PG, Kroenke K**. Evaluation of acute knee pain in primary care. Ann Intern Med. 2003;139:575-88. [PMID: 14530229]

Item 98   Answer: E

Acute hearing loss in patients with an otherwise-normal neurologic examination with no mechanical obstruction (for example, foreign body or cerumen impaction) on examination of the auditory canal is usually idiopathic. These patients may benefit from prompt systemic corticosteroids and require emergent referral. The evidence base for empiric corticosteroids in acute idiopathic hearing loss is small but suggests benefit if given promptly. Administration of empiric corticosteroid therapy should coincide with emergent otorhinolaryngologic referral to rule out other causes of acute hearing loss.

Other causes of acute hearing loss include acoustic neuroma, temporal bone fracture, meningitis, viral or suppurative labyrinthitis, systemic or local inflammatory disease, and drugs, such as cisplatin or aminoglycosides. Presbycusis is usually not associated with acute hearing loss and is frequently bilateral, although one ear may be more severely affected than the other. Without evidence of bacterial infection, empiric oral antibiotics are not indicated for resolving viral upper respiratory infections. A formal hearing test in 1 week without empiric corticosteroids and emergent referral will delay the diagnosis and cause the patient to miss the window of opportunity for corticosteroid treatment. A CT of the head for possible acoustic neuroma or meningioma should be performed, but after simultaneous corticosteroid therapy and initial evaluation by an otorhinolaryngologist.

KEY POINT

- **Patients with acute hearing loss and an otherwise-normal neurologic examination with no mechanical obstruction usually benefit from prompt systemic corticosteroids and require emergent referral.**

Bibliography

1. **Yueh B, Shapiro N, MacLean CH, Shekelle PG**. Screening and management of adult hearing loss in primary care: scientific review. JAMA. 2003;289:1976-85. [PMID: 12697801]

Item 99   Answer: C

Acute angle-closure glaucoma occurs when folds of the iris block the acute angle and inhibit drainage of aqueous humor, resulting in rapidly increased intraocular pressure and pain. Halos appear around lights because of corneal edema. The eye is firm on palpation as compared with the uninvolved eye, there is diffuse erythema that is most pronounced in the limbic or circumcorneal area, and the pupil is moderately dilated and fixed. Acute angle-closure glaucoma typically occurs in older persons; farsighted individuals are particularly susceptible. Symptoms often occur in the evening due to decreased ambient light and result in mydriasis, causing the iris folds to block the angle and prevent aqueous drainage.

Anterior uveitis presents with red, painful eye and blurred vision or vision loss. It usually occurs in young or middle-aged persons. As with acute angle-closure glaucoma, there is diffuse erythema prominent at the limbus, but light reflex is sluggish or unreactive and the pupil is constricted. Diagnosis usually requires slit-lamp examination; hypopyon or hyphema may be visible at the base of the anterior chamber. In hyperacute bacterial conjunctivitis, the eye is red but not painful, and there is no vision loss. The conjunctivitis progresses rapidly, and there is abrupt onset of copious purulent discharge, bright red conjunctiva, and marked lid swelling and pain. The conjunctivitis is usually gonococcal and requires both topical and systemic antibiotics. Vitreous hemorrhage is commonly associated with diabetes or trauma; the eye is not red or painful, but there is decreased visual acuity. The red reflex and retinal detail are obscured on direct ophthalmoscopy. All of these eye conditions require emergency referral to an ophthalmologist.

KEY POINT

- **Acute angle-closure glaucoma results in rapidly increased intraocular pressure, pain, diffuse erythema, and a moderately dilated, fixed pupil.**

Bibliography

1. **Leibowitz HM**. The red eye. N Engl J Med. 2000;343:345-51. [PMID: 10922425]
2. **Shingleton BJ, O'Donoghue MW**. Blurred vision. N Engl J Med. 2000;343:556-62. [PMID: 10954765]

Item 100   Answer: C

Lipodermatosclerosis is a fibrosing panniculitis of subcutaneous tissue present in patients with advanced chronic venous insufficiency. Patients have circumferential areas of fibrosis extending proximally from above the ankles (with the overall appearance of an inverted champagne bottle), with pitting edema above the area of fibrosis and over the feet. Cellulitis and venous ulceration often complicate this condition. Lipedema, which occurs almost exclusively in women, appears as bilateral leg swelling due to accumulation of fatty substances in subcutaneous tissue. The swelling extends between the pelvis and ankles but spares the feet. Lymphedema is characterized by nonpitting edema, involvement of the toes, with thickened skin and a peau d'orange appearance. In developed countries, lymphedema frequently occurs secondary to lymph node dissection and/or radiation therapy for malignancy. Although this patient has a slightly elevated serum thyroid-stimulating hormone level, pretibial myxedema is an uncommon complication of hyperthyroidism (Graves' disease)—not hypothyroidism—that is initially characterized by asymmetric, firm, nonpitting, skin-colored or violaceous nodules or plaques. These lesions can eventually coalesce to involve the entire lower leg and dorsa of the foot with a peau d'orange appearance.

KEY POINT

- Lipodermatosclerosis can occur in patients with advanced chronic venous insufficiency and involves circumferential areas of fibrosis extending proximally from above the ankles, with pitting edema above the area of fibrosis and over the feet.

Bibliography

1. **Rockson SG**. Lymphedema. Am J Med. 2001;110:288-95. [PMID: 11239847]

Item 101   Answer: A

This patient has social anxiety disorder and probably has had this disorder for many years. Because she has good insight, most experts would recommend psychotherapy for this patient at this point, with continuation of the current antidepressant regimen, to produce synergism between the two modalities. Clonazepam would be a good complementary treatment choice in this patient to provide immediate relief while she awaits the results of therapy. Benzodiazepines are very effective in patients with social anxiety disorder, with up to 80% improvement, although these patients often have difficulty in tapering or discontinuing these agents; therefore, benzodiazepines should be reserved for patients at low risk for substance abuse and given at minimum therapeutic doses for immediate relief of symptoms in conjunction with anticipated improvement from antidepressant therapy or psychotherapy.

Because she has responded well to her current medication regimen, increasing her dosage of sertraline or substituting it for another selective serotonin reuptake inhibitor is not likely to be more effective for treating her symptoms of social anxiety disorder. Given the recurrent nature of depression in patients who do not take their medication, weaning sertraline would not be appropriate.

KEY POINT

- Clonazepam is an appropriate complementary treatment choice in patients with social anxiety disorder for providing immediate relief while they await the results of psychotherapy.

Bibliography

1. **Rowa K, Antony MM**. Psychological treatments for social phobia. Can J Psychiatry. 2005;50:308-16. [PMID: 15999944]
2. **Gross R, Olfson M, Gameroff MJ, Shea S, Feder A, Lantigua R, et al**. Social anxiety disorder in primary care. Gen Hosp Psychiatry. 2005;27:161-8. [PMID: 15882762]

Item 102   Answer: E

This patient has a case of contact dermatitis due to poison ivy resulting from contact with the plant and causing vesicles. Although smoke from the burning plant is harmless, dermatitis can occur if particulate matter in the smoke comes in contact with the skin. Severe poison ivy dermatitis, including cases with extensive involvement and edema, can be treated with oral prednisone (about 1 mg/kg/d), tapering the dosage slowly over 2 to 3 weeks. Although high-potency topical corticosteroids may reduce the erythema that sometimes surrounds vesicles, this treatment is not recommended on the face, neck, or intertriginous areas, where corticosteroid atrophy is more likely to occur. When these areas are involved with blisters, topical treatment is ineffective and oral treatment is more appropriate.

Treatment of poison ivy dermatis with pimecrolimus was not helpful when compared with placebo cream in one study. Contrary to popular belief, vesicles from active lesions do not cause spread of the dermatitis. No studies support length of treatment with oral corticosteroids. However, clinical experience has shown that rapid tapering often results in rebound dermatitis.

The main allergic component of the poison ivy plant is urushiol, a sap found in the leaves, stems, and roots of poison ivy, poison sumac, and poison oak. Once the resin is on the skin, dermatitis can be prevented if the skin is washed with soap and water soon after contact.

KEY POINT

- Severe cases of poison ivy can be treated with oral prednisone.

Bibliography

1. **Amrol D, Keitel D, Hagaman D, Murray J**. Topical pimecrolimus in the treatment of human allergic contact dermatitis. Ann Allergy Asthma Immunol. 2003;91:563-6. [PMID: 14700441]

Item 103   Answer: E

Surgery is recommended as a treatment option for patients with class III obesity, defined as those with a BMI of 40 or greater and who have been unable to maintain weight loss with exercise and diet with or without drug therapy and who have obesity-related comorbid conditions, such as hypertension, impaired glucose tolerance, diabetes mellitus, hyperlipidemia, and obstructive sleep apnea. This patient meets these criteria. Gastric bypass surgery has proven efficacy in weight loss, with one meta-analysis demonstrating a 61.2% loss of excess weight (95% CI, 58.1 to 64.4). The effects of sibutramine and orlistat are significantly more modest than gastric bypass surgery, resulting in less than a 5-kg (11-lb) weight loss at 1 year in clinical trials. Low-carbohydrate and fat-restricted diets have limited evidence to support long-term efficacy and safety. Other benefits of gastric bypass surgery include improved social and economic status and improved control of chronic diseases, but no cardiovascular mortality benefit from gastric bypass has been established. Patients considering gastric bypass surgery should receive counseling about the long-term side effects of this procedure, including the possibility for re-operation, gall bladder disease, and malabsorption. In addition, surgical risks include a 30-day postoperative mortality rate of 2%.

KEY POINT

- Surgery is a recommended treatment option for patients with class III obesity, defined as those with a BMI of ≥40 and who cannot maintain weight loss with exercise and diet with or without drug therapy and who have obesity-related comorbid conditions.

Bibliography

1. Buchwald H, Avidor Y, Braunwald E, Jensen MD, Pories W, Fahrbach K, et al. Bariatric surgery: a systematic review and meta-analysis. JAMA. 2004;292:1724-37. [PMID: 15479938]

Item 104   Answer: A

Antihistamines, which decrease bladder contractility, can exacerbate lower urinary tract symptoms in men with enlarged prostates. Similarly, oral decongestants can precipitate urinary retention by increasing smooth muscle tone in the prostate and bladder neck. Avoiding these medications is an appropriate first step for reducing symptoms. Although transurethral resection of the prostate may ultimately be required, one episode of urinary retention with a reversible cause is not sufficient justification for surgery. Aside from recurrent urinary retention, other indications for surgery include renal insufficiency, recurrent urinary tract infections, bladder stones, or persistent gross hematuria. Finasteride is helpful for treating lower urinary tract symptoms and preventing disease progression but takes months to work and is most effective with larger prostates (>60 mL). α-Blockers quickly and effectively reduce lower urinary tract symptoms and increase urinary flow. However, neither finasteride nor terazosin would be necessary unless the patient were to have persistent bothersome symptoms after stopping the antihistamine. Although saw palmetto is safe, a large, well-designed, randomized trial reported no significant differences between saw palmetto and placebo in reducing urinary symptoms or improving urinary flow.

KEY POINTS

- Antihistamines can exacerbate lower urinary tract symptoms in men with enlarged prostates.
- Oral decongestants can precipitate urinary retention by increasing smooth muscle tone in the prostate and bladder neck.

Bibliography

1. McConnell JD, Roehrborn CG, Bautista OM, Andriole GL Jr, Dixon CM, Kusek JW, et al. The long-term effect of doxazosin, finasteride, and combination therapy on the clinical progression of benign prostatic hyperplasia. N Engl J Med. 2003;349:2387-98. [PMID: 14681504]
2. Bent S, Kane C, Shinohara K, Neuhaus J, Hudes ES, Goldberg H, et al. Saw palmetto for benign prostatic hyperplasia. N Engl J Med. 2006;354:557-66. [PMID: 16467543]

Item 105   Answer: B

Wearing below-knee elastic compression stockings during the day for 2 years or longer has been shown to reduce the incidence of postphlebitic syndrome by approximately 50% (21.1% vs. 40.0%) compared with no treatment in patients with symptomatic proximal deep venous thrombosis (DVT). Both custom-fitted and off-the-rack compression stockings are effective. However, compression stockings have not been effective in preventing postphlebitic syndrome in patients with asymptomatic proximal DVT. Diuretics may help reduce edema but have not been evaluated in the prevention of postphlebitic syndrome. Intermittent pneumatic compression is used to treat venous leg ulcers and limb swelling from lymphedema, but it has not been evaluated for preventing postphlebitic syndrome. Prolonged oral anticoagulation therapy would be recommended for reducing the risk of recurrent thromboembolic events in patients with permanent risk factors; however, this therapy would not prevent postthrombotic syndrome and is not appropriate in the setting of postoperative DVT.

KEY POINT

- Wearing below-knee elastic compression stockings during the day for 2 years or longer reduces the risk for postphlebitic syndrome by approximately 50% in patients with symptomatic proximal deep venous thrombosis.

Bibliography

1. Prandoni P, Lensing AW, Prins MH, Frulla M, Marchiori A, Bernardi E, et al. Below-knee elastic compression stockings to prevent the post-thrombotic syndrome: a randomized, controlled trial. Ann Intern Med. 2004;141:249-56. [PMID: 15313740]

Item 106   Answer: D

The presence of a red reflex, central opacity, and visible fundus is consistent with an immature nuclear cataract.

Cataract extraction is indicated when visual deficits impair quality of life, but this patient has only minimal visual problems and well-corrected visual acuity; therefore, monitoring the patient for progressive visual impairment is an appropriate strategy. Randomized trials have shown that vitamin E supplements do not prevent the development or progression of senile cataracts. β-Carotene supplements reduce the risk of cataracts in smokers; however, this intervention is not recommended because several randomized cancer prevention trials in smokers found that β-carotene supplements increase the risk for lung cancer. Topical ophthalmic prostaglandins are first-line therapy for primary open-angle glaucoma. Although a mature cataract can rarely cause secondary glaucoma, patients with primary open-angle glaucoma usually present with a red, painful eye.

KEY POINTS

- The presence of a red reflex, central opacity, and visible fundus is consistent with an immature nuclear cataract.
- Cataract extraction is indicated when visual deficits impair quality of life.

Bibliography

1. Asbell PA, Dualan I, Mindel J, Brocks D, Ahmad M, Epstein S. Age-related cataract. Lancet. 2005;365:599-609. [PMID: 15708105]

Item 107   Answer: A

The patient meets the criteria for acute bacterial rhinosinusitis: duration of symptoms longer than 1 week and worsening symptoms after initial improvement, maxillary tenderness, purulent drainage, and poor response to decongestants. Generally, antibiotics should be reserved for patients who meet these criteria or for those with severe symptoms of rhinosinusitis (high fever, periorbital swelling, and severe facial pain) of any duration. Antibiotics targeting *Streptococcus pneumoniae* and *Haemophilus influenzae* reduce symptom duration. A 3- to 10-day course of a narrow-spectrum antibiotic, such as amoxicillin, trimethoprim–sulfamethoxazole, or doxycycline, is the preferred initial treatment. Broad-spectrum antibiotics (amoxicillin–clavulanate) are no more effective than narrow-spectrum antibiotics in treating acute sinusitis. However, broad-spectrum antibiotics are more expensive, more likely to cause adverse reactions, and potentially more likely to increase antibiotic resistance. Although oral nonsedating antihistamines may be effective in patients with chronic sinusitis related to allergic rhinitis, there is insufficient evidence for recommending their use in patients with acute bacterial rhinosinusitis. Sinus radiography and sinus CT are not recommended for acute, uncomplicated cases. CT is more sensitive than plain radiography, but neither test can distinguish bacterial from viral infection.

KEY POINTS

- The criteria for acute bacterial rhinosinusitis are duration of symptoms longer than 1 week and worsening symptoms after initial improvement, maxillary tenderness, purulent drainage, and poor response to decongestants.
- Antibiotics should be reserved for patients who meet the criteria for acute bacterial rhinosinusitis.

Bibliography

1. Williams JW Jr, Aguilar C, Cornell J, Chiquette ED, Makela M, Holleman DR, et al. Antibiotics for acute maxillary sinusitis. Cochrane Database Syst Rev. 2003:CD000243. [PMID: 12804392]
2. Snow V, Mottur-Pilson C, Hickner JM, et al. Principles of appropriate antibiotic use for acute sinusitis in adults. Ann Intern Med. 2001;134:495-7. [PMID: 11255527]

Item 108   Answer: B

Osteomalacia and osteoporosis are common in celiac disease and can occur even in patients who have no gastrointestinal symptoms. Bone loss is related to secondary hyperparathyroidism due to prolonged vitamin D deficiency not normalized with a gluten-free diet. Most patients are asymptomatic; very few have bone pain. The incidence of osteoporosis is 27% to 36% in patients with celiac disease; men are more severely affected than women. Routine screening for osteoporosis with a dual X-ray absorptiometry (DXA) scan for bone density is important in this high-risk population. In one study, bone mineral density did not differ between patients on a gluten-free diet and patients who had not begun therapy. Another study demonstrated an increased prevalence of celiac disease among persons with osteoporosis (3.4%) as compared with persons without osteoporosis (0.2%).

Other risk factors for osteoporosis include age older than 65 years, family history of fracture, prolonged use of corticosteroids, hyperthyroidism (including intentional suppression in treatment of thyroid cancer), and other chronic diseases associated with bone loss.

Celiac sprue does not increase this patient's risk for colon cancer. Routine screening for colon cancer is not recommended until age 50 years in patients at average risk. Risk factors for colon cancer include history of a first-degree relative with colorectal cancer younger than age 60 years, history suggestive of familial polyposis or hereditary nonpolyposis colorectal cancer, or personal history of ulcerative colitis.

Because the patient is older than 25 years and monogamous, she is at very low risk for sexually transmitted infections, including *Chlamydia trachomatis*. Some organizations recommend routine screening for diabetes beginning at age 45 years, but the U.S. Preventive Services Task Force recommends screening only in patients with other cardiac risk factors, such as hyperlipidemia and hypertension, or in persons with a strong family history of diabetes. Screening asymptomatic persons for thyroid disease is controversial. Some guidelines recommend obtaining a thyroid-stimulating hormone level in postmenopausal and postpartum women, in patients with diabetes or Down's syndrome, and in elderly patients. The evidence for treating subclinical (asymptomatic) thyroid disease is inconclusive. This patient has no symptoms of thyroid disease that would support the need for screening.

KEY POINT

- Osteomalacia and osteoporosis are common in celiac disease and can occur even in patients who have no gastrointestinal symptoms.

Bibliography

1. Meyer D, Stavropolous S, Diamond B, Shane E, Green PH. Osteoporosis in a North American adult population with celiac disease. Am J Gastroenterol. 2001;96:112-9. [PMID: 11197239]
2. Stenson WF, Newberry R, Lorenz R, Baldus C, Civitelli R. Increased prevalence of celiac disease and need for routine screening among patients with osteoporosis. Arch Intern Med. 2005;165:393-9. [PMID: 15738367]

Item 109   Answer: A

The inactivated influenza vaccine is recommended for patients with chronic medical conditions, including heart failure, kidney disease, lung disease, diabetes, asthma, HIV/AIDS, cancer, and chronic corticosteroid therapy. It is also recommended for infants 6 to 23 months old, persons 65 years or older, residents of long-term care facilities, women who will be pregnant during flu season, and household contacts or caretakers of infants and people at serious risk from influenza. The vaccine is provided as an intramuscular injection every fall.

Chronic warfarin therapy is not a contraindication to the inactivated influenza vaccine, but attention to strong compression at the injection site is warranted. In general, warfarin therapy does not complicate skin or dental procedures, lumbar punctures, or ophthalmologic interventions. A milk allergy is also not a contraindication to the inactivated influenza vaccine, but persons with egg allergy should avoid the inactivated vaccine because it contains egg.

The live intranasal formulation of the influenza vaccine is approved for persons aged 5 to 49 years, but should be avoided in persons over 50 years and in all those with chronic medical conditions. Although there has not been a head-to-head trial of the live intranasal formulation versus the inactivated influenza vaccine in chronically ill persons, animal models and immunologic studies are inconclusive about whether the formulations are equally effective. For now, the Centers for Disease Control and Prevention recommend limiting intranasal live vaccination to persons younger than 50 years who do not have a chronic medical condition.

Prevention of influenza is more effective than treatment with neuraminidase inhibitors. If given within 48 hours of onset of symptoms, a 5-day course of neuraminidase inhibitors can decrease duration of symptoms by 1 day as compared with placebo. Cost-effectiveness studies support limiting use of neuraminidase inhibitors to those individuals most likely to have significant benefit from avoiding pneumonia or hospitalization, including unvaccinated individuals at high risk for complications or residents in a long-term care facility with an outbreak of influenza.

KEY POINT

- The inactivated influenza vaccine is recommended for patients with chronic medical conditions, including heart failure, kidney disease, lung disease, diabetes, asthma, HIV/AIDS, cancer, and chronic corticosteroid therapy.

Bibliography

1. Lee PY, Matchar DB, Clements DA, Huber J, Hamilton JD, Peterson ED. Economic analysis of influenza vaccination and antiviral treatment for healthy working adults. Ann Intern Med. 2002;137:225-31. [PMID: 12186512]
2. Rothberg MB, Bellantonio S, Rose DN. Management of influenza in adults older than 65 years of age: cost-effectiveness of rapid testing and antiviral therapy. Ann Intern Med. 2003;139:321-9. [PMID: 12965940]

Item 110   Answer: C

The patient's history of trauma and the evidence of significant injury point to hemothorax as the most likely cause of his dyspnea. Hemothorax is most commonly due to trauma, either blunt or penetrating (including iatrogenic). Examination should include auscultation and percussion with the patient in the upright position. (Examination of the patient in the supine position will obscure findings.) Nontraumatic causes of blood in the pleural space are less common. They include malignancy, blood dyscrasia, pulmonary embolism, bullous emphysema, and necrotizing infection, including tuberculosis. Cases have been reported of endometriosis causing hemothorax.

Delayed hemothorax from blunt thoracic trauma is not common but should be considered when appropriate, given its 18% mortality in adults. It tends to occur most often in older adults; acute hemothorax is more likely in younger patients. In one retrospective series, two thirds of all patients with hemothorax were male. Rib fracture occurred in 75% of cases. All cases of delayed hemothorax involved men, all of whom had rib fractures. Patients with hemothorax ≥1.5 cm on CT scan were four times more likely to require drainage than were patients with hemothorax ≤1.5 cm.

Pneumonia usually presents with cough and evidence of infection (fevers, chills, or sweats). Chest pain is common, as is abdominal pain with lower-lobe pneumonias. Cough is also a strong clinical factor in atypical pneumonias. This patient describes primarily dyspnea and orthopnea and shows no other evidence of pneumonia or infection.

Pulmonary embolism must be considered in all patients with dyspnea and could have a similar presentation. However, this patient's symptoms began the night of the injury and progressively worsened, and he does not have the marked hypoxia associated with pulmonary embolism. Sinus tachycardia is the most common electrocardiographic finding in patients with pulmonary embolism. This patient also has no known predisposing factors for pulmonary embolism (obesity, immobilization, recent surgery, or known cancer).

Pleural effusion as a result of heart failure must be considered because of the patient's orthopnea. However, his examination does not support such a diagnosis because of the lack of S_3 gallop, rales, and elevated jugular venous distension.

Chylothorax is drainage of lymphatic fluid into the pleural space secondary to disruption or blockage of the thoracic duct. It is usually associated with malignancy (non-Hodgkin's lymphoma accounts for almost 60% of cases), but it can also be idiopathic or due to cirrhosis, tuberculosis, or filariasis. About 25% of cases of chylothorax are preceded by cardiothoracic procedures. Nonsurgical traumatic chylothorax is rare and not consistent with this patient's history and clinical findings.

KEY POINT

- **Hemothorax is most commonly due to trauma, either blunt or penetrating (including iatrogenic).**

Bibliography

1. **Sharma OP, Hagler S, Oswanski MF**. Prevalence of delayed hemothorax in blunt thoracic trauma. Am Surg. 2005;71:481-6. [PMID: 16044926]

2. **Bilello JF, Davis JW, Lemaster DM**. Occult traumatic hemothorax: when can sleeping dogs lie? Am J Surg. 2005;190:841-4. [PMID: 16307931]

Item 111   Answer: B

Because this patient's symptoms fall in the C7 distribution and the Spurling maneuver is positive (pain with neck flexion toward the affected side), he most likely has degenerative arthritis with foramenal encroachment and subsequent radiculopathy. Treatment of choice for radiculopathy is anti-inflammatory medications and moist heat; a soft collar may also be helpful by limiting extreme movement of the neck. Cervical traction combined with physical therapy may also be useful, although evidence to support its value is limited. The natural history of cervical radiculopathies indicates that most patients improve with nonsurgical interventions, so conservative management will relieve the symptoms for most patients. Once acute symptoms diminish, patients should be encouraged to begin a stretching and strengthening program to prevent further episodes.

High-dose, short courses of prednisone may be useful as second-line treatment for cervical radiculopathy to reduce the associated inflammation from compression, but there has been no controlled study to support this use of oral corticosteroids. Translaminar and transforamenal epidural injections of corticosteroids may provide relief; however, these are associated with rare but serious complications. To date, there have been no placebo-controlled trials to confirm the safety and efficacy of this option.

Plain radiography is usually the initial diagnostic test. It is most useful in detecting fractures and subluxations in patients with a history of neck trauma, but has low specificity and sensitivity. CT provides good visualization of the bony elements and may help identify fractures. CT myelography is best for assessing and localizing spinal cord compression and underlying atrophy. For soft-tissue visualization, though, CT is being replaced by MRI. MRI can detect ligament and disk disruption not seen on other studies, but because of its high sensitivity, it should be used only if the history and physical examination support significant disease.

Electromyography is valuable in identifying physiologic abnormalities of the nerve root. Its primary use is to diagnose nerve root dysfunction when the diagnosis is uncertain. It may be useful in this patient if he does not respond to conservative management after 6 to 8 weeks of treatment.

KEY POINT

- **The diagnosis of cervical radiculopathy is supported by increased pain with neck flexion toward the affected side.**

Bibliography

1. **Carette S, Fehlings MG**. Clinical practice. Cervical radiculopathy. N Engl J Med. 2005;353:392-9. [PMID: 16049211]

Item 112   Answer: D

Alopecia areata is common in thyroid disease, vitiligo, diabetes, atopy, and Down's syndrome. The affected skin generally has no signs of inflammation, desquamation, or scarring. Typically, there are one or more rounded, denuded patches in hair-bearing areas. Evaluating the hair bulbs under microscopy reveals tapering of the proximal end or "exclamation point" hairs, which are pathognomonic of this condition. It can also be valuable to do a "pull test" to see how many hairs come out with gentle traction. A positive result consisting of 25 to 50 hairs removed indicates that the disease is active, and further hair loss should be anticipated. For limited disease, a topical corticosteroid or minoxidil is effective in delaying hair loss, and for more extensive disease, oral or pulse intravenous corticosteroids are effective in delaying hair loss; however, neither corticosteroids nor minoxidil has an effect on ultimate outcome in patients with hair loss. New biologic therapies to selectively inhibit the immune response are being studied for alopecia areata.

Telogen effluvium is nonpermanent hair loss that can be related to drug effect, acute illness, or stress. Hair shifts into the shedding or "telogen" phase instead of the growth phase, which creates increased hair loss. On examination, 25 to 50 hairs can be removed with a gentle pull.

Microscopy demonstrates a white bulb on the shaft. It is usually self-limited and requires only reassurance to the patient.

Trichotillomania is habitual pulling out of hair. It can be isolated or associated with mental health problems, especially compulsion or impulse-control behaviors, and is difficult to treat. Behavioral therapy alone or in combination with pharmacologic therapy has been studied for this condition.

Tinea capitis is a superficial fungal infection of the skin, commonly affecting the scalp, eyebrows, and eyelashes. Lesions generally show evidence of active infection with exudates, inflamed crusts, matted hair, and even debris. In severe cases, it can develop into a patch with hair loss and scarring alopecia. Most, but not all, pathogens in tinea capitis cause the infected hairs to fluoresce in "black" ultraviolet light with Wood's light examination. Microscopy and culture can also aid the diagnosis. Treatment is with griseofulvin or an antifungal "azole" medication. Topical treatment is usually ineffective.

KEY POINTS

- **Alopecia areata is common in thyroid disease, vitiligo, diabetes, atopy, and Down's syndrome.**
- **The affected skin in alopecia areata generally has no signs of inflammation, desquamation, or scarring.**

Bibliography

1. **Norris D**. Alopecia areata: current state of knowledge. J Am Acad Dermatol. 2004;51:S16-7. [PMID: 15243493]

Item 113   Answer: B

Chronic pelvic pain that lasts years is a complex syndrome related to neurologic, psychologic, musculoskeletal, and endocrinologic factors. Affected women frequently have a history of sexual victimization, so screening for posttraumatic stress disorder is recommended. Generally, patients with posttraumatic stress disorder require a multidisciplinary approach with psychotherapy, physical therapy, and medication to achieve long-term symptomatic relief.

Domestic violence and sexual abuse are frequently under-recognized by practitioners, yet physician awareness of the problem has the biggest impact on helping victims. Physicians should screen all patients and work to overcome the barriers (such as patient comfort and safety) associated with disclosure of these problems. Physicians also need to understand the many stages involved in behavioral change of the victim. Informed, active physicians have the greatest potential to improve these patients' lives, reduce the long-term effects of violence, and improve their survival. Victims often go to the emergency room, where practitioners must have a high index of suspicion and vigilantly screen for abuse.

The primary manifestation of adult attention deficit disorder (AADD) is disinhibition. Other characteristics of this disorder are distractibility, poor concentration, impulsivity, and elevated motor activity. Patients with AADD often have a lifelong history of such symptoms, which are not present in this patient.

Conversion disorder is characterized by the acute onset of a symptom, usually neurologic, in response to overwhelming stress. However, this patient's symptoms are chronic in onset and are not neurologic in nature; therefore, conversion disorder is not likely in this scenario.

Malingering patients purposefully feign symptoms and are often engaged in ongoing legal battles or have substance abuse problems, a profile that does not match the symptoms, history, and findings in this patient.

Hypochondriasis is a state of constant, deep fear of developing a serious medical condition, with misattribution of physical symptoms. Nothing in this patient's history is suggestive of this somatic disorder.

KEY POINT

- **Screening for posttraumatic stress disorder is recommended in women with chronic pelvic pain, who frequently have a history of sexual victimization.**

Bibliography

1. **Poleshuck EL, Dworkin RH, Howard FM, Foster DC, Shields CG, Giles DE, et al**. Contributions of physical and sexual abuse to women's experiences with chronic pelvic pain. J Reprod Med. 2005;50:91-100. [PMID: 15755045]
2. **Director TD, Linden JA**. Domestic violence: an approach to identification and intervention. Emerg Med Clin North Am. 2004;22:1117-32. [PMID: 15474785]

Item 114   Answer: A

This patient has chronic, progressive metastatic cancer–induced pain that is not alleviated by standard short-term pain management. He requires high-dose, escalating, long-acting narcotic analgesia, and in this setting, morphine would be appropriate.

There is no evidence that any long-acting narcotic is better than another such agent. In particular, the efficacy of oxycodone is similar to that of morphine and is appropriate for use in patients with cancer-related pain. However, oxycodone is considerably more expensive than morphine, and because there is no evidence of its improved efficacy or a better side-effect profile compared with morphine, it would be appropriate to first use the lowest-cost alternative of agents with comparable efficacy.

Transdermal fentanyl is also a useful long-acting narcotic but is considerably more expensive than long-acting morphine and is often used in patients who have limitations on oral intake or intolerance to other long-acting narcotics.

Duloxetine is a new antidepressant drug with an approved indication for some chronic pain syndromes but would not be an appropriate alternative to long-acting narcotic analgesia for the treatment of severe, progressive, cancer-related pain.

Methadone is another effective long-acting narcotic that is comparable in cost and efficacy to morphine and, therefore, would be an appropriate cost-effective alternative.

> **KEY POINT**
>
> • Patients with progressive pain that ceases to respond to short-term pain management may require high-dose, escalating, long-acting narcotic analgesia.

Bibliography
1. Reid CM, Martin RM, Sterne JA, Davies AN, Hanks GW. Oxycodone for cancer-related pain: meta-analysis of randomized controlled trials. Arch Intern Med. 2006;166:837-43. [PMID: 16636208]
2. Bruera E, Palmer JL, Bosnjak S, Rico MA, Moyano J, Sweeney C, et al. Methadone versus morphine as a first-line strong opioid for cancer pain: a randomized, double-blind study. J Clin Oncol. 2004;22:185-92. [PMID: 14701781]

Item 115   Answer: B

This patient has probable musculoskeletal chest pain, and, more specifically, costochondritis, which can be treated with an NSAID and avoidance of strenuous activity. Because obstructive coronary artery disease (CAD) is often of primary concern given the ramifications of missing such a diagnosis, it would be reasonable to assess for this type of disease; however, there are validated methods for assessing such probability using only simple clinical information, obtainable from a telephone history. In this case, the low probability of obstructive CAD (based on this patient's symptoms, which are atypical for angina because they have occurred at rest without progression over 4 weeks and have not been exacerbated by exertion or relieved with rest), the lack of factors indicating high risk for acute coronary syndrome (the lack of dyspnea or progressive tempo), and the more likely competing diagnosis of musculoskeletal chest pain, which commonly occurs in the setting of recent heavy lifting or exercise, allow for the outpatient management of this undifferentiated syndrome. The patient should be thoroughly counseled that if the symptoms do not improve in the ensuing week after empiric NSAID therapy and rest, he should undergo evaluation in the office or, if the symptoms worsen significantly, he should go to the emergency department.

Although the differential diagnoses responsible for chest pain depend on several clinical variables, particularly age and sex, the general order of prevalent causes of chest pain in ambulatory general medical settings are roughly the same. In one study of the causes of chest pain in a primary care setting, musculoskeletal chest pain, including costochondritis, accounted for 33.4% of all diagnoses, followed by reflux esophagitis (13.4%). Stable angina pectoris was the primary diagnosis in only 10.3% of episodes, and unstable angina or possible myocardial infarction in 1.5%. In this study, most resources used to evaluate chest pain were devoted to ruling out cardiac causes.

Other common causes of chest pain include esophageal spasm, herpetic neuralgia, anxiety (including panic disorder), and reactive airways. Panic disorder is present in more than 30% of patients evaluated in the emergency department for chest pain and who are found to have no evidence of CAD. Therefore, in situations in which the cause of chest pain cannot be determined, a thorough evaluation for panic disorder should occur; this disorder is highly amenable to treatment with either benzodiazepines or selective serotonin reuptake inhibitors.

Because gastroesophageal reflux disease is the second most common cause of chest pain in primary care settings, and empiric treatment with high-dose proton pump inhibitors is an effective way to diagnose this disorder, this would be a reasonable next step in the management of this syndrome if the initial strategy were unsuccessful.

> **KEY POINTS**
>
> • Validated methods exist for assessing the probability of coronary artery disease using only simple clinical information, obtainable from a telephone history.
> • Symptoms atypical of angina, an absence high-risk factors for acute coronary syndrome, and the higher likelihood for musculoskeletal chest pain in the setting of recent strenuous activity allow for the outpatient management of noncardiac chest pain.

Bibliography
1. Morise AP. Comparison of the Diamond-Forrester method and a new score to estimate the pretest probability of coronary disease before exercise testing. Am Heart J. 1999;138:740-5. [PMID: 10502221]
2. Klinkman MS, Stevens D, Gorenflo DW. Episodes of care for chest pain: a preliminary report from MIRNET. Michigan Research Network. J Fam Pract. 1994;38:345-52. [PMID: 8163958]

Item 116   Answer: D

Orlistat, a lipase inhibitor that increases fecal fat loss, would be an appropriate treatment in this patient to aid in her attempts at modest weight loss. Orlistat is Food and Drug Administration (FDA) approved for weight loss in obese patients, and meta-analysis has demonstrated a mean weight loss of 2.89 kg (6.37 lb) at 12 months. Side effects of orlistat are related to malabsorption of fat in the gastrointestinal tract and include steatorrhea, bloating, and oily discharge. In addition to lipase inhibitors, medications for weight loss consist of appetite suppressants. Sibutramine is an appetite suppressant that works through combined norepinephrine and serotonin reuptake inhibition. The side effects include a modest increase in heart rate and blood pressure, nervousness, dry mouth, headache, and insomnia. A meta-analysis of sibutramine reported a mean difference in weight loss of 4.45 kg (95% CI, 3.62 to 5.29) at 12 months compared with placebo groups. Sibutramine is not recommended for patients with poorly controlled hypertension.

Phentermine, a sympathetic amine, is an appetite suppressant found to be effective for achieving modest weight loss (3 to 5 kg [6.62 to 11.03 lb]) in a meta-analysis of pharmacologic therapy for obesity. However, it is not FDA approved for the treatment of obesity. Mirtazapine is a tetracyclic atypical antidepressant medication that has some serotonin 5-HT$_2$ and 5-HT$_3$ receptor antagonist properties. Although there is some evidence to support the use of the selective serotonin reuptake inhibitor fluoxetine in achieving modest weight loss, mirtazapine is associated with weight gain and increased appetite and is not an appropriate pharmacologic treatment for obesity.

KEY POINT

- **Sibutramine is not recommended for weight loss in patients with poorly controlled hypertension.**

Bibliography

1. Li Z, Maglione M, Tu W, Mojica W, Arterburn D, Shugarman LR, et al. Meta-analysis: pharmacologic treatment of obesity. Ann Intern Med. 2005;142:532-46. [PMID: 15809465]

Item 117   Answer: D

This patient has tinea versicolor, otherwise known as *Pityriasis versicolor*. This is a superficial mycotic (or fungal) infection of young and middle-aged adults caused by the lipophilic yeast *Malassezia furfur*. The infection is usually noticed because involved areas do not tan, and there is resulting hypopigmentation. There is also a hyperpigmented form of tinea versicolor. In patients with tinea versicolor, large, blunt hyphae and thick-walled budding spores in a "spaghetti and meatballs" pattern are evident on examination of scale with 10% potassium hydroxide. Topical ketoconazole cream is an effective therapy for these patients. Ketoconazole is also effective as a systemic treatment in an oral form or as a shampoo.

Although oral terbinafine is not effective in treating tinea versicolor, topical terbinafine is effective in treating this infection. Itraconazole, although an effective treatment for this infection, is contraindicated in patients who use statins. Corticosteroids are not an effective treatment for fungal infections. Griseofulvin in the topical or oral form is not effective in treating tinea versicolor. Selenium sulfide shampoos are also effective treatments for patients with tinea versicolor. The infection commonly recurs, and prophylaxis and/or periodic courses of treatment may be necessary in these patients.

KEY POINT

- **Topical ketoconazole cream is an effective therapy for patients with tinea versicolor.**

Bibliography

1. Schwartz RA. Superficial fungal infections. Lancet. 2004;364:1173-82. [PMID: 15451228]
2. Loo DS. Cutaneous fungal infections in the elderly. Dermatol Clin. 2004;22:33-50. [PMID: 15018008]

Item 118   Answer: D

The most appropriate management of patients with suspected chronic sinusitis who have not responded to medical treatment is to perform imaging studies, and this patient should receive sinus CT. Chronic rhinosinusitis is defined clinically by the presence of nasal and paranasal sinus inflammation lasting for at least 12 consecutive weeks. This patient presents with the characteristic symptoms of sinus headache, nasal congestion, and mucopurulent postnasal drainage, and his deviated septum is a risk factor for chronic rhinosinusitis. Although he did not respond to trimethoprim–sulfamethoxazole or doxycycline, bacterial resistance to these antibiotics is common. However, his condition was also refractory to long-term intensive medical treatment with a broad-spectrum antibiotic. Although he could also have an anaerobic or fungal infection, the role of these pathogens in chronic rhinosinusitis is uncertain, and empiric therapy is not recommended. A noncontrast-enhanced sinus CT can best define the extent and location of chronic sinusitis and identify bony abnormalities—particularly obstructions of the ostiomeatal complex, which drains the frontal, maxillary, and ethmoid sinuses—that might benefit from surgical management. Sinus CT has a sensitivity of 85% to 94% and a specificity of 41% to 59%, depending on the radiographic staging score cutoff for diagnosing chronic rhinosinusitis. Otolaryngologic referral for nasal endoscopy should be considered for patients with an abnormal sinus CT scan.

Referral for allergy testing should be considered in patients with atopic symptoms, which are not present in this patient, or if there is no evidence of obstruction on CT. Performing a culture of the paranasal sinuses with cotton swabs is difficult. Furthermore, nasal cultures correlate poorly with cultures obtained from sinus aspiration because nasal cultures are frequently contaminated by *Staphylococcus aureus* colonization. An otolaryngologist can collect secretions with nasal endoscopy for aerobic, anaerobic, and fungal cultures. Sinus MRI provides better imaging of soft-tissue structures than CT but is limited by poor bony imaging and high false-positive rates. Sinus radiography is less sensitive than CT for detecting chronic sinusitis, particularly for ostiomeatal complex obstruction.

KEY POINT

- **Imaging studies are appropriate in patients with suspected chronic sinusitis who have not responded to medical treatment.**

Bibliography

1. Bhattacharyya N, Fried MP. The accuracy of computed tomography in the diagnosis of chronic rhinosinusitis. Laryngoscope. 2003;113:125-9. [PMID: 12514395]

Item 119   Answer: A

The best method for transporting an avulsed tooth to the dentist is by replacing it in its socket. If dental care is immediately attained after the injury (within 30 minutes), and there are no other significant injuries, the likelihood is high that the tooth can be successfully replanted, with successful replantation rates exceeding 90%. Although 1 tablespoon of table salt mixed in a pint of water results in a solution that has the same salinity as blood, this is not as good a transport medium as replacement of the avulsed tooth in its socket. If the tooth cannot be placed immediately back in its socket, the second-best transport medium is whole milk. There are special dental transport media available in some emergency departments; however, they are still not as effective as the original socket for transporting avulsed teeth. Packing the avulsed tooth in ice is not an effective method for transport because freezing can damage the tooth.

KEY POINT

- If dental care is immediately attained within 30 minutes of injury, successful replantation rates of avulsed teeth exceed 90%.

Bibliography

1. Krasner PR. Emergency treatment of avulsed teeth. Emerg Med Serv. 2004;33:114, 116-7. [PMID: 15651257]
2. Chappuis V, von Arx T. Replantation of 45 avulsed permanent teeth: a 1-year follow-up study. Dent Traumatol. 2005;21:289-96. [PMID: 16149925]

Item 120   Answer: A

This patient has major depression and generalized anxiety disorder and should receive paroxetine. All the selective serotonin reuptake inhibitors and the serotonin norepinephrine reuptake inhibitors are effective for depression and generalized anxiety disorder and have Food and Drug Administration (FDA) approval for these indications. Bupropion is a proven antidepressant and clonazepam is a proven anxiolytic, but neither is FDA approved for treating depressive disorder. The atypical antipsychotic agents, such as risperidone, olanzapine, and quetiapine, are sometimes added to antidepressant therapy to augment response in patients with treatment-resistant major depressive disorder but are not indicated as monotherapy for major depression and dysthymia or generalized anxiety disorder.

Patients with depression commonly have some symptoms of anxiety also, and approximately one third meet the criteria for a concomitant anxiety disorder. Depressive symptoms often respond more quickly to treatment than do anxiety symptoms, and it is not uncommon for anxiety to be "unmasked" during the first few weeks of antidepressant treatment.

KEY POINTS

- All the selective serotonin reuptake inhibitors and the serotonin norepinephrine reuptake inhibitors are effective for depression and generalized anxiety disorder and have Food and Drug Administration approval for these indications.
- Depressive symptoms often respond more quickly to treatment than do anxiety symptoms, and it is not uncommon for anxiety to be "unmasked" during the first few weeks of antidepressant treatment.

Bibliography

1. Kroenke K, West SL, Swindle R, Gilsenan A, Eckert GJ, Dolor R, et al. Similar effectiveness of paroxetine, fluoxetine, and sertraline in primary care: a randomized trial. JAMA. 2001;286:2947-55. [PMID: 11743835]

Item 121   Answer: C

This patient has allergic rhinitis based on characteristic symptoms of nasal congestion, rhinorrhea, postnasal drainage, and sneezing; clinical findings of pale turbinates with watery secretions; and positive results on allergen skin testing. Nasal corticosteroids are the most effective and well-tolerated treatments for improving nasal symptoms and quality of life in patients with allergic rhinitis. Meta-analyses of randomized trials have shown nasal corticosteroids to be more effective than either leukotriene inhibitors or oral antihistamines—both sedating and non-sedating—in treating patients with allergic rhinitis. Nasal decongestants are highly effective for treating nasal congestion but should not be used for more than 3 to 5 days due to the risk of rhinitis medicamentosa. Oral decongestants show some benefit in reducing nasal congestion but not for treating other symptoms of allergic rhinitis. Oral decongestants can modestly increase systolic blood pressure and heart rate and should be used cautiously in patients with cardiovascular disease.

KEY POINTS

- Symptoms of allergic rhinitis consist of nasal congestion, rhinorrhea, postnasal drainage, and sneezing; clinical findings of pale turbinates with watery secretions; and positive results on allergen skin testing.
- Nasal corticosteroids are more effective than either leukotriene inhibitors or oral antihistamines—both sedating and non-sedating—in treating patients with allergic rhinitis.

Bibliography

1. **Long A, McFadden C, DeVine D, Chew P, Kupelnick B, Lau J**. Management of allergic and nonallergic rhinitis. Evid Rep Technol Assess (Summ). 2002:1-6. [PMID: 12173440]

2. **Salerno SM, Jackson JL, Berbano EP**. Effect of oral pseudoephedrine on blood pressure and heart rate: a meta-analysis. Arch Intern Med. 2005;165:1686-94. [PMID: 16087815]

Item 122   Answer: D

The evidence is good that routine postoperative lung expansion (for example, incentive spirometry or deep-breathing exercises) prevents postoperative pulmonary complications. Based on current evidence, no modality is clearly superior to the other, but nasal continuous positive airway pressure may be particularly useful in patients who are not able to perform incentive spirometry. The evidence is insufficient to determine whether prophylactic corticosteroids or antibiotics prevent pneumonia.

Multiple trials have shown that routine intravenous or enteral hyperalimentation in malnourished patients does not prevent postoperative pulmonary complications except perhaps in the severely malnourished or in those expected to be without oral intake for an extended period (for example, 2 or 3 weeks). There is emerging evidence suggesting that enteral nutrition especially formulated to enhance the immune system may prevent postoperative infection.

KEY POINT

- **The evidence is good that routine postoperative lung expansion (for example, incentive spirometry or deep-breathing exercises) prevents postoperative pulmonary complications.**

Bibliography

1. **Lawrence VA, Cornell JE, Smetana GW**. Strategies to reduce postoperative pulmonary complications after noncardiothoracic surgery: systematic review for the American College of Physicians. Ann Intern Med. 2006;144:596-608. [PMID: 16618957]

2. **Qaseem A, Snow V, Fitterman N, Hornbake ER, Lawrence VA, Smetana GW, et al**. Risk assessment for and strategies to reduce perioperative pulmonary complications for patients undergoing noncardiothoracic surgery: a guideline from the American College of Physicians. Ann Intern Med. 2006;144:575-80. [PMID: 16618955]

Item 123   Answer: C

Patients with a history of cancer and new skeletal complaints should be evaluated for metastasis. Cancers that most commonly spread to bone include prostate, breast, lung, thyroid, and renal cell carcinomas. Pain in two contiguous joints is common because patients realign themselves and their gait, causing strain to another area as they protect the affected joint. Bone scan or scintigraphy is the gold standard for detecting bone metastases, showing a "hot spot" where there is osteoblastic activity. It can detect lesions as small as 2 mm. CT and MRI can define soft-tissue and bone abnormalities but at considerably

greater expense. Plain radiography is not very sensitive. Lesions must be at least 1 cm to be visible, or there must be considerable bone destruction or sclerosis before the plain film will be positive.

Scanning with positron emission tomography (PET) is being studied in breast, lung, and esophageal cancer with mixed results. It may be valuable in following response to treatment of patients with bone metastases. PET scans are more likely to detect osteoclastic than osteoblastic lesions.

CT-guided arthrocentesis might be indicated in a patient with a high suspicion for infectious arthritis, which is not the case in this scenario. There is no history of fever, chills, or recent instrumentation of the genitourinary tract to suggest septic arthritis. CT-guided arthrocentesis is invasive and costly, and should be used only when there are strong clinical indications.

This patient may be at risk for gout or pseudogout, especially in light of his age and because he takes a thiazide diuretic for hypertension, but his history of cancer suggests a different, more pressing issue. There is also usually more evidence of acute inflammation on examination than described. Gout affects the first metatarsophalangeal joint in at least 70% of cases and seldom affects the central joints (hips, shoulders, and spine). Pseudogout has a predilection for knees and wrists and usually is associated with chondrocalcinosis on radiography, with pathognomonic pyrophosphate crystals in the synovial fluid. When gout or pseudogout is suspected, joint fluid analysis for crystals is essential for definitive diagnosis.

KEY POINTS

- **Cancers that most commonly spread to bone include prostate, breast, lung, thyroid, and renal cell carcinomas.**

Bibliography

1. **Langer C**. Management of bone metastases: 2005 update. J Natl Compr Canc Netw. 2005;3 Suppl 1:S59-63. [PMID: 16280117]

Item 124   Answer: D

This woman most likely has benign memory loss of aging. This process occurs commonly in patients as they age and is almost universally present in patients by 70 years of age. There are several reversible causes of memory problems, including depression, hyper- or hypothyroidism, liver or renal dysfunction, hypercalcemia, and B_{12}/folate deficiency. In her case, the B_{12}/folate and rapid plasma reagin are the only tests not recently ordered and would be the most appropriate management option at this time. Interestingly, some patients with B_{12} deficiencies with neurologic manifestations have no abnormalities on hematologic studies, and a normal mean corpuscular volume should not preclude an assessment for B_{12} deficiency. Benign memory loss can be distinguished from mild cognitive impairment by lack of evidence of cognitive impairment on objective tests (for example, her normal Mini–Mental State Examination score).

Although approximately 12% of patients with mild cognitive impairment progress to dementia, age-related forgetfulness does not increase the risk for developing dementia.

Among patients with mild cognitive impairment, donepezil had no effect on progression to Alzheimer's disease during 3 years of treatment in a randomized-controlled trial. Asking patients about depression or anhedonia is a sufficient screening method for ruling out depression in the absence of any signs suspicious for these disorders. Because there are no worrisome findings on physical examination, MRI or CT of the head is not indicated.

KEY POINTS

- **Benign memory loss can be distinguished from mild cognitive impairment by lack of evidence of cognitive impairment on objective tests.**
- **Although approximately 12% of patients with mild cognitive impairment progress to dementia, age-related forgetfulness does not increase the risk for developing dementia.**

Bibliography

1. **Budson AE, Price BH**. Memory dysfunction. N Engl J Med. 2005;352:692-9. [PMID: 15716563]
2. **Schonknecht P, Pantel J, Kruse A, Schroder J**. Prevalence and natural course of aging-associated cognitive decline in a population-based sample of young-old subjects. Am J Psychiatry. 2005;162:2071-7. [PMID: 16263846]
3. **Petersen RC, Thomas RG, Grundman M, Bennett D, Doody R, Ferris S, et al**. Vitamin E and donepezil for the treatment of mild cognitive impairment. N Engl J Med. 2005;352:2379-88. [PMID: 15829527]

Item 125 Answer: E

A trial involving weekly fluconazole treatment may benefit this patient, who is experiencing recurrent vaginal yeast infections. In a recent study, 373 women with at least four documented episodes of yeast vaginitis during the previous year were treated with fluconazole, 150 mg weekly for 6 months, or placebo. At 6 months, more patients in the treatment group (90.8%) were free of recurrent yeast vaginitis than those in the placebo group (35.9%). During a 6-month observation period following treatment, fewer treatment and placebo patients were recurrence free (21.9% and 42.9%, respectively). Although this therapy did not result in a long-term cure of yeast vaginitis, it was an effective short-term treatment.

No evidence supports the treatment of recurrent vaginal infections with lactobacillus, douching, or avoidance of simple sugars. (Women with diabetes experience more episodes of candidiasis, so it is advisable to measure fasting plasma glucose in women with recurrent vaginal yeast infections.) Additionally, no evidence suggests that treatment of the patient's partner is beneficial.

Vaginal yeast infections occur in about 5% of women. *Candida albicans* infections occur without a known cause.

Besides diabetes, however, the infections can be associated with pregnancy or the use of broad-spectrum antibiotics or corticosteroids. Heat, moisture, and occlusive clothing contribute to occurrence of infection. Symptoms include pruritus, external and internal erythema and nonodorous white curd-like discharge. Because vaginal yeast is found in 10% to 20% of normal women, the existence of *Candida* without symptoms does not require treatment.

KEY POINT

- **Weekly oral fluconazole reduces the short-term incidence of yeast vaginitis in patients with recurrent infection.**

Bibliography

1. **Sobel JD, Wiesenfeld HC, Martens M, Danna P, Hooton TM, Rompalo A, et al**. Maintenance fluconazole therapy for recurrent vulvovaginal candidiasis. N Engl J Med. 2004;351:876-83. [PMID: 15329425]

Item 126 Answer: E

This patient is likely experiencing myalgias from fluvastatin, but he may not have the same problem with another statin or when taking fluvastatin at a lower dose. If the patient's muscle symptoms were tolerable, he would not need to change his medication. Because his symptoms are bothersome, it is advisable to discontinue the fluvastatin and, after he becomes completely asymptomatic, try another statin.

Common dose-related muscle symptoms that can occur with the use of statins include in 1% to 5% of cases focal or diffuse myalgia and creatine kinase (CK) elevations that are less than 10 times the upper limit of normal levels. Myopathy, indicated by a serum CK level more than 10 times the upper limit of normal, occurs in 0.1% to 0.5% of patients treated with statins in clinical trials. Some medications increase the risk of statin-associated myopathy, including fibrates, cyclosporine, macrolide antibiotics, various antifungal drugs, and cytochrome P-450 inhibitors. The Medical Letter consultants recommend measuring CK levels before starting a statin and again on development of muscle pain. However, other expert panels do not recommend this approach. In general, the statin should be discontinued if the CK value is more than 3 to 10 times the upper limit of the normal range.

Cholestyramine is not recommended in this patient because it might increase his serum triglyceride level, which is already elevated. Although a fibric acid derivative would lower his triglyceride level, the more important objective is to lower his serum low-density lipoprotein cholesterol level to reduce his risk for coronary artery disease. Pentoxifylline may help treat symptoms of vascular disease, but this patient's symptoms are not likely caused by vascular disease. He does not have exercise-induced leg symptoms, and physical examination indicates normal peripheral pulses.

- It is advisable to discontinue a statin in patients with bothersome symptoms and try another statin once symptoms have resolved.
- Some medications increase the risk for statin-associated myopathy, including fibrates, cyclosporine, macrolide antibiotics, various antifungal drugs, and cytochrome P-450 inhibitors.

Bibliography

1. Drugs for lipids. Treat Guidel Med Lett. 2005;3:15-22. [PMID: 15726011]
2. **Thompson PD, Clarkson P, Karas RH**. Statin-associated myopathy. JAMA. 2003;289:1681-90. [PMID: 12672737]

Item 127   Answer: A

This patient has nonspecific dyspepsia, of which there are a limited number of causes and for which the clinical history does not accurately distinguish between organic and functional (or nonulcer) dyspepsia. In patients without alarm symptoms suggestive of serious disease (age of onset >50 years, anemia, weight loss, and positive fecal occult blood testing results), one decision analysis concluded that a "test-and-treat" approach using urea breath testing (UBT) (or serum *Helicobacter pylori* antibody testing if UBT is not available) followed by *H. pylori* eradication in patients with positive results, was the most cost-effective strategy to produce a symptomatic cure compared with initial endoscopy, double-contrast barium, empirical eradication therapy, or empirical antisecretory therapy. This analysis was sensitive to the efficacy of eradication therapies for *H. pylori* infection in patients with nonulcer dyspepsia. A meta-analysis of the effect of eradicating *H. pylori* in patients with nonulcer dyspepsia showed a small effect (9% relative risk reduction) on persistent symptoms.

Endoscopy would be an appropriate initial strategy for patients with warning signs of a more serious underlying condition but is too costly as an initial step for use in all patients with dyspepsia.

Double-contrast barium imaging does not facilitate evaluation for *H. pylori*, which is responsible for many cases of dyspepsia for which a cure is available.

Although empiric acid suppression, particularly with a proton pump inhibitor (PPI), would lead to symptomatic improvement in this patient, lifelong therapy would be required in many patients who might otherwise be cured with a simpler, short-term *H. pylori* eradication regimen. An empirical trial of acid suppression with a PPI for 4 to 8 weeks may be an initial option in situations in which the prevalence of *H. pylori* infection is low (<10%), followed by the test-and-treat strategy in patients who respond or relapse rapidly after cessation of antisecretory therapy. In patients who respond to initial therapy, treatment should be stopped after 4 to 8 weeks, and if symptoms recur, another course of this treatment is justified. Chronic use of PPIs is only marginally effective in improving symptoms of nonulcerative dyspepsia.

- In patients with nonspecific dyspepsia and no alarm symptoms, a "test-and-treat" approach with urea breath testing followed by *Helicobacter pylori* eradication in patients with positive results is the most cost-effective strategy for curing symptoms.

Bibliography

1. **Makris N, Barkun A, Crott R, Fallone CA**. Cost-effectiveness of alternative approaches in the management of dyspepsia. Int J Technol Assess Health Care. 2003;19:446-64. [PMID: 12962332]
2. **Moayyedi P, Soo S, Deeks J, Delaney B, Harris A, Innes M, et al**. Eradication of Helicobacter pylori for non-ulcer dyspepsia. Cochrane Database Syst Rev. 2006:CD002096. [PMID: 16625554]
3. **Delaney B, Ford AC, Forman D, Moayyedi P, Qume M**. Initial management strategies for dyspepsia. Cochrane Database Syst Rev. 2005:CD001961. [PMID: 16235292]

Item 128   Answer: B

This patient has fulminant keratitis in the setting of a recent corneal ulcer. Corneal abrasions are often caused by contact lens use, particularly the soft, extended-wear type. Additionally, there is an increased risk for fulminant keratitis caused by pseudomonal infection in contact lens users who develop corneal abrasions. Gram-negative bacteria (particularly *Pseudomonas* and *Serratia* species) are relatively common contaminants of contact lens solutions, and when they infect disrupted corneal tissue, can cause rapid corneal destruction, ulceration, and even eye perforation. Soft contact users are more susceptible to these gram-negative infections than are hard contact lens users. Thus, given the association between contact lens use and fulminant progression of this condition, close monitoring, usually consisting of daily follow-up to assure resolution, is required in patients with symptoms of corneal abrasion, and early intervention with antibiotics is indicated in patients with evidence of progression.

Patients with diabetes mellitus and swimmers are at higher risk for developing pseudomonal ear infections than those without these factors, but there is no evidence that they are at higher risk for microbial keratitis in the setting of corneal abrasions. Similarly, chronic conjunctivitis and autoimmune disease, such as systemic lupus erythematosus, have not been associated with progressive keratitis in the setting of corneal abrasions.

- Corneal abrasions are often caused by contact lens use, particularly the soft, extended-wear type.
- There is an increased risk for fulminant keratitis caused by pseudomonal infection in contact lens users who develop corneal abrasions.

Bibliography

1. **Mah-Sadorra JH, Yavuz SG, Najjar DM, Laibson PR, Rapuano CJ, Cohen EJ**. Trends in contact lens-related corneal ulcers. Cornea. 2005;24:51-8. [PMID: 15604867]

2. **Cheng KH, Leung SL, Hoekman HW, Beekhuis WH, Mulder PG, Geerards AJ, et al**. Incidence of contact-lens-associated microbial keratitis and its related morbidity. Lancet. 1999;354:181-5. [PMID: 10421298]

Item 129   Answer: E

This patient is at very low risk for group A β-hemolytic streptococcus (GABHS) because her Centor score is 1 (based on the presence of a fever). Conservative management to reduce her symptoms is sufficient.

Antibiotic treatment is recommended for patients with GABHS pharyngitis to prevent rheumatic fever, acute glomerulonephritis, and suppurative complications and to reduce contagion and symptom duration. Pharyngitis is one of the most common symptoms in adult primary care, but the prevalence of GABHS is only 5% to 15%. However, approximately 75% of adults presenting with pharyngitis receive a prescription for antibiotics, most targeting GABHS. Consequently, clinical-prediction rules have been developed to efficiently guide antibiotic treatment and testing for GABHS. The validated Centor prediction score assigns one point to each of four clinical findings: fever, tonsillar exudates, tender anterior cervical lymphadenopathy, or absence of cough. The probability of GABHS in the original study of adults evaluated in an urban emergency room was 2.5% for a Centor score of 0, 6.5% for a score of 1, 15% for a score of 2, 32% for a score of 3, and 56% for a score of 4, with associated likelihood ratios for GABHS of 0.16, 0.3, 0.75, 2.1, and 6.3, respectively.

Although a narrow-spectrum antibiotic such as penicillin is more appropriate than a broad-spectrum antibiotic such as amoxicillin–clavulanate for treating GABHS, empirical antibiotic therapy and further diagnostic testing (rapid streptococcal testing or throat culture) are inappropriate in this case because the probability of GABHS is so low.

KEY POINT

- **Antibiotic treatment is recommended for patients with group A β-hemolytic streptococcal pharyngitis to prevent rheumatic fever, acute glomerulonephritis, and suppurative complications and to reduce contagion and symptom duration.**

Bibliography

1. **Ebell MH, Smith MA, Barry HC, Ives K, Carey M**. The rational clinical examination. Does this patient have strep throat? JAMA. 2000;284:2912-8. [PMID: 11147989]

2. **Cooper RJ, Hoffman JR, Bartlett JG, Besser RE, Gonzales R, Hickner JM, et al**. Principles of appropriate antibiotic use for acute pharyngitis in adults: background. Ann Intern Med. 2001;134:509-17. [PMID: 11255530]

Item 130   Answer: B

This patient has a somatization disorder, for which the optimal initial management strategy is cognitive behavioral therapy (CBT). Somatization disorder criteria include several years of many physical complaints beginning before age 30 years that result in treatment being sought or significant impairment in social, occupational, or other important areas of functioning. To meet the criteria for this disorder, patients must have experienced two gastrointestinal tract symptoms, one sexual symptom, and one pseudoneurologic symptom, none of which can be explainable by another medical diagnosis. Although there is some evidence that CBT is helpful in treating patients with somatization disorder, these patients often are reluctant to undergo CBT. Reorienting them by suggesting that CBT may help them cope better by allowing them to live more productively with their symptoms can be helpful, particularly when patients trust that their physicians do not believe the problems to be "in their heads."

Because recent results of exhaustive diagnostic tests have been negative, repeated testing is not indicated in this patient at this time. Venlafaxine and nortriptyline both inhibit uptake of norepinephrine; therefore, it is unlikely that switching from one agent to another with a similar mechanism of action will provide relief to this patient.

KEY POINTS

- **Somatization disorder criteria include several years of many physical complaints beginning before age 30 years that result in treatment being sought or significant impairment in social, occupational, or other important areas of functioning.**
- **To meet the criteria for somatization disorder, the patient must have experienced two gastrointestinal tract symptoms, one sexual symptom, and one pseudoneurologic symptom, with none of these symptoms explained by another medical diagnosis.**

Bibliography

1. **Smith RC, Lyles JS, Gardiner JC, Sirbu C, Hodges A, Collins C, et al**. Primary care clinicians treat patients with medically unexplained symptoms: a randomized controlled trial. J Gen Intern Med. 2006;21:671-7. [PMID: 16808764]

2. **Smith RC, Lein C, Collins C, Lyles JS, Given B, Dwamena FC, et al**. Treating patients with medically unexplained symptoms in primary care. J Gen Intern Med. 2003;18:478-89. [PMID: 12823656]

3. **Kroenke K**. The interface between physical and psychological symptoms. J Clin Psychiatry Primary Care Companion. 2003;5[suppl 7]:11-18.

Item 131   Answer: D

Severe urinary incontinence is one of the most serious adverse outcomes of radical prostatectomy. The rates of postprostatectomy incontinence requiring treatment range from 3% to 60% in the literature depending on the definition of incontinence and the method for obtaining data. The cause of urinary incontinence in most cases is intrinsic sphincteric incompetence, for which the treatment options are anticholinergic therapy, collagen injections, sling procedures, and artificial urinary sphincter implantation. Incontinence due to the serotonergic antidepressant agents has been described but is rare. In addition, because the use of sertraline predated the onset of this patient's symptoms, discontinuing sertraline is unlikely to be an effective intervention. The patient did not respond to tolterodine and is therefore unlikely to respond to oxybutynin. There is no evidence of efficacy for behavioral therapy in patients with postprostatectomy urinary sphincter incontinence.

KEY POINT

- **The cause of urinary incontinence in most cases is intrinsic sphincteric incompetence, for which the treatment options are anticholinergic therapy, collagen injections, sling procedures, and artificial urinary sphincter implantation.**

Bibliography

1. **Madersbacher H, Madersbacher S**. Men's bladder health: urinary incontinence in the elderly (Part II): Management. J Mens Health Gend. 2005;2(1):31-37.

2. **Stern JA, Clemens JQ, Tiplitsky SI, Matschke HM, Jain PM, Schaeffer AJ**. Long-term results of the bulbourethral sling procedure. J Urol. 2005;173:1654-6. [PMID: 15821529]

Item 132   Answer: B

This patient's skin examination findings are consistent with moderate-to-severe inflammatory acne. The combination of a topical comedolytic agent (a retinoid) and the topical antibiotic have not been effective. The next step in management would be concomitant use of an oral antibiotic with a topical antibiotic. Oral antibiotics, particularly in the tetracycline group, are efficacious and relatively safe for treating moderate-to-severe acne. Oral antibiotic treatment generally requires 6 to 8 weeks before efficacy can be determined, but consensus is lacking on the appropriate length of oral antibiotic treatment courses. Prolonged use of topical or oral antibiotics can lead to bacterial resistance. Combined oral contraceptives can be used as a treatment for women with acne; ethinyl estradiol and norgestimate (Ortho Tri-Cyclin®) and ethinyl estradiol and norethindrone (Estrostep®) are Food and Drug Administration (FDA) approved for this indication. Discontinuing oral contraceptives would not improve, and may worsen, acne. Oral isotretinoin is FDA approved only for recalcitrant nodular acne and is associated with an 80% remission rate. However, this agent is also frequently associated with mucocutaneous side effects and teratogenicity. Physicians who prescribe isotretinoin must have evidence of a recent negative pregnancy test, provide counseling regarding pregnancy prevention, and obtain informed patient consent. Oral isotretinoin has also been linked with depression,

suicidal ideation, suicide attempts, and suicide, but there is no clear causal relationship between these events and isotretinoin. A rare adverse effect of oral isotretinoin is acne fulminous, which requires treatment with systemic corticosteroids. Oral corticosteroids are not a treatment for, and may cause, acne.

KEY POINT

- **Oral isotretinoin is Food and Drug Administration approved only for recalcitrant nodular acne and is associated with an 80% remission rate.**

Bibliography

1. **Haider A, Shaw JC**. Treatment of acne vulgaris. JAMA. 2004;292:726-35. [PMID: 15304471]

2. PIER: Physicians' Information and Education Resource [database online]. Philadelphia: American College of Physicians; 2006. Updated February 27, 2006. Available at http://online.statref.com/Document/Document.aspx?DocId=19&FxId=50&Scroll=1&Index=0&SessionId=67A87EVZTNIUCVBJ.

Item 133   Answer: D

This patient requires further evaluation by breast ultrasonography or fine-needle aspiration. She has several risk factors for breast cancer, including a family history of breast cancer in a first-degree relative, older age at first childbirth, and no history of breast-feeding. However, the risk-factor profile should not influence the approach to the evaluation of a breast mass because 75% of patients with breast cancer have no identifiable risk factors. Once a clinician confirms the presence of a dominant mass on physical examination, a methodic approach must be taken until the mass is fully evaluated. Bilateral diagnostic mammography is useful because it can identify other breast abnormalities that are not palpable on examination. A mammogram that is suspicious for malignancy in the area of the palpable mass can also be helpful in localizing the area for biopsy; however, a negative mammogram should not deter the physician from completing the workup of a dominant breast mass, which requires further evaluation by breast ultrasonography or fine-needle aspiration.

Repeated mammography in 6 months is not an adequate evaluation for patients with a palpated dominant breast mass because it may delay diagnosis. Repeating the clinical breast examination in 4 to 6 weeks or 3 months after a change in dietary habits is also not appropriate because it may delay the diagnosis. Performing a repeated clinical breast examination in 4 to 6 weeks would be adequate only following cyst aspiration if the mass were to be identified as a simple cyst. MRI is now being considered as part of a screening protocol for women at high risk for breast cancer; however, MRI is not appropriate as part of a workup for a dominant mass. Breast ultrasonography could be performed to determine whether the mass is cystic or solid. A solid or complex mass would then require a tissue diagnosis from fine-needle aspiration biopsy (FNAB), a core-needle biopsy, or an excisional biopsy. The American

College of Radiology has established the Breast Imaging Reporting and Data System (BIRADS), in which mammograms are rated in six categories: 0 (needs additional imaging); 1 (negative); 2 (benign finding); 3 (probably benign finding); 4 (suspicious abnormality); and 5 (highly suggestive of malignancy).

KEY POINT

- **Patients with a negative mammogram in the setting of a dominant mass on clinical breast examination require further evaluation by breast ultrasonography or fine-needle aspiration.**

Bibliography

1. **Kerlikowske K, Smith-Bindman R, Ljung BM, Grady D**. Evaluation of abnormal mammography results and palpable breast abnormalities. Ann Intern Med. 2003;139:274-84. [PMID: 12965983]

Item 134   Answer: A

Several clues in this patient's history and findings suggest bulimia nervosa. She has excoriations at the back of her throat from self-induced vomiting and hypertrophy of the parotid glands. Chronic purging can lead to mild electrolyte abnormalities, including hypokalemia and slightly elevated serum bicarbonate and slightly decreased serum chloride levels. Other signs suspicious for this disorder include oropharyngeal ulcers, dental erosions, and bite marks or scars on the back of the hand. Anorexia nervosa is another eating disorder but is not as likely as bulimia in this patient because she is slightly overweight and has maintained her normal body weight despite trying to lose weight; patients with anorexia usually have difficulty maintaining weight within 15% of an ideal body weight and often appear emaciated on physical examination. This clinical scenario does not support a diagnosis of surreptitious ingestion of diuretics or renal tubular acidosis.

KEY POINT

- **Bulimia may be characterized by excoriations at the back of the throat caused by self-induced vomiting, hypertrophy of the parotid glands, and mild electrolyte abnormalities.**

Bibliography

1. **Wilson GT, Shafran R**. Eating disorders guidelines from NICE. Lancet. 2005;365:79-81. [PMID: 15639682]
2. **Devlin MJ, Goldfein JA, Petkova E, Jiang H, Raizman PS, Wolk S, et al**. Cognitive behavioral therapy and fluoxetine as adjuncts to group behavioral therapy for binge eating disorder. Obes Res. 2005;13:1077-88. [PMID: 15976151]

Item 135   Answer: C

This patient would benefit if his regimen were to include a higher-potency statin such as atorvastatin to lower his serum low-density lipoprotein (LDL) cholesterol level to less than at least 100 mg/dL (2.59 mmol/L). He is at the very highest risk for coronary artery disease (CAD) based on his history of diabetes and known cardiovascular disease. The National Cholesterol Education Program (NCEP) recommends lowering LDL cholesterol levels to <70 mg/dL (1.81 mmol/L) as a therapeutic option, with a goal of <100 mg/dL (2.59 mmol/L) as a strong recommendation in patients at the very highest risk for CAD. Ongoing clinical trials may more clearly define whether LDL levels should be uniformly decreased to <70 mg/dL (1.81 mmol/L) in all high-risk patients. No trials clearly show clinical benefit in patients with stable CAD.

This patient's lovastatin is already at the maximum recommended dose; increasing the dose would not likely help. Monitoring cholesterol levels periodically would be appropriate once cholesterol values have been reduced to recommended levels. Prescribing a fibric acid derivative with a statin would not be recommended because of the increased risk of myopathy. A fibric acid derivative would lower triglyceride levels, which would not be necessary for this patient because his triglyceride levels are acceptable. Adding a bile acid sequestrant or ezetimibe to lovastatin is also an acceptable alternative to substituting atorvastatin for lovastatin.

KEY POINT

- **In patients with the very highest risk for coronary artery disease, lowering LDL cholesterol levels <70 mg/dL is recommended as a therapeutic option, with a goal of <100 mg/dL strongly recommended.**

Bibliography

1. **Grundy SM, Cleeman JI, Merz CN, Brewer HB Jr, Clark LT, Hunninghake DB, et al**. Implications of recent clinical trials for the National Cholesterol Education Program Adult Treatment Panel III guidelines. Circulation. 2004;110:227-39. [PMID: 15249516]
2. Drugs for lipids. Treat Guidel Med Lett. 2005;3:15-22. [PMID: 15726011]

Item 136   Answer: D

Symptoms of bacterial vaginosis include increased malodorous discharge without irritation or pain. On physical examination, clinical criteria for bacterial vaginosis include homogenous, white discharge that smoothly coats the vaginal walls, without the presence of vaginal erythema; presence of clue cells; vaginal pH >4.5; and vaginal discharge that develops a fishy odor either before or after the addition of 10% potassium hydroxide slide preparation. Symptomatic patients who have at least three of these criteria should be treated with metronidazole or clindamycin, either orally or vaginally.

Patients with candidal vaginitis are likely to have vaginal irritation, inflammation, and lack of odor on physical examination. Patients with *Trichomonas vaginalis* often note a discharge that is typically yellow–green. Physiologic discharge is not usually malodorous and would not likely change as suddenly as this patient's history suggests.

- Symptoms of bacterial vaginosis include increased malodorous discharge without irritation or pain.

Bibliography

1. Anderson MR, Klink K, Cohrssen A. Evaluation of vaginal complaints. JAMA. 2004;291:1368-79. [PMID: 15026404]

Item 137   Answer: C

Recent memory loss is a common presenting symptom of dementia. The most frequently used mental state examination in this country is the Folstein Mini–Mental State Examination (MMSE). The MMSE can be performed in the office and requires patients to complete a range of cognitive tasks, including short-term memory tests, reading, following directions, drawing, and writing a sentence. A score of less than 23 (of 30) is considered to be a positive screening result for dementia. This patient could have Alzheimer's disease, vascular dementia, or a mixed dementia. The Katz Index of Activities of Daily Living and the Barthel Index are used to assess activities of daily living, such as eating, dressing, toileting, and washing. Although important parts of geriatric assessment, they are not used to establish a diagnosis of cognitive impairment. The Geriatric Depression Scale is a five-item scale, and a score of 2 or higher is a positive screening result for depression. This patient does not have symptoms of depression because she is sleeping and eating well and has no mood complaints.

- A score of less than 23 (of 30) on the Mini–Mental State Examination is considered to be a positive screening result for dementia.

Bibliography

1. Strub R. Vascular dementia. South Med J. 2003;96:363-6. [PMID: 12916555]
2. Adelman AM, Daly MP. Initial evaluation of the patient with suspected dementia. Am Fam Physician. 2005;71:1745-50. [PMID: 15887453]

Item 138   Answer: A

This patient has atopic dermatitis, most commonly associated with a rash in the creases of the skin and on the hands. Topical corticosteroids are best suited to treat moderate to severe symptoms of this condition when the patient is already using topical moisturizers (emollients), the typical first-line treatment. Severity is determined by involvement of more than one location, presence of sleep disturbance, and poor response to topical moisturizers. For the face, neck and intertriginous areas, only mild topical corticoster-

oids should be used. For the rest of the body, the lowest effective potency should be used intermittently, such as twice per week, to avoid thinning of the skin from regular topical corticosteroid use.

Topical tacrolimus may as effective as topical corticosteroids, but topical tacrolimus is indicated only for moderate to severe dermatitis that is unresponsive to topical corticosteroids, or for patients who cannot tolerate topical corticosteroids. Topical tacrolimus might also help where only the lowest-potency topical corticosteroids can be used, such as on the face, neck, and intertriginous areas. In March 2005, the Food and Drug Administration released an alert establishing a potential connection between the use of topical tacrolimus and lymphomas and skin cancers, based on case reports and studies in animals. For this reason, tacrolimus should be used only for short-term and intermittent treatment.

Oral antibiotics and topical antifungals cannot be used to effectively treat atopic dermatitis.

Oral corticosteroids are recommended only for a severe flare-up of dermatitis that is unresponsive to topical treatments. The support of a specialist, if available, is also recommended. No randomized trials support the use of oral corticosteroids; the optimal dose and length of treatment are unknown.

The criteria for the diagnosis of atopic dermatitis includes evidence of itchy skin plus three or more of the following: 1) involvement of the skin creases, including areas around the neck or eyes, elbows, knees, and ankles; 2) history of asthma or hay fever; 3) history of dry skin during the past year; 4) onset in a child younger than 2 years of age; and 5) visible dermatitis of skin flexures.

- Topical corticosteroids are the best treatment for atopic dermatitis in patients who are already using topical moisturizers.

Bibliography

1. Williams HC. Clinical practice. Atopic dermatitis. N Engl J Med. 2005;352:2314-24. [PMID: 15930422]

Item 139   Answer: C

Two sources, the North American Menopause Society (NAMS) and the American College of Physicians' Information and Education Resource (PIER, pier.acponline.org), conclude that some short-term studies show that black cohosh effectively reduces hot flushes compared with placebo and conjugated equine estrogens. All studies do not consistently show the same results, however. The mechanism for black cohosh's effects is unknown. Patients should be advised to use this treatment for 6 months or less because no data on effects of long-term treatment exist. Side effects of treatment with black cohosh include nausea, vomiting, headache, and dizziness.

Many women use topical progesterone or combination estrogen and progesterone creams for treatment of hot flushes. Dosages, formulations, and additional ingredients vary widely and are prepared by a compounding pharmacist. Results of studies on these topical formulations are mixed, showing a benefit or equivalent reduction in hot flushes compared with placebo, and data on safety and side effects are lacking. Patients might have heard that these agents are safer than conventional hormone treatment, but no data support these claims. There is insufficient evidence to recommend either dong quai or vitamin E as effective or safe alternative treatments for hot flushes. Studies have shown mixed results for both treatments.

KEY POINT

- **Short-term studies have shown that black cohosh is effective in reducing hot flushes.**

Bibliography

1. Treatment of menopause-associated vasomotor symptoms: position statement of The North American Menopause Society. Menopause. 2004;1:11-33. [PMID: 14716179]
2. **Col N, Cyr M, Miller M, Wheeler C**. Menopause and hormone therapy. Physicians' Information and Education Resource (PIER, pier.acponline.org) Updated Dec. 22, 2005. Editorial changes made Aug. 7, 2006.

Item 140   Answer: C

This patient has symptoms and findings suggestive of proliferative diabetic retinopathy. The most effective treatment is laser photocoagulation. The efficacy of laser photocoagulation in the treatment of diabetic retinopathy is well established. Aspirin inhibits platelet secretion and aggregation but has not been found to influence the progression of retinopathy. ACE inhibitors have been found to decrease the rate of progression of diabetic nephropathy but not diabetic retinopathy. Although this patient requires improved hypertension control, treatment of his diabetic retinopathy is a more important immediate priority. Vitrectomy is an effective treatment in patients with symptoms of advanced retinal disease who have had non-clearing vitreous hemorrhages or retinal detachments but would not be the initial treatment indicated in this patient. This patient has poorly controlled diabetes with a hemoglobin A_{1C} of 7.9%. Glucose and blood pressure control are important preventive measures for diabetic retinopathy, and insulin may eventually be indicated. However, this patient with visual changes and findings consistent with proliferative diabetic retinopathy first requires laser photocoagulation therapy rather than initiation of insulin. In addition, a transient worsening of retinopathy has been described in 10% of patients who have preexisting retinopathy and in whom tight insulin control is instituted.

KEY POINT

- **The most effective treatment for proliferative diabetic retinopathy is laser photocoagulation.**

Bibliography

1. **Frank RN**. Diabetic retinopathy. N Engl J Med. 2004;350:48-58. [PMID: 14702427]
2. **Harvey PT**. Common eye diseases of elderly people: identifying and treating causes of vision loss. Gerontology. 2003;49:1-11. [PMID: 12457044]

Item 141   Answer: C

This patient has conversion disorder, which is manifested by the acute onset of a symptom, usually neurologic, in the face of overwhelming stress. One relatively common setting for conversion disorders is among new recruits at military basic training camps. Blindness is a common form of conversion disorder; others include loss of hearing, sensation, or motor function. The history in patients with conversion disorder often includes components that make no physical sense, such as color vision loss followed by total vision loss, and neurologic findings that conflict with the patient's description of symptoms, such as normally reactive pupils in the case of sudden blindness. This patient's history and physical examination findings are not suggestive of optic neuritis, temporal arteritis, macular edema, compression of optic chiasm, or multiple sclerosis.

Patients with conversion disorder are not consciously "faking" their symptoms; the symptoms are real, and this patient is truly unable to see, despite the proper functioning of her neurologic mechanisms.

KEY POINTS

- **Conversion disorder is manifested by the acute onset of a symptom, usually neurologic, in the face of overwhelming stress.**
- **Blindness is a common form of conversion disorder; others include loss of hearing, sensation, or motor function.**

Bibliography

1. **Bourgeois JA, Chang CH, Hilty DM, Servis ME**. Clinical Manifestations and Management of Conversion Disorders. Curr Treat Options Neurol. 2002;4:487-497. [PMID: 12354375]
2. **Hurwitz TA**. Somatization and conversion disorder. Can J Psychiatry. 2004;49:172-8. [PMID: 15101499]

Item 142   Answer: B

This patient has mild, comedonal acne with an absence of inflammatory lesions. For comedonal-only acne, topical retinoids are the mainstay of treatment. Retinoids are derivatives of vitamin A and prevent comedone formation by normalizing desquamation of follicular epithelium. Topical retinoid therapies may be combined with other topical agents, including antibiotics or keratolytic agents, but there is no evidence that combined-agent topical therapy is better than single-agent topical therapy for treating comedonal-only acne. Combined-agent therapy with a topical antibiotic may be helpful if there are inflammatory lesions (pustules) in addition to comedonal lesions. There is no evidence that avoidance of certain foods, including fried foods or chocolate, will prevent or treat acne. Oral corticosteroids are not a treatment for, and may cause, acne. Oral antibiotics are indicated for moderate-to-severe inflammatory acne and are not required in this case. Topical tretinoin is not teratogenic. In contrast, oral tretinoin is teratogenic and requires registration in an FDA iPLEDGE program by prescribing physicians. The iPLEDGE program requires a recent negative pregnancy test, counseling regarding pregnancy prevention, and informed patient consent.

KEY POINT

- **For comedonal-only acne, topical retinoids are the mainstay of treatment.**

Bibliography

1. **Haider A, Shaw JC**. Treatment of acne vulgaris. JAMA. 2004;292:726-35. [PMID: 15304471]

2. PIER: Physicians' Information and Education Resource [database online]. Philadelphia: American College of Physicians; 2006. Updated February 27, 2006. Available at http://online.statref.com/Document/Document.aspx?DocId=19&FxId=50&Scroll=1&Index=0&SessionId=67A87EVZTNIUCVBJ.

Item 143   Answer: C

This patient meets Rome II criteria for irritable bowel syndrome (IBS). Treatment for IBS is largely symptomatic. For diarrhea-predominant IBS, loperamide has been found effective. Antidepressants, both tricyclic agents and selective serotonin reuptake inhibitors, have been shown to improve overall well being and pain levels, but have no impact on other IBS symptoms. Alosetron is Food and Drug Administration approved for diarrhea-predominant IBS; however, its use should be restricted to patients with severe, diarrhea-predominant IBS who have not responded to other symptomatic measures, because it has been associated with ischemic colitis in approximately 1 in 700 patients who take this drug. Physicians who prescribe alosetron must register with the manufacturer, and patients must sign a consent form before beginning therapy. Adding fiber to the diet is a common approach to treating IBS. Although safe, fiber was found to be no more beneficial in treating global IBS symptoms than placebo in a recent meta-analysis. Finally, although clinical trials suggest that antispasmodic agents, such as dicyclomine and hyoscyamine, may be helpful in managing pain in patients with IBS, a recent meta-analysis suggests the benefit is weak.

KEY POINTS

- **For diarrhea-predominant irritable bowel syndrome (IBS), loperamide has been found effective.**
- **Although safe, fiber was found to be no more beneficial in treating global IBS symptoms than placebo in a recent meta-analysis.**

Bibliography

1. **Quartero AO, Meineche-Schmidt V, Muris J, Rubin G, de Wit N**. Bulking agents, antispasmodic and antidepressant medication for the treatment of irritable bowel syndrome. Cochrane Database Syst Rev. 2005:CD003460. [PMID: 15846668]

2. **Lesbros-Pantoflickova D, Michetti P, Fried M, Beglinger C, Blum AL**. Meta-analysis: The treatment of irritable bowel syndrome. Aliment Pharmacol Ther. 2004;20:1253-69. [PMID: 15606387]

3. **Chey WD, Chey WY, Heath AT, Dukes GE, Carter EG, Northcutt A, et al**. Long-term safety and efficacy of alosetron in women with severe diarrhea-predominant irritable bowel syndrome. Am J Gastroenterol. 2004;99:2195-203. [PMID: 15555002]

Item 144   Answer: B

This patient with a red eye and tearing most likely has viral conjunctivitis. This is a self-limited process that is expected to resolve spontaneously. No further treatment is required. The key aspects of the history that are used to establish this patient's diagnosis are the presence of a red eye, the absence of ocular pain, and the absence of visual changes. The patient can be reassured but told that the process may spread to the other eye and could be contagious for 2 weeks.

The absence of purulent discharge indicates that this is not bacterial conjunctivitis, and, therefore, topical antibiotics are not needed. Allergic conjunctivitis is an unlikely diagnosis in this patient given the absence of pruritus and the unilateral distribution of symptoms. Therefore, topical antihistamines are not indicated. An urgent referral to an ophthalmologist for red eye is needed only in patients who have ocular pain and visual loss, symptoms of which may be suggestive of scleritis, acute angle-closure glaucoma, anterior uveitis, or viral or bacterial keratitis. Treatment with topical corticosteroids is indicated in the case of anterior uveitis, which is characterized by red eye but is also associated with ocular pain and visual loss, symptoms not found in this patient. Topical corticosteroids are generally not recommended without an evaluation by an ophthalmologist because they may worsen some types of eye conditions, specifically herpes keratitis. Patients with signs suspicious for anterior uveitis require urgent referral to an ophthalmologist.

KEY POINT

- **Viral conjunctivitis is characterized by subacute appearance of a red eye without ocular pain or change in visual acuity.**

Bibliography
1. **Leibowitz HM**. The red eye. N Engl J Med. 2000;343:345-51. [PMID: 10922425]

Item 145   Answer: C

Recommended prophylaxis for elective total knee replacement before the patient is ambulating consists of high-dose low-molecular-weight heparin (subcutaneous enoxaparin, 30 mg twice daily), fondaparinux, adjusted-dose warfarin with a target INR of 2.5, or use of a continuous SCD. High-dose low-molecular-weight heparin is currently the only specifically recommended venous thromboembolism prophylaxis among the options listed above for patients who have begun ambulating after knee arthroplasty. Other options include fondaparinux and adjusted-dose warfarin with a target INR of 2.5. Low-dose low-molecular-weight heparin (subcutaneous enoxaparin, 40 mg daily) and low- or high-dose unfractionated heparin (5000 U subcutaneously twice or three times daily) are effective prophylaxis for patients undergoing general surgery but are not adequate for those undergoing knee-replacement surgery.

Single-modality use of unfractionated heparin, foot SCD, or compression stockings is not recommended. Compared with higher-gradient, fitted compression hose, lower-gradient standard-issue support hose offer protection only when patients are supine because the elastic does not have a sufficient pressure gradient to override gravity once patients sit or stand. Patient compliance with SCDs is variable, and the devices are effective only if worn continuously while patients are not ambulating. Unfractionated heparin is less effective than low-molecular-weight heparin for prophylaxis in major orthopedic surgery. Although prophylaxis is not recommended for patients who have undergone elective knee arthroplasty after discharge, the risk for deep venous thrombosis is increased for months after elective hip arthroplasty or hip fracture repair surgery, and extended prophylaxis is recommended for approximately 1 month after these procedures.

KEY POINTS

- Recommended prophylaxis for elective total knee replacement before the patient is ambulating consists of high-dose low-molecular-weight heparin, fondaparinux, adjusted-dose warfarin with a target INR of 2.5, or use of a continuous SCD.
- Low-dose low-molecular-weight heparin (subcutaneous enoxaparin, 40 mg daily) and low- or high-dose unfractionated heparin (5000 U subcutaneously twice or three times daily) are effective prophylaxis for patients undergoing general surgery but are not adequate for those undergoing knee-replacement surgery.

Bibliography
1. **Geerts WH, Pineo GF, Heit JA, Bergqvist D, Lassen MR, Colwell CW, et al**. Prevention of venous thromboembolism: the Seventh ACCP Conference on Antithrombotic and Thrombolytic Therapy. Chest. 2004;126:338S-400S. [PMID: 15383478]

Index

Note: Page numbers followed by f indicate figures; those followed by t indicate tables; and those preceded by Q indicate test questions.